Pharmaceutical Chartbook

Abraham G. Hartzema
Editor

LEWIS PUBLISHERS

Library of Congress Cataloging-in-Publication Data

Pharmaceutical services chartbook.

Includes bibliographical references.
Includes index.
1. Pharmaceutical services--United States--Statistics. 2. Pharmaceutical services--United States--Tables. I. Hartzema, Abraham G. II. Hirsch, Jan D. III. Perfetto, Eleanor M. [DNLM: 1. Drug Utilization--United States--statistics. 2. Fees, Pharmaceutical--United States--statistics. 3. Insurance, Pharmaceutical Services--United States--statistics. 4. Pharmacies--United States--statistics. QV 16 P5364]
RS92.P47 1990 362.1′782′0973 90-6410
ISBN 0-87371-173-4

LEWIS PUBLISHERS, INC.
121 South Main Street, P.O. Drawer 519, Chelsea, Michigan 48118

PRINTED IN THE UNITED STATES OF AMERICA

Preface

The pharmaceutical industry, the pharmaceutical distribution system, pharmaceutical services as well as pharmacotherapy itself are in a rapid transition. Even for use by those who are deeply involved in pharmacy it is often difficult to keep up with these rapid developments. This Chartbook is meant to provide a bird's eye view of significant trends in the pharmaceutical industry, including manufacturers, wholesalers, retail drugstores, pharmacists, prescribers, drugs, health care delivery organizations, third party payers, and others.

Major trends are placed in the context of changing population demographics, developments in research productivity and intensity in the pharmaceutical industry and increasing constraints in the financing of pharmaceutical services and organization of pharmaceutical services delivery and other factors that impinge on the pharmaceutical market. The Chartbook is divided in different chapters, each referring to a set of charts centered around a defined content area.

In Chapter 1, charts are provided offering insights in the changing population demographics that are of importance to future drug use levels, payment mechanism for drugs, and human resources issues in the pharmaceutical distribution system.

Chapter 2 presents drug utilization data, total, by category, and by population groups. It further lists new drugs that are coming to the market and their status in the drug approval process.

Chapter 3 highlights trends in drug costs, drug expenditures, drug insurance penetration and other trends. It contains also a major section on the catastrophic health bill and its impact on the pharmaceutical distribution system.

Chapter 4 displays issues in drug reimbursement and financing, out of pocket payments, third party payments, private insurance and insurance of drugs by Medicaid and Medicare.

Chapter 5 details drug development and production, new drugs on the market, drug lag, drug production, and export.

Chapter 6 addresses the organization of the pharmaceutical distribution system, statistics on manufactures, wholesalers, and retailers are included.

Chapter 7, pharmacy human resources, trends in pharmacy graduates, Ph.D. graduates, degree mix, dropout rates, and productivity trends are displayed.

Finally, pharmacy policy developments, federal laws, and changes in legislation are reviewed in Chapter 8, which is the last chapter of the Chartbook.

This book will provide individuals involved in policy making, in management, in education, or in research, convenient access to statistical data and their sources on the pharmaceutical distribution system. It enables one to have and keep the finger on the pulse of the pharmaceutical industry in its broadest context. In other applicatons, the Chartbook can serve as a teaching tool by providing illustration material for educational purposes, meetings, proposals, or for making a point in a presentation.

The author enjoyed the development of the Chartbook and hopes that the readers have as much satisfaction in reviewing the charts as it has given him compiling the information. We like to thank the many organizations, companies, and individuals whose data and information we have used. It was not possible to individually approach all data sources used to extend our gratitude. The source of the data, if available, has been placed in a footnote for each chart.

To collect the information, many data sources are utilized. These sources vary in the methods of data collection and analysis. Because of the different methods used in data collection, the information displayed in the graphs may vary in reliability and vailidity. Thus any interpretation of the data should be handled with care.

As in any endeavor, where a lot of information has to be abstracted or distilled in a simple format, we may have made errors. Although the graphs and the data were carefully reviewed, the data errors may originate from our data entry or from the many primary and secondary data sources employed.

The Chartbook would not have been possible without the help of many individuals that assisted in the development of the book, our graduate students preliminary work, colleague faculty for their useful advise, our student assistant So Yon Yu who did a great job compling the graphs, Carol Vanscoy for maintaining the extensive correspondence that was involved in the preparation of the Chartbook, our publisher who so patiently guided us in its production, and the University of North Carolina at Chapel Hill for the resources made available to the project.

Last but not least, I have to thank Christine who had to share the authors attention for this project with one that may have been closer to her heart and for her patience. We would like to thank all who contributed in making this Chartbook become a reality.

Abraham G. Hartzema

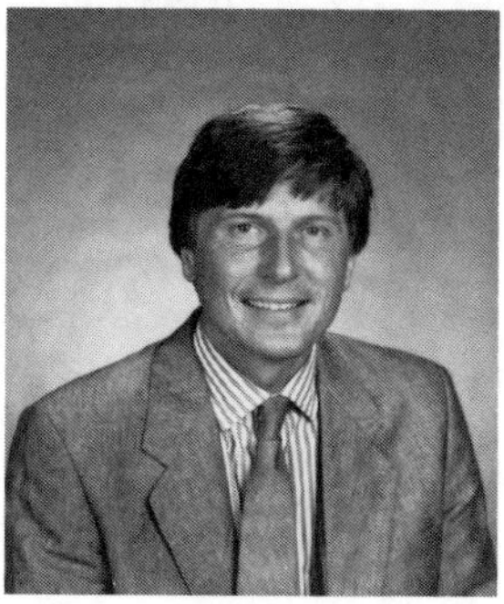

Dr. Abraham G. Hartzema received his M.Sc. of Public Health in Health Services Research from the University of Washington and a Ph.D. in Pharmacy Administration from the University of Minnesota. Presently he is an associate professor in Pharmacy Administration and Health Policy and Administration in the Schools of Pharmacy and Public Health at the University of North Carolina at Chapel Hill.

He has a longstanding interest in health care delivery and the pharmaceutical distribution system. His current interests are the U.S. pharmaceutical market, the organization of pharmaceutical care, and drug reimbursement issues. He has been principal investigator for several grants. Three books and more than fifty book chapters, abstracts, and articles have resulted from his work.

Table of Contents

CHAPTER 1: DEMOGRAPHICS

1. Projected U.S. Population Growth 2
2. Projections of the Total U.S. Population 3
3. Percent Population Change by Age Group: 1980—1990 4
4. Live Births and Deaths 5
5. Infant Mortality Rates 6
6. Expectation of Life at Various Ages in the United States: 1987 7
7. U.S. Life Expectancy for Males and Females at Birth: 1950—1987 8
8. Population 65 Years Old and Over as a Percent of Total Population 9
9. Mortality Rates: Males vs. Female 10
10. U.S. Deaths per 100,000 Population from Selected Diseases, 1986 11
11. Reduction in Reported U.S. Cases of Infectious Diseases: 1940—1985 12
12. Acute Conditions, by Age: 1986 13
13. AIDS Cases Reported from 1981—1988 14
14. AIDS Patients — Hospital Days of Care: 1984—1986 15
15. AIDS Patients — Hospital Discharges: 1984—1986 16
16. Marital Status of the Population 17
17. 1987 Income Distribution as a Percent of Households 18
18. Income Distribution of Households with Residents Age 70 and Over 19
19. Sources of Income for the Elderly 20
20. Living Arrangements for Non-Institutionalized Elderly 21
21. Contributions Toward Medical Benefits for Retirees 22

CHAPTER 2: DRUG UTILIZATION

1. Current Trends in the Number of Prescriptions Dispensed: 1978—1987 24
2. Total New and Refill Prescriptions 25

3. National Prescription Audit: New Rx 26
4. Decline in the Percentages of Total New and Refill Prescriptions of the Top 200 Drugs, 1980—1987 27
5. Percent of Prescriptions Filled by Chains 28
6. U.S. Prescription Volume: 1977—1987 29
7. New Prescription Volume: Product Source 30
8. Top 25 Prescription Drugs — New and Refill Rxs Dispensed by Drugstores 31
9. Top 25 Prescription Drugs: New Rxs Dispensed in Drugstores 32
10. Top Ten Retail Drugs: 1987—1988 33
11. 1988's Biggest Gainers 34
12. Ranking of the Leading Products: 1986 and 1987 35
13. Ranking of the Leading Products for Hospitals: 1986 and 1987 36
14. The Top Ten Therapeutic Classes Worldwide 37
15. 1988 New Product Launches: U.S. Retail Market 38
16. Use of Psychotropic Drugs: Total U.S. Population 39
17. Use of Psychotropic Drugs: Persons with at least One Psychotropic Drug Prescription 40
18. Use of Psychotropic Drugs: Psychotropic Drugs as Percent of All Prescribed Medicines 41
19. Annual Expenses and Sources of Payment for Psychotropic Drugs: Mean Expense per Person with Expense 42
20. Top Ten Diagnostic Related Groups 43
21. Ten Most Frequently Performed Surgical Procedures in 1986 44
22. Use of Prescribed Medicines by Age 45
23. Average Rate of Adverse Drug Reaction Reports in Nine Major Countries 46
24. Patients' Rating of Communication on Medication 47

CHAPTER 3: DRUG COST EXPENDITURE

1. Expenditures for Total Medical Care in the United States 50
2. United States Total Health Care Expenditures 51
3. Comparison of Annual Growth Rates of Gross National Product and National Health Expenditures, 1970—1987 52
4. National Health Expenditures Aggregate 53
5. Expenditures for Medical Care in the United States 54
6. Medical Care Price Changes 55
7. National Health Expenditures as a Percent of Gross National Product: 1970—1986 56
8. Health Expenditures as Percent of Gross Domestic Product, 1986 57
9. U.S. Total Health Care Expenditure: How the Bill is Paid 58
10. The Nation's Health Dollar: 1986 59

11. National Health Expenditures 60
12. U.S. Total Health Care Expenditure: Where the Money Goes 61
13. 1986 Health Care Expenditures 62
14. Spending on Health Care: A Look at Eight Countries: 1986 63
15. Health Care Cost-Containment Measures 64
16. Consumer Price Index for Medical Care Items in the United States: 1967—1988 65
17. Trends in Pharmaceuticals 66
18. Consumer Price Index for Drugs and Prescriptions in the United States, 1967—1988 67
19. Per Capita Expenditure on Medicines by Country 68
20. International Drug Price Comparison 69
21. Range of Market Prices Paid for Brand Name Prescription Drugs, Spring 1989 70
22. Pharmaceutical Preparations-Producer Price Indexes 71
23. Pharmaceutical Preparations-Producer Price Indexes (comparison of selected OTC categories) 72
24. Pharmaceutical Preparations-Producer Price Indexes (comparison of selected therapeutic categories) 73
25. Pharmaceutical Preparations-Producer Price Indexes (comparison of selected prescription drugs) 74
26. Annual Percent Change in the Consumer Price Index for Urban Consumers 75
27. Antiulcer Products—Total Sales in Retail Market 76
28. Antiulcer Products: Number of Total Prescriptions 77
29. Antiarthritic Drug Retail Sales 78
30. ACE Inhibitors—Retail Market 79
31. ACE Inhibitors—Retail Market 80
32. Oral Calcium Channel Blockers: Retail Market 81
33. Total Retail Sales: Cardiovascular Drugs 82
34. Antilipemics—Retail Market 83
35. Antilipemics—Total Prescriptions 84
36. Consumer Price Index for Drugs and Prescriptions in the United States, 1967—1988 85

CHAPTER 4: THIRD PART COVERAGE, REIMBURSEMENT, AND FINANCING

1. Sources of Prescription Payment 88
2. Third-Party Prescriptions: 1987 89
3. Third-Party Prescription Ratios—1987 90
4. Drug Distribution to Members by Third Parties 91
5. Percentage Distribution of U.S. Ethical Pharmaceutical Sales by Class of Customer 92
6. Health Insurance Coverage Status: 1985 93

7. National Health Insurance Coverage Rates: 1987 94
8. Dollar Outlay by Employers for Employee Insurance Coverage: 1987 95
9. Major Health Care Service Provider Companies 96
10. Growth in Life Insurance Companies' Pension Reserves in the U.S. 97
11. Health Insurance Claims Payments in the United States 98
12. Ratio of Insurance Premiums to Disposable Personal Income 99
13. Life Insurance Policy Value and Disposable Personal Income per Household in the U.S. 100
14. Average Size Life Insurance Policy in Force in the United States 101
15. Percent Change in Average Total Professional and Liability Insurance Expenses of Self-Employed Physicians 102
16. Estimated Health Insurance Premiums to Increase for 1989 103
17. Medicare Enrollment 1977—1986 104
18. Distribution of Medicare Enrollees, by Census Region: 1966 and 1987 105
19. Number and Percent Distribution of Medicare Enrollees, 1966 and 1987 106
20. Growth of Medicare, Selected Years 107
21. Medicare Physician Services per User 108
22. Mean Total Medicare and Mean Total Patient Visits per Week in Selected Specialties: 1987 109
23. Medicare Average Allowed Charge per User 110
24. Mean Annual Utilization of Medicare Services 111
25. Mean Annual Reimbursement for Medicare Services 112
26. Annual Expenditures for Noninstitutionalized Medicare Beneficiaries, 1987 113
27. Annual Prescription Drug Expenditures for Noninstitutionalized Medicare Beneficiaries, 1987 114
28. Prescription Use by Elderly Medicare Beneficiaries, 1980 and 1987 (average charge per prescription) 115
29. Prescription Use by Elderly Medicare Beneficiaries, 1980 and 1987 (average annual prescription expenditures) 116
30. Prescription Use by Elderly Medicare Beneficiaries, 1980 and 1987 (average annual Prescriptions per beneficiary) 117
31. Prescription Use by Elderly Medicare Beneficiaries, 1980 and 1987 (percent with at least one prescription during year) 118
32. Elderly Prescription Drug Use by Medicare Beneficiaries: 1967—1980 119
33. Medicaid Rx Product Cost as a Percentage of Total Rx Price 120
34. The Impact of Cutting Pharmacy Reimbursement (Medicaid Rx Drug Reimbursement Components) 1982—1987 121

35. Labor-Intensive vs. Product-Intensive Industries: Distribution of Expenses 122
36. Pharmacy Fee Increases 123
37. Minutes Worked to Pay for an Average Prescription 124
38. Predicted Effect of the Catastrophic Drug Insurance Program on Medicare Expenditures 125
39. Insurers Step Up Efforts to Reduce Use of Free-Choice Health Plans 126
40. Expected Growth of Managed Care 127
41. Total HMO Membership: 1978—1987 128
42. Number of HMO Plans: 1978—1987 129
43. Changes in the Total Number of HMOs and PPOs 130
44. Health Maintenance Organizations and Preferred Provider Organizations by Region as of 2/28/89 131
45. New HMO Data: Counts of HMO Organizations 132
46. Unduplicated Provider Counts on the HMO/PPO Census Database File 133
47. Information on Preferred Provider Organization 134
48. HMO Enrollment: Top Ten States 135
49. States with Lowest HMO Enrollment 136
50. HMO Enrollment as a Percentage of State Population 137
51. HMO Enrollments 138
52. Distribution of HMO Membership: 1988 139
53. Rating Method of HMO Plan Enrollees: 1988 140
54. HMO Ownership: 1988 141
55. Corporate Owned and Managed HMOs by Region, 1988 142
56. Ten Largest Medicare HMOs 143
57. HMO Diversification Activities: 1988 144
58. Selected Characteristics of HMO Accounts 145
59. Coverage of Various Preventive Services in Best Selling Benefit Package: 1988 146
60. Percent of Plans Using Copayments for Selected Basic Benefits, by Plan Age 147
61. Percentage of HMO Enrollment in Best Selling Benefit Package, Distribution of Plans (plans over three years old), 1988 148
62. Extent of Agreement with Other HMOs to Address Employer Needs (plans over three years old) 1988 149
63. Transplant Coverage by Type: 1988 150
64. Factors Cited as Contributions to Rising HMO Premiums: 1988—1989 151
65. Monthly HMO Premium Increases: 1988—1989 152
66. Average HMO Premium Increase 153
67. Average HMO Premium Increase: 1987—1988 154
68. Generic vs. Branded Drugs by Model Type 155

69. Major Health Care Service Provider Companies........................156
70. Anticipated Growth of Freestanding Ambulatory Centers 157
71. Percent Ambulatory Encounters by Provider 158

CHAPTER 5: DRUG DEVELOPMENT AND PRODUCTION

1. The Steps Toward Drug Approval.......................................160
2. National Support for Health R&D by Source: 1977—1987 161
3. U.S. Pharmaceutical R&D Expenditures as a Percentage of U.S. Pharmaceutical Sales 162
4. R&D Expenditures for Human Use Ethical Pharmaceuticals 1974—1987...163
5. U.S. Pharmaceutical R&D Expenditures by Product Class: 1986...164
6. U.S. Patents for Drugs and Medicines 165
7. Number of New U.S. Patents for Drugs and Medicines by Origin: 1973—1986...166
8. New single Chemical-Entity Drugs Introduced to U.S. Market 1940—1987 by Country of Origin 167
9. Top 10 Companies Worldwide in R&D Compounds: 1987..............168
10. Listing of Important (''A''-Rated) New Drugs Introduced by the Top 25 U.S. Drug Manufacturers: 1981—1988....................169
11. Top 25 Manufacturers' Annual Production of New Drugs by FDA Therapeutic Classification 170
12. New Drugs from Top 25 Drug Companies as Proportion of New Drugs from All Companies, 1981—1988.........................171
13. Individual Drug Manufacturer Track Record: Number of Therapeutic Breakthroughs Between 1981—1988.......................172
14. Average Development Time: New Molecular Entities First Approved Abroad: 1987..173
15. New Molecular Entities Marketed Abroad Prior to U.S. Approval 174
16. Number of New Drug Applications (NDA) and New Molecular Entities (NME) Approved: 1975—1987..............................175
17. New Molecular Entities (NMEs) Introduced by 25 Largest U.S. Rx Drug Manufacturers, 1981—1988.................................176
18. U.S. New Molecular Entity Approvals per Year 177
19. New Molecular Entity Backlog...178
20. New Single Entity Drug Introductions to U.S. Markets 179
21. Patent Expirations on Prescription Drugs..............................180
22. Total Value of Drug Imports and Exports: 1980—1989................181
23. Value of Drug Imports by Category: 1980—1989 182
24. Value of Drug Exports by Category: 1980—1989 183
25. Pharmaceutical Imports as Percentage of Total Supply: 1977—1986...184

26. Exports as a Percent of Total Shipments 185
27. Value of Biological Products Produced: 1979—1988 186
28. Value of Medicinals and Botanicals Produced from 1979—1988 187
29. Value of Shipments Sold by the Drugs Industry 188

CHAPTER 6: PHARMACEUTICAL

1. U.S. and Foreign Pharmaceutical Sales: PMA Member Firms 190
2. Manufacturers' Domestic Sales of Ethical Drugs for Human Use by Product Class 191
3. Foreign Sales of Ethical Drugs for Human Use by Product Class 192
4. Foreign Sales of Ethical Pharmaceuticals by U.S.-Owned PMA Member Firms 193
5. Relative Profitability Trends as Measured by After-Tax Return on Net Worth, 1980—1988 194
6. Biotech Firms: Product Plans 195
7. Estimated Total Wholesale Industry Sales Growth, 1981—1988 196
8. Expense Trends for Wholesalers: 1981—1988 197
9. Wholesalers' Gross Margin and Operating Expense Trends, 1982—1988 198
10. Percentage Net Profit Margin Trend for Pharmaceutical Wholesalers 199
11. Operating Profit Margin Trend for Pharmaceutical Wholesalers, 1982—1988 200
12. Return on Net Worth Trend for National Wholesale Druggists' Association Firms: 1981—1988 201
13. Financial Leverage Trend for Wholesalers Total Assets to Net Worth, 1981—1988 202
14. Total Operating Expenses as a Percent of Gross Profit for Pharmaceutical Wholesalers 203
15. Total Asset Turnover Trend for Wholesalers, 1981—1988 204
16. Return of Total Assets for All National Wholesale Druggists' Association Firms, 1981—1988 205
17. Average Collection Period and Average Days' Sales in Inventory Trends for Wholesalers, 1980—1988 206
18. Pharmaceutical Wholesalers: Customer Sales Mix 207
19. Pharmaceutical Wholesalers: Prodcut Sales Mix 208
20. U.S. Retail Prescription Drug Sales: 1976—1987 209
21. Retail Sales Figures for Chain Drug Stores 210
22. Top 10 American Drug Chains: 1988 Store Totals 211
23. Top 10 American Drug Chains: 1988 Dollar Volume 212
24. 1988 Drug Chains: Sales per Average Store 213
25. Top Deep Discounters 214

26. 1988 Drug Chains: Growth in Units....215
27. Average Sales Gain for Chain Drug Stores....216
28. Ethical Pharmaceutical Sales: Leading Companies for Drug Stores....217
29. Top Ten Companies: U.S. Retail Sales to Drug Stores....218
30. Ethical Pharmaceuticals: Leading Product for Drug Stores....219
31. Breakout of 1988 Chain Drug Sales: 1988 Total Chain Sales....220
32. Chain Drug Store Average Sales Mix: 1987....221
33. Percent of Prescriptions Filled by Chains....222
34. Total Dollar Sales: Independent vs. Chain....223
35. Total Number of Independent and Chain Pharmacies, 1978—1987....224
36. U.S. Retail Drug Store Sales Chain vs. Independent....225
37. U.S. Retail Drug Store Sales Chain vs. Independent....226
38. Daily Prescription Output: 1st. Qtr. 1989....227
39. Prescription Output (1st Qtr. 1989) Total No. Scripts Filled: 420 million....228
40. 1988 Drug Chains: Net-to-Sales Ratio....229
41. 1988 Drug Chains: Expense Ratio....230
42. Pharmacy Sales by Number of Prescriptions Dispensed Daily in 1987....231
43. 10-Year Sales Trends....232
44. Drug Store Pharmaceutical Purchases: Total Rx vs. Total OTC....233
45. Sales Growth in Independent Community Pharmacies: 1970—1988....234
46. Retail Pharmacies' Shrinking Share of the Nation's Prescription Sales: 1985 and 1988....235
47. Prescription Sales Dollar Distribution....236
48. Pharmaceutical Purchases: Drug Stores vs. Hospitals....237

CHAPTER 7: HOSPITALS AND LONG TERM CARE

1. U.S. Hospitals....240
2. Allocation of Beds According to Hospital Size: 1987....241
3. Total Expenditures of Community Hospitals by Bed-Size....242
4. Trends Among Noncommunity Hospitals....243
5. Hospital Staffing by Type of Hospital....244
6. Percent of Beds Occupied in Average Private Nonprofit Hospitals....245
7. Length of Stay for Private Nonprofit Hospitals....246
8. Average Hospital Discharges per Week and Length of Stay of Discharged Patients (in days) for All Physicians....247
9. Hospital Operating Statistics: Average Bed Capacity: 1987....248
10. Average Hospital Prescription Cost: 1988....249
11. Pharmacy Services Offered in Hospitals....250

12. Average Hospital Pharmacy Admissions 251
13. Hospital Pharmacy Inventory and Purchases by Bed Capacity: 1988 252
14. Average Hospital Pharmacy: Inventory and Purchases 1978—1987 253
15. Hospital Pharmacy: Nonparenteral and Parenteral Orders/Week: 1987 254
16. Chemical Entities Most Frequently Dispensed in Hospitals, Patients Ages 65 Years and Older: 1987 255
17. Ethical Pharmaceutical Sales: Leading Companies for Hospitals 256
18. Trends in Hospital Surgery 257
19. Trends in Hospital Surgery by Age Group 258
20. Source of Payment for Hospital Surgery 259
21. Planned Involvement of Hospitals in Retirement Communities 260
22. Hospitals and Nursing Homes 261
23. Nursing Homes by Type of Ownership 262

CHAPTER 8: PHARMACEUTICAL HUMAN RESOURCES

1. U.S. Health Industry Personnel 264
2. Total Health Care Employment: No Direct Patient Care 265
3. Health Care Employment: Direct Patient Care 266
4. Food and Drug Administration Staffing Levels 267
5. Pharmacy Manpower: 1975—1990 268
6. Pharmacist Employment (1st. Qtr. 1989) 269
7. Pharmacists — Sex of Pharmacist 270
8. Chain Drug Store Personnel: 1987 271
9. Pharmacists — Licensing Status Trends 272
10. Pharmacists — Total Number Licensed 273
11. Licensed Pharmacies: 1983—1987 274
12. Pharmacists — Total Number by Practice 275
13. Bachelor of Science Degrees Conferred 276
14. Doctor of Pharmacy as the First Professional Degree Conferred, 1960—1987 277
15. Master of Science Degrees Conferred 278
16. Doctor of Philosophy Degrees Conferred 279
17. Total Pharmacy Degrees Conferred 280
18. Pharmacy Degrees Conferred by Ethnic Group, 1976—1987 281
19. Entry Level Degrees Conferred in the Northeast, South, Midwest and West Regions, 1976—1987 282
20. Pharmaceutical Science Graduate Studies: Enrollment of Pharmacists 283
21. Pharmaceutical Science: Ph.D. Degrees Granted to Non-Americans as a Percent of Total Degrees 284
22. Total Pharmaceutical Science Ph.D. Degrees Granted 285

23. Average Base Salaries for Pharmacists: How the Practice Settings Stack Up 286
24. Average Total Compensation 287
25. Average Overtime Earnings of Employee Pharmacists 288
26. Total Average Compensation by Region: 1989 289
27. Hours Worked by Employed Pharmacists: 1986 and 1987 290
28. Fringe Benefits: How Widespread Are They? 291
29. Hospital Pharmacy: Pharmacist, Technician, and Support Personnel Hours/Week, 1987 292
30. Pharmacy Personnel Hours in Average Private Nonprofit Hospital 293
31. Average Hourly Earnings of Health Care Production and Nonsupervisory Workers 294
32. Average Hourly Earnings of Health Care Production and Nonsupervisory Workers: Health Services 295
33. Indexes of Productivity: U.S. Pharmaceutical Industry and U.S. Private Non-Farm Business 296
34. Annual Percent Change in Employment 297
35. Annual Percent Change in Workhours 298
36. Annual Percent Change in Earnings 299
37. Physician, Dentists and Nurses: 1960 to 1986 300
38. Active U.S. Physician Population 301
39. Active U.S. Physician Population for Selected Years: 1970—1986 302
40. Projected Percent Distribution of U.S. Active Physician Population: 1986—2010 303
41. Projected Percent Distribution of Active Physician Population by Specialty 304
42. Post-Resident U.S. Physician Population in Direct Patient Care by Specialty 305
43. Post-Resident U.S. Physician Population in Direct Patient Care 306
44. Physician and Dental Visits per Person by Sex: 1970—1986 307
45. Percent Change in Average Fees for Physician Visits: 1982—1986 308
46. Mean Expenditure on Medical Suplies per Self-Employed Physician: 1986 309
47. Distribution of Average Professional Expenses of Self-Employed Physicians: 1982 and 1986 310
48. Office-Based Physicians' Net Earnings from Practice by Specialty: 1986 311
49. Companies with Flexible Benefit Plans by Size 312
50. Flexible Benefit Plan Coverage 313
51. Percent of Employers Providing Retiree Health Coverage (by employer size) 314

Chapter 1

DEMOGRAPHICS

Population demographics of importance to future drug consumption levels and human resource issues

Projected U.S. Population Growth

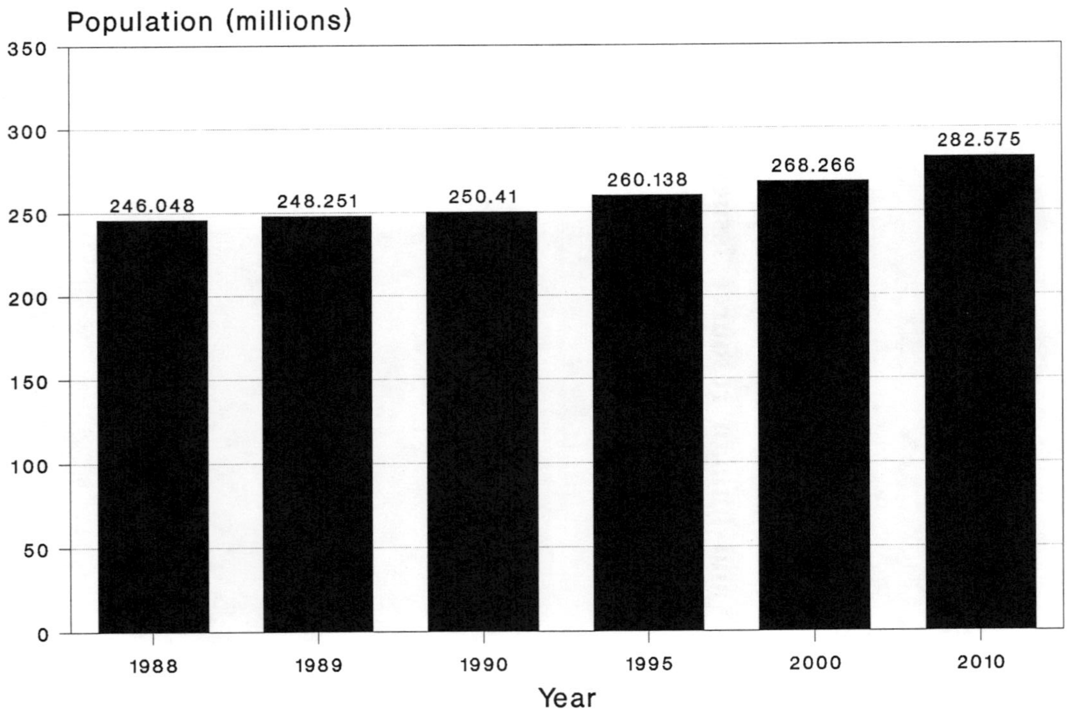

Source: U.S. Bureau of the Census, Current Population Reports, Series P-25 No. 1018.

Projections of the Total U.S. Population

(by age group)

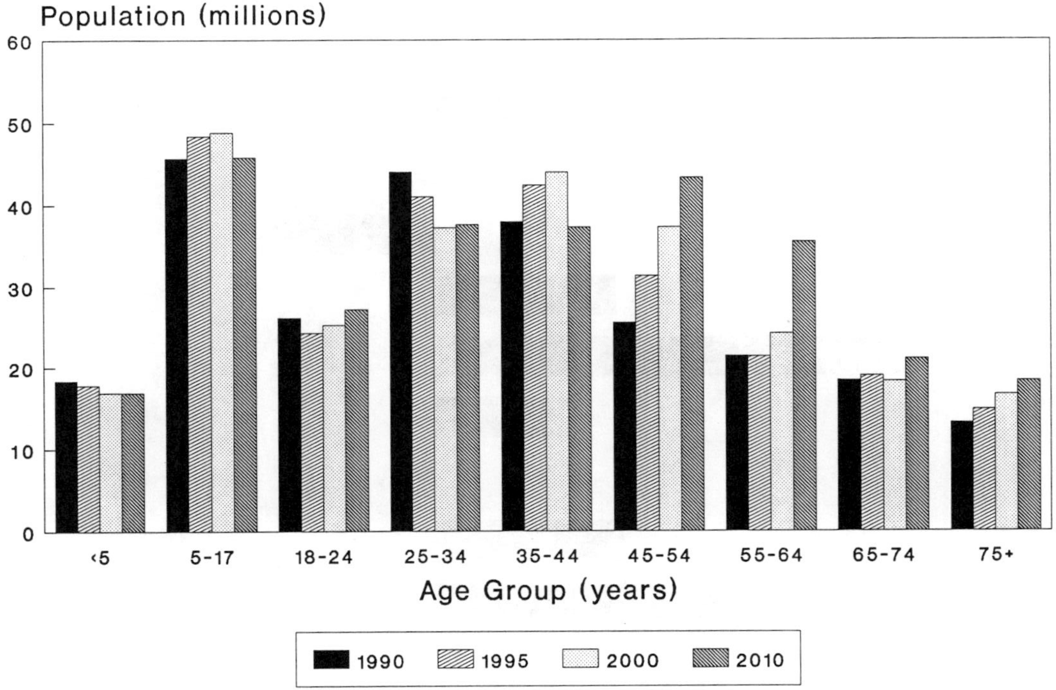

Source: U.S. Bureau of the Census, Current Population Reports, series P-25, No. 1018.

Percent Population Change by Age Group 1980-1990

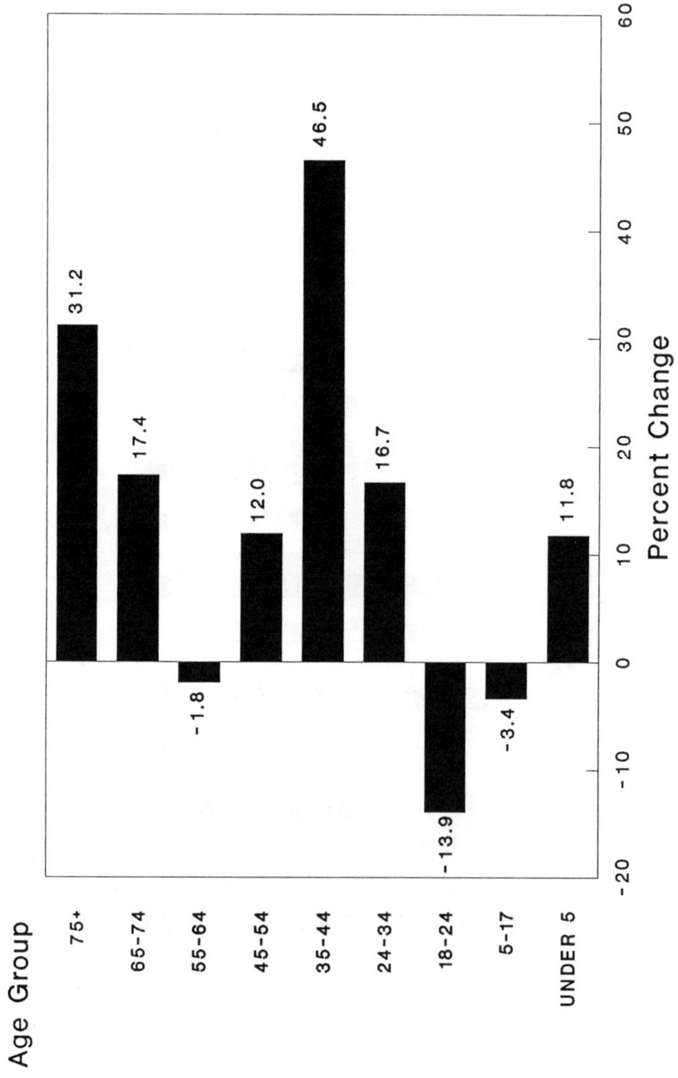

Source: U.S. Bureau of the Census
Current Population Reports, series P-25,
No. 1018.

Live Births and Deaths

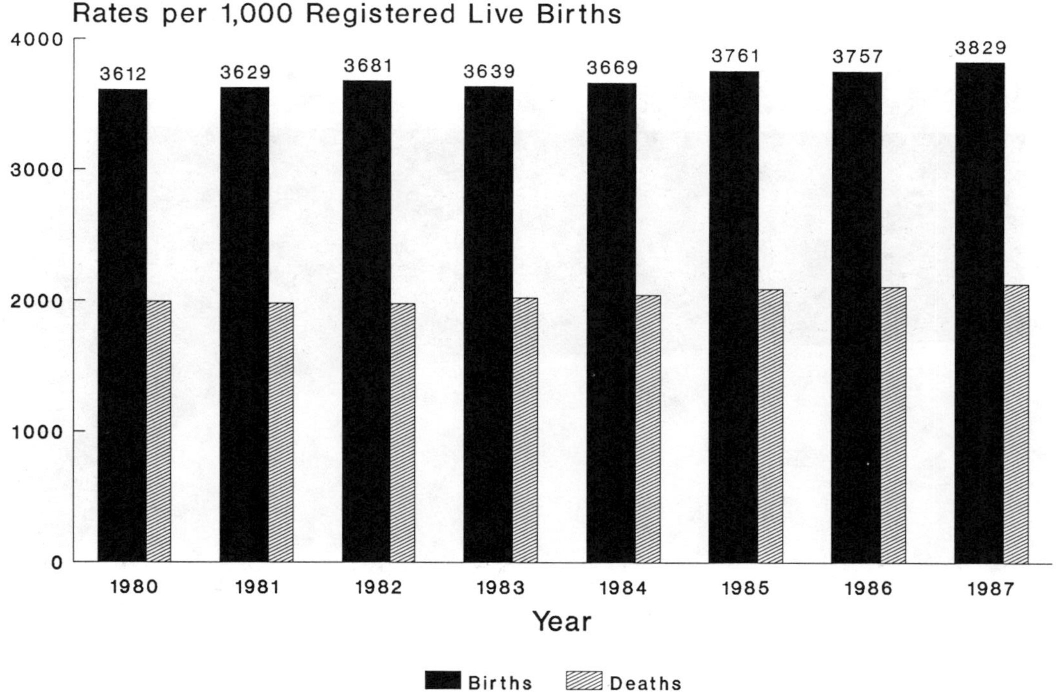

Source: U.S. National Center for Health Statistics, Vital Statistics of the U.S. Annual, 1987.

Infant Mortality Rates

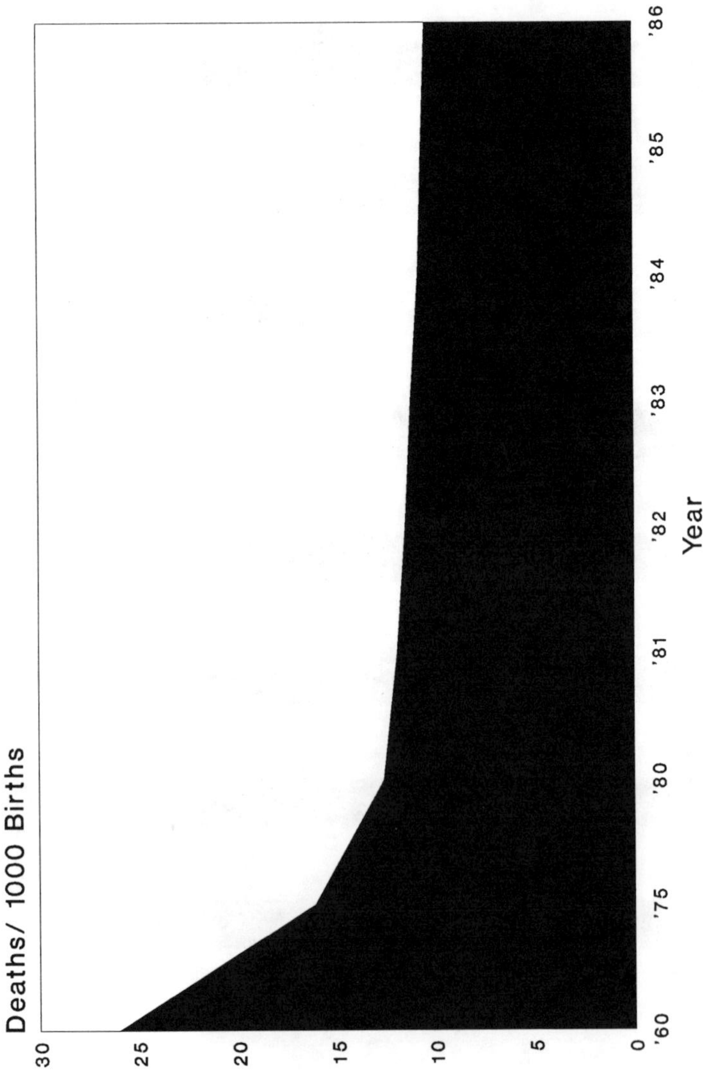

Source: U.S. National Center for Health Statistics, Vital Statistics of the U.S., annual, 1989.

Expectation of Life at Various Ages in the United States 1987

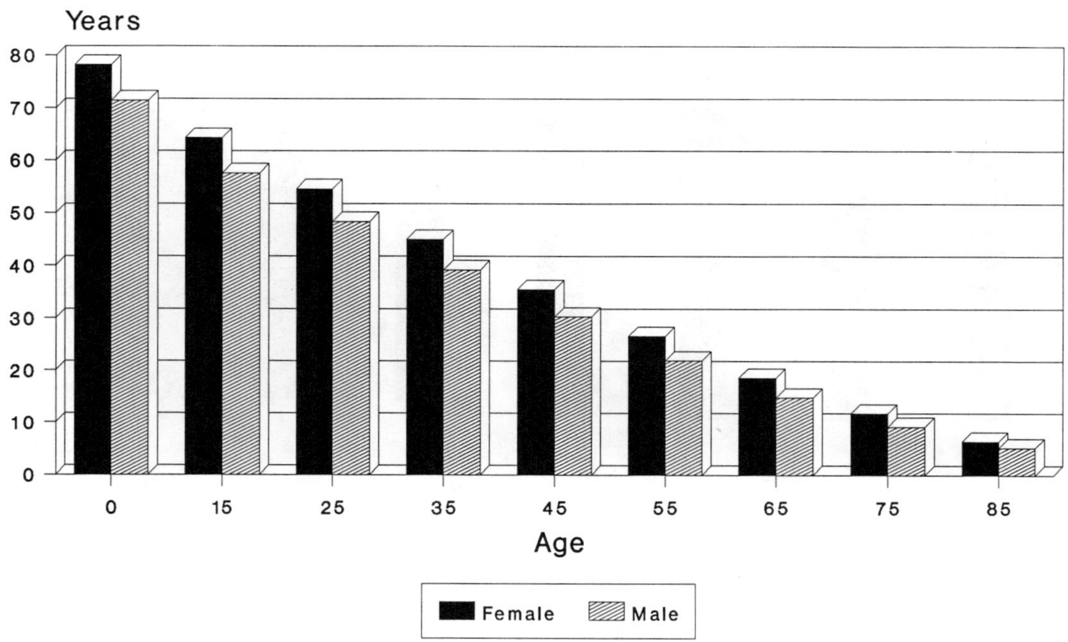

Source: National Center for Health Statistics, Vital Statistics of the U.S. annual, 1987.

U.S. Life Expectancy for Males and Females at Birth 1950-1987

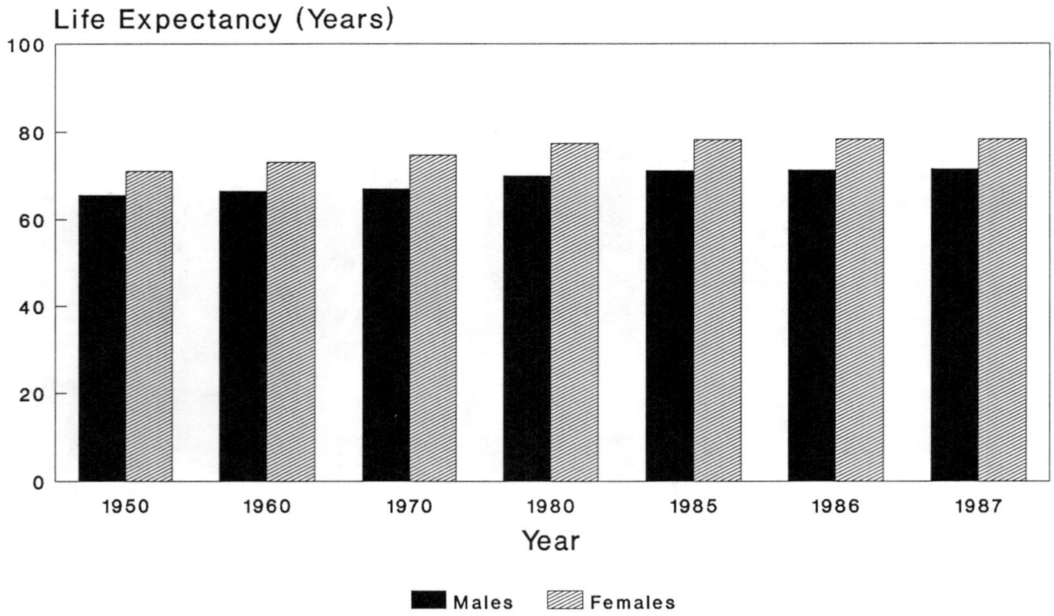

Source: U.S. National Center for Health Statistics, Vital Statistics of the U.S. Annual, 1987.

Population 65 Years Old and Over as a Percent of Total Population

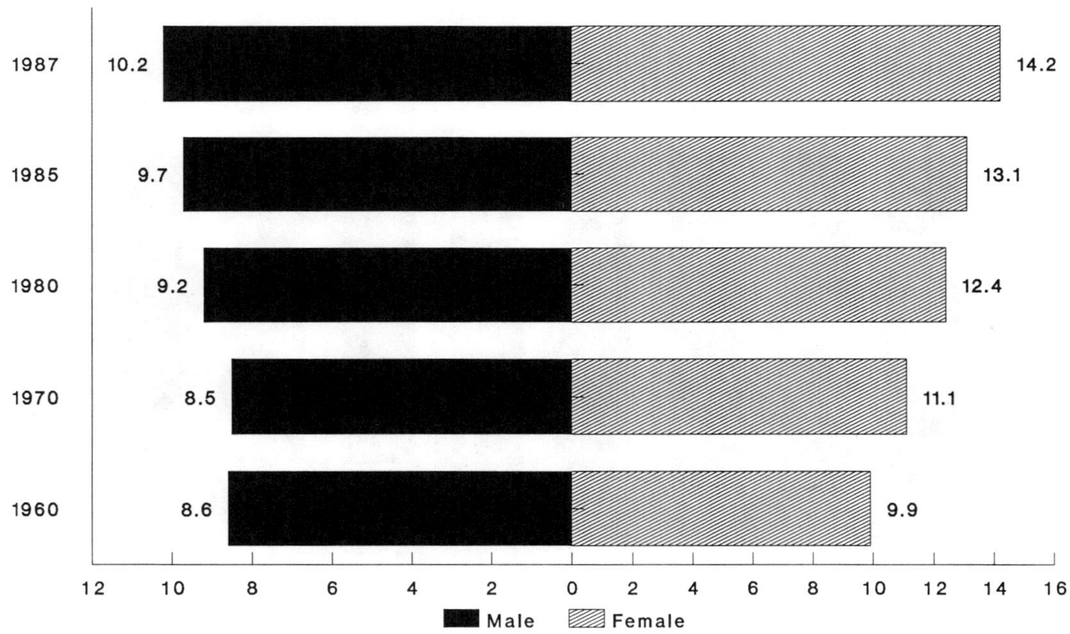

Source: U.S. Bureau of the Census, Current Population Reports, series P-25, No. 1018, 1987.

Mortality Rates: Male vs. Female

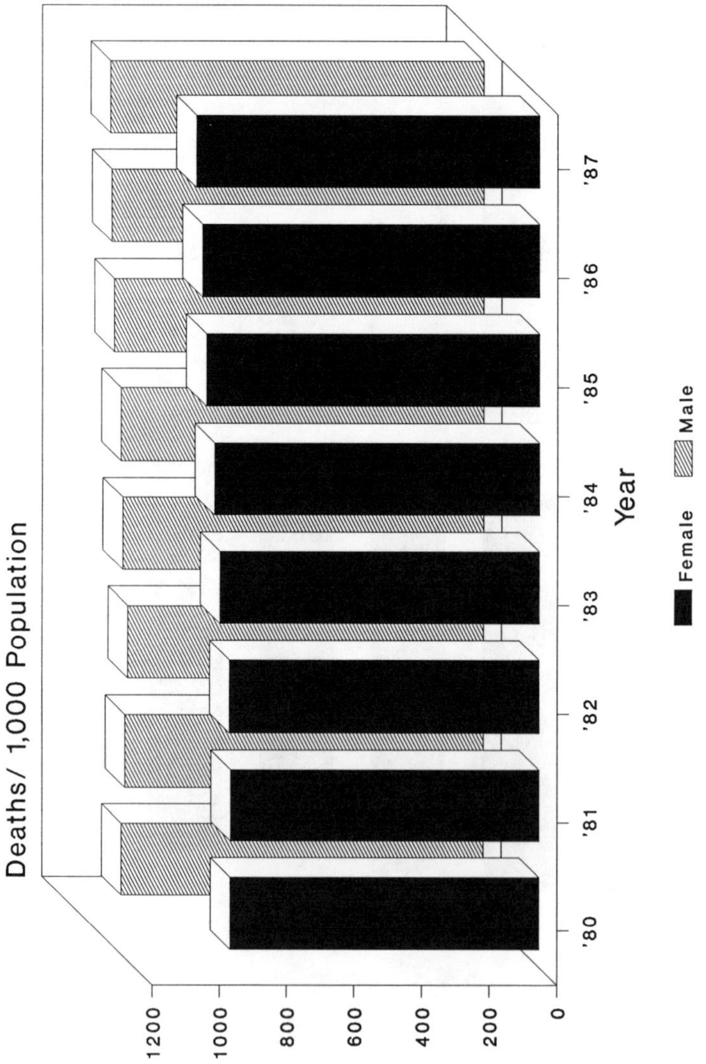

Source: U.S. National Center for Health Statistics, Vital Statistics of the U.S. annual, 1987.

U.S. Deaths per 100,000 Population from Selected Diseases, 1986

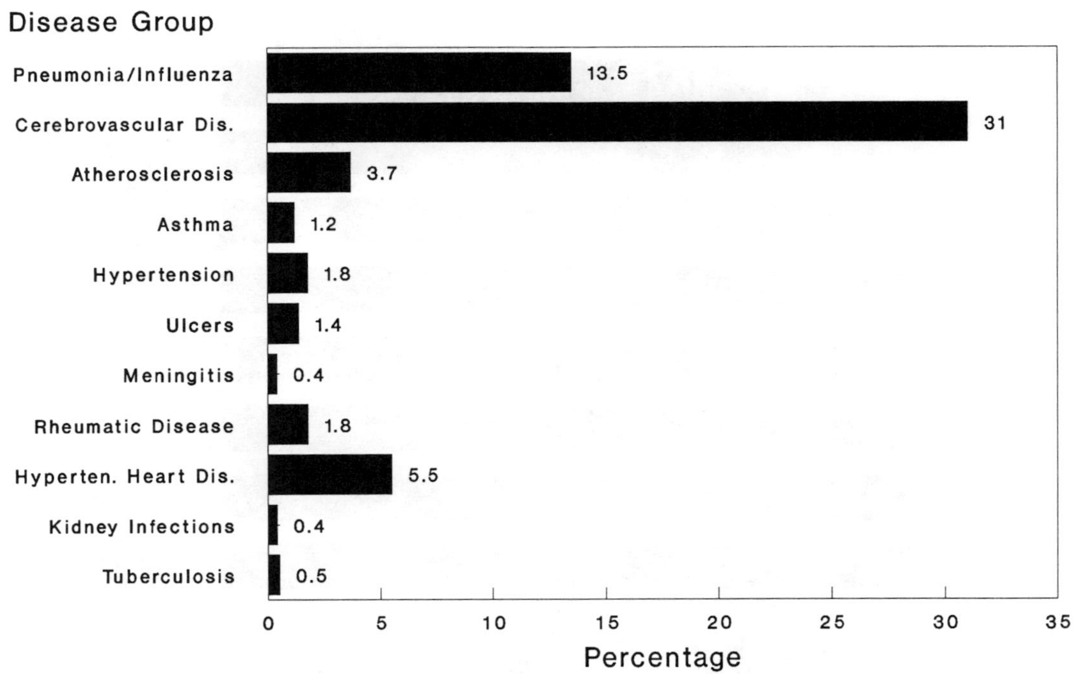

Source: U.S. National Center for Health Statistics, Vital Statistics of the U.S., annual, 1989.

Reduction in Reported U.S. Cases of Infectious Diseases: 1940-1985

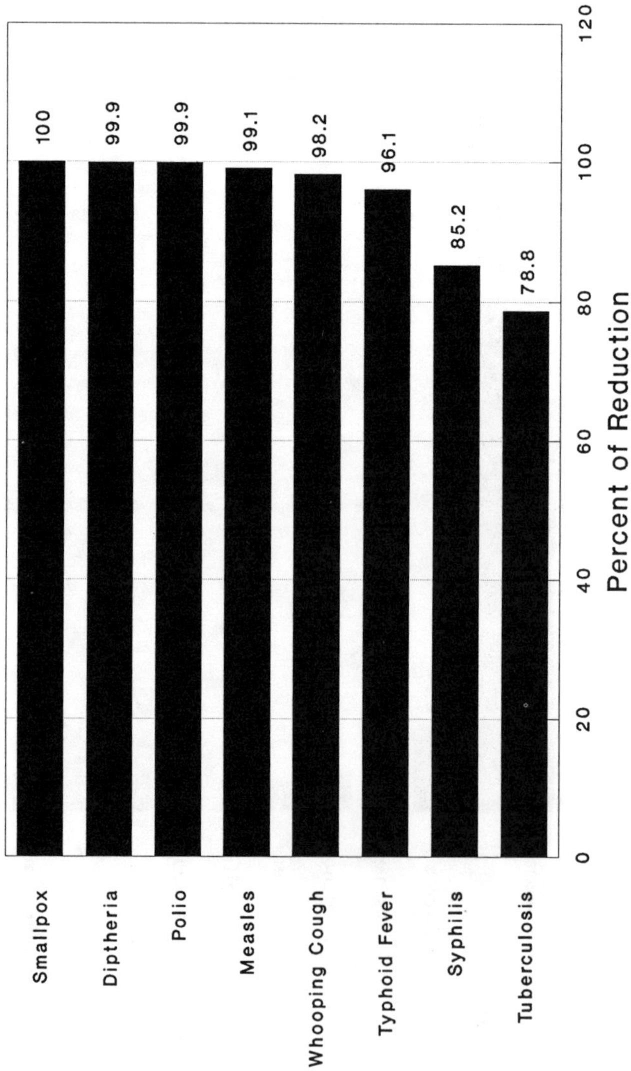

Source: Morbidity and Mortality Weekly Report, Annual Summary, 1984, U.S. Dept. of Health and Human Services

Acute Conditions, by Age: 1986

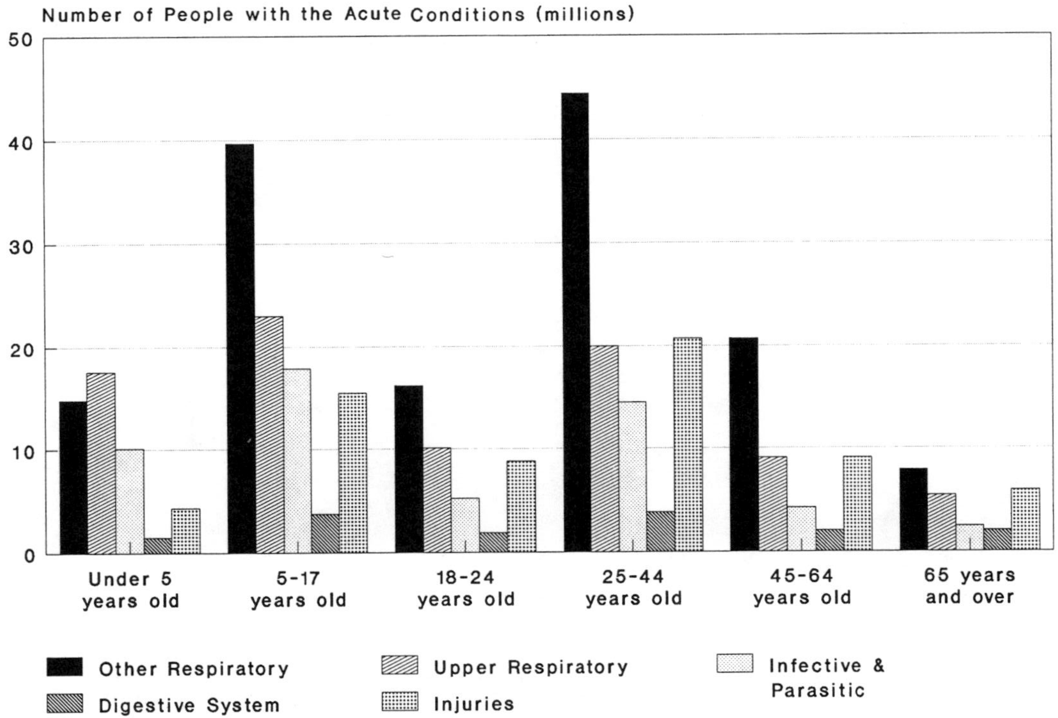

Source: U.S. National Center for Health Statistics, Vital and Health Statistics, series 10, and unpublished data, 1989.

AIDS Cases Reported from 1981-1988

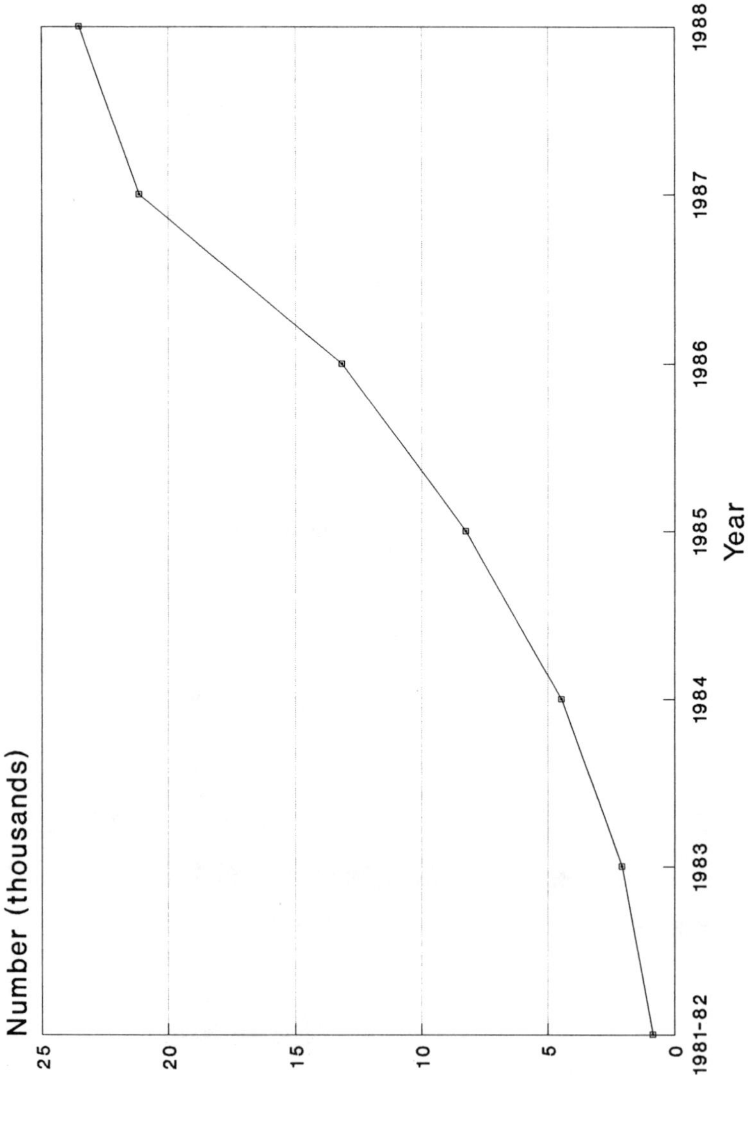

Source: U.S. Centers for Disease Control
Atlanta, GA, unpublished data, 1989.

AIDS Patients - Hospital Days of Care 1984-1986

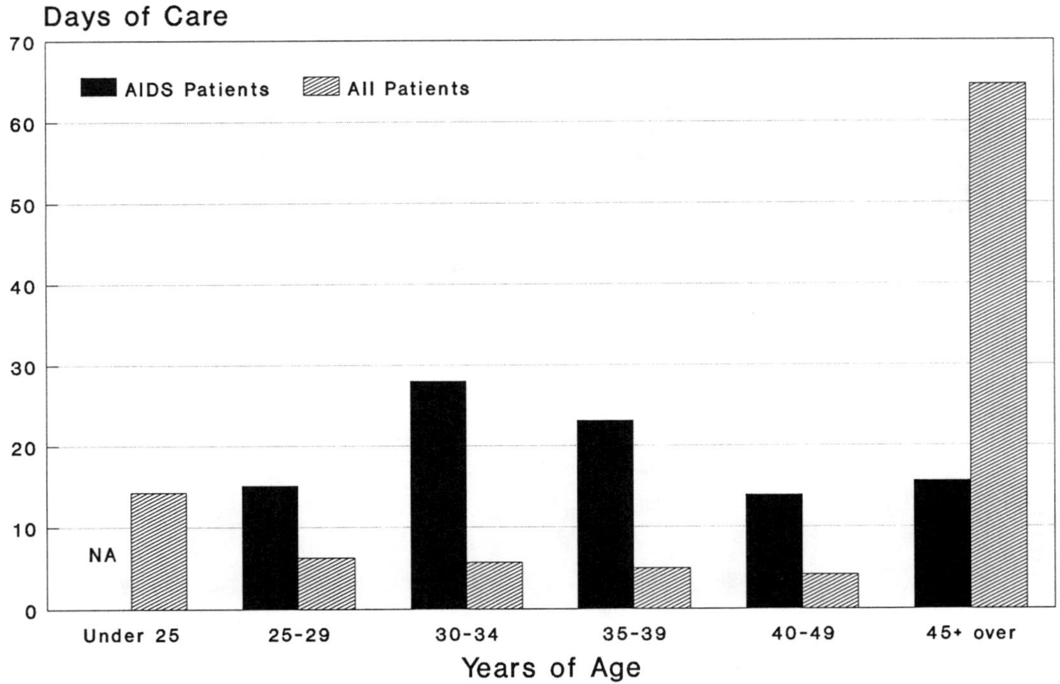

Source: U.S. National Center for Health Statistics, Advance Data from Vital and Health Statistics, No.156, 1989.

AIDS Patients - Hospital Discharges: 1984-1986

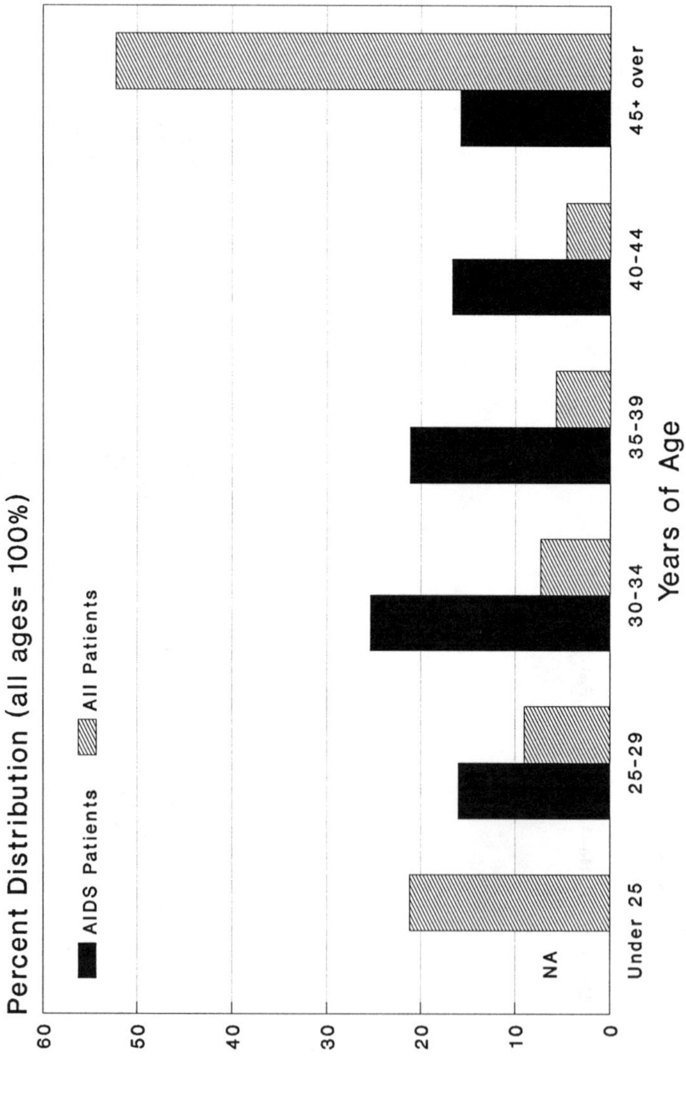

Source: U.S. National Center for Health Statistics, Advance Data from Vital and Health Statistics, No. 156, 1989.

Marital Status of the Population

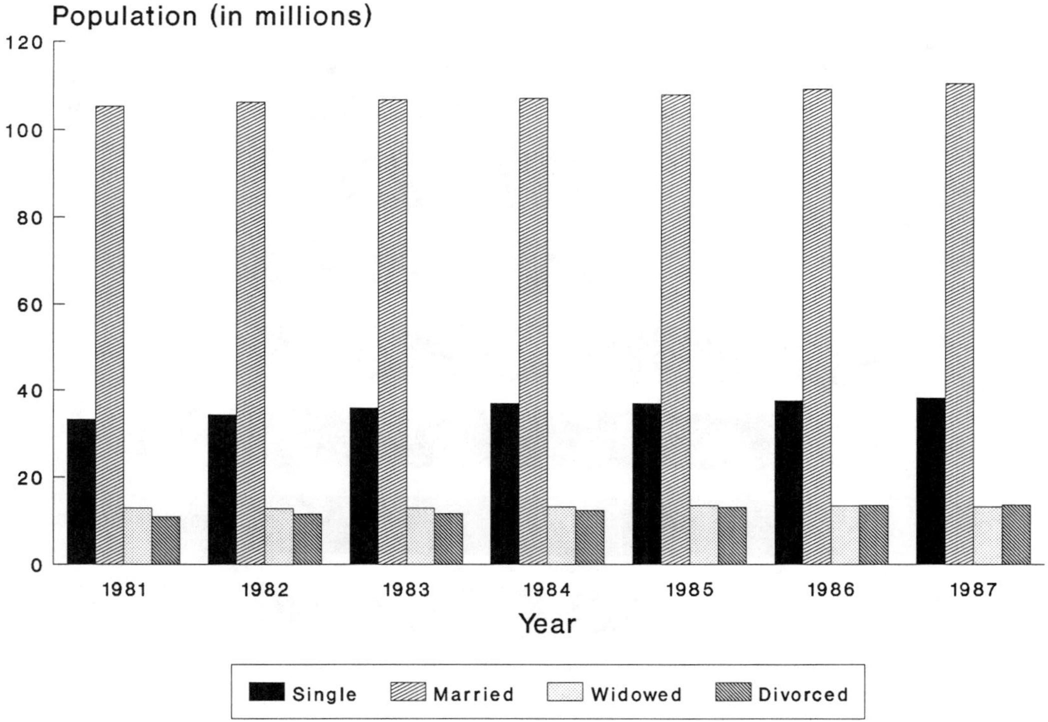

Source: U.S. Bureau of the Census,
Current Population Reports, Series P-20
No.423 and earlier reports, 1989.

1987 Income Distribution as a Percent of Households

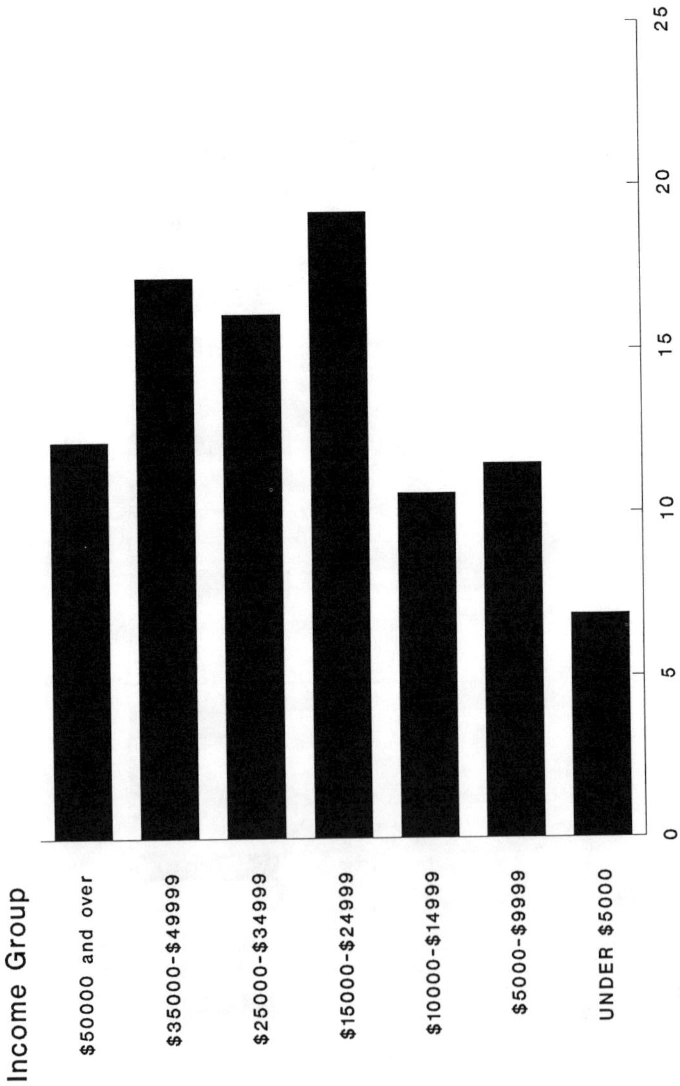

Source: U.S. Bureau of the Census

Income Distribution of Households with Residents Age 70 and Over

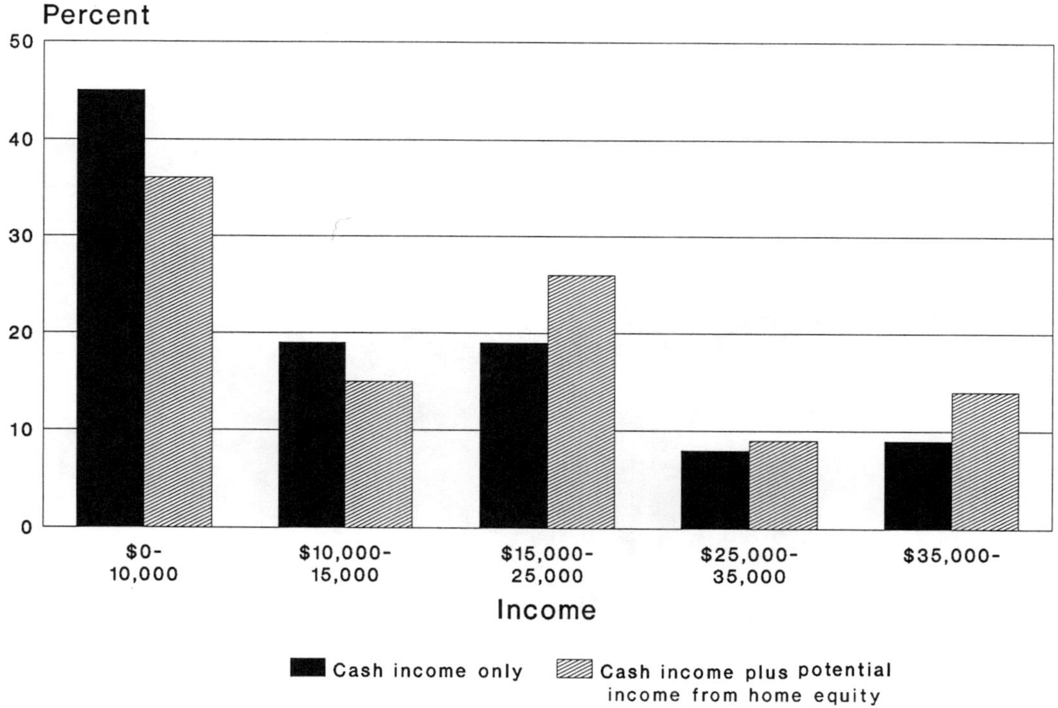

Source: Elderly Housing
Gimmy and Boehm, 1988.

Sources of Income for the Elderly

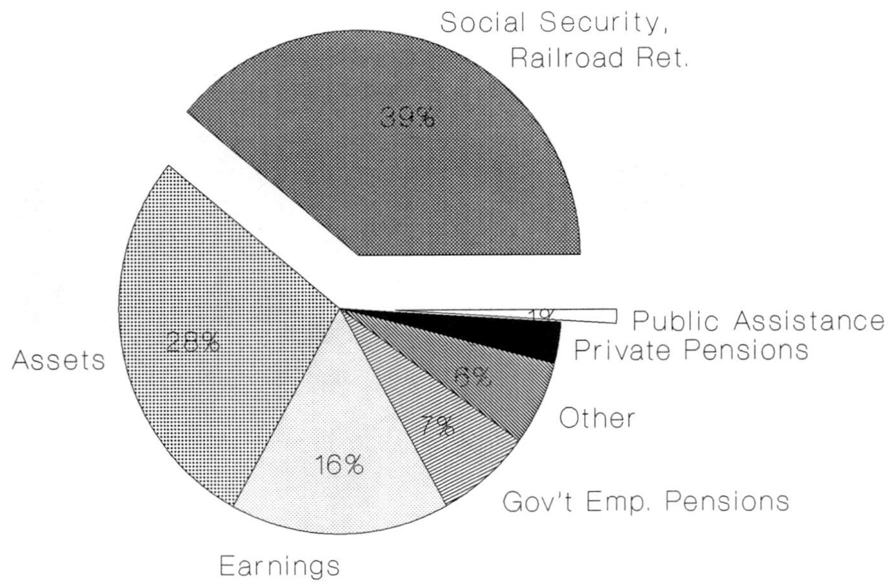

Source: Social Security Bulletin, 1986.

Living Arrangements for Non-Institutionalized Elderly

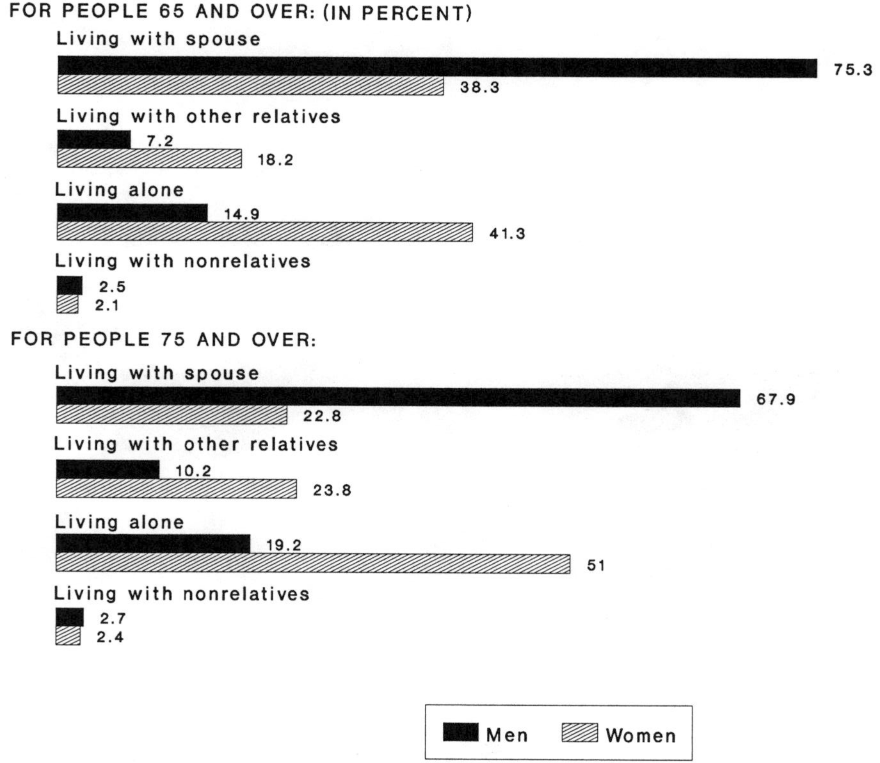

Source: Census Bureau, 1986.

Contributions Toward Medical Benefits for Retirees

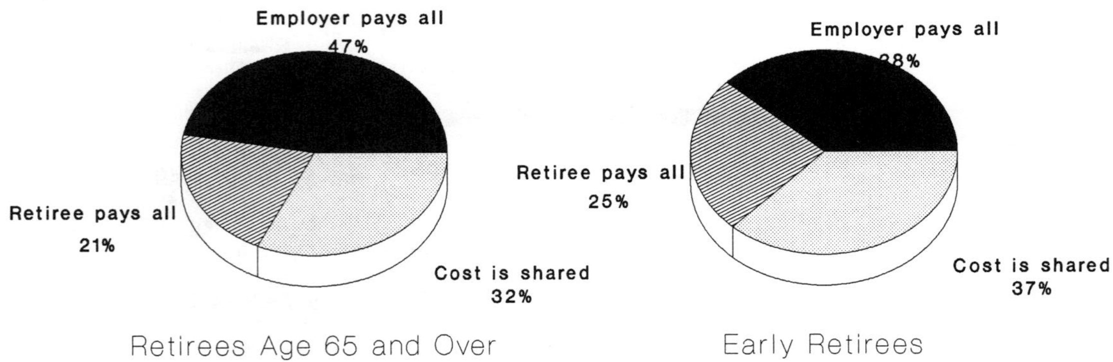

Source: Foster Higgins, 1988

Chapter 2

DRUG UTILIZATION

Drug utilization data, overall, by category, population group. New drug categories, etc., generic vs. brand name use

Current Trends in the Number of Prescriptions Dispensed 1978-1987

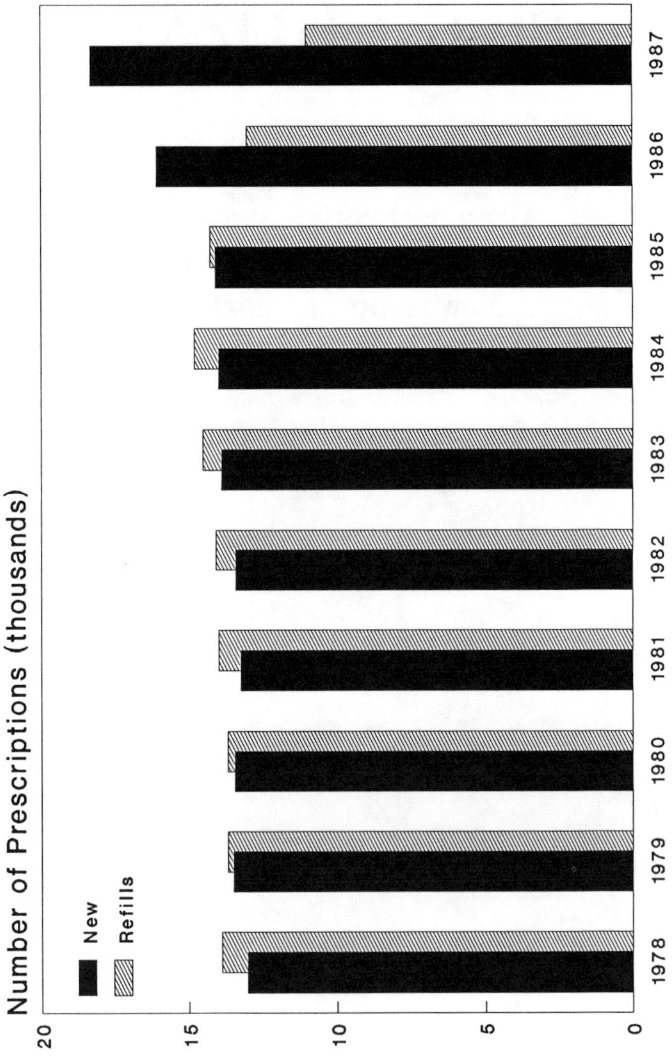

Source: Lilly Digest, 1979-1988

Total New and Refill Prescriptions

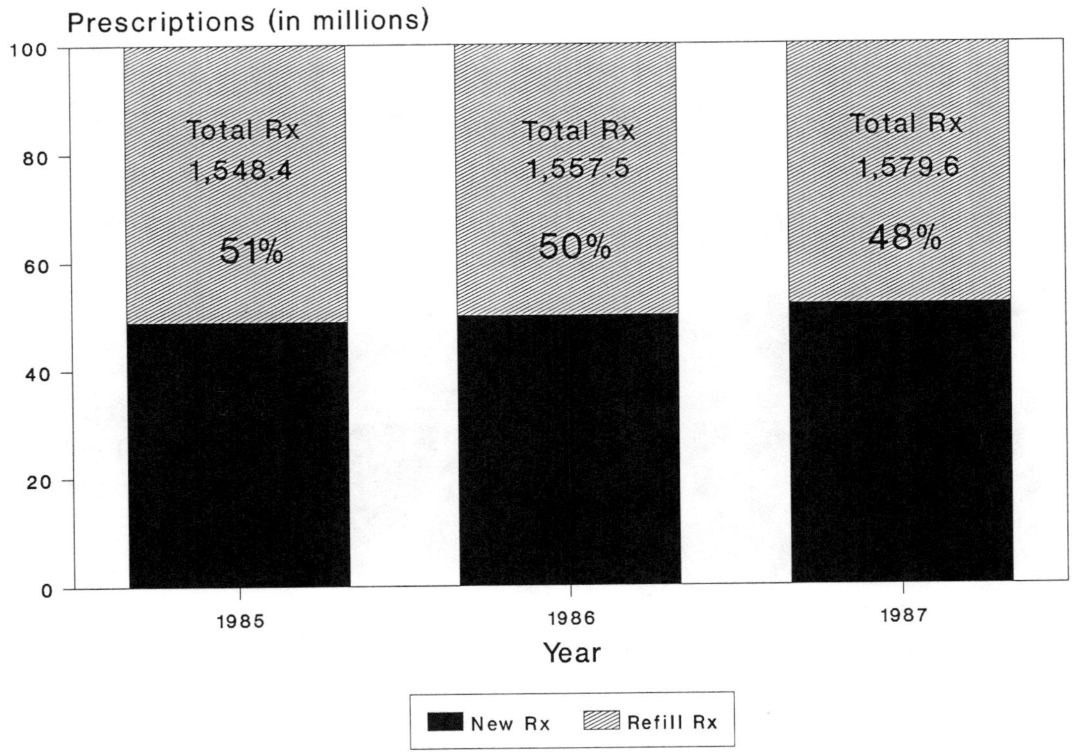

Source: Year-in-Review, 1987
IMS America, LTD., 1988.

National Prescription Audit: New RX

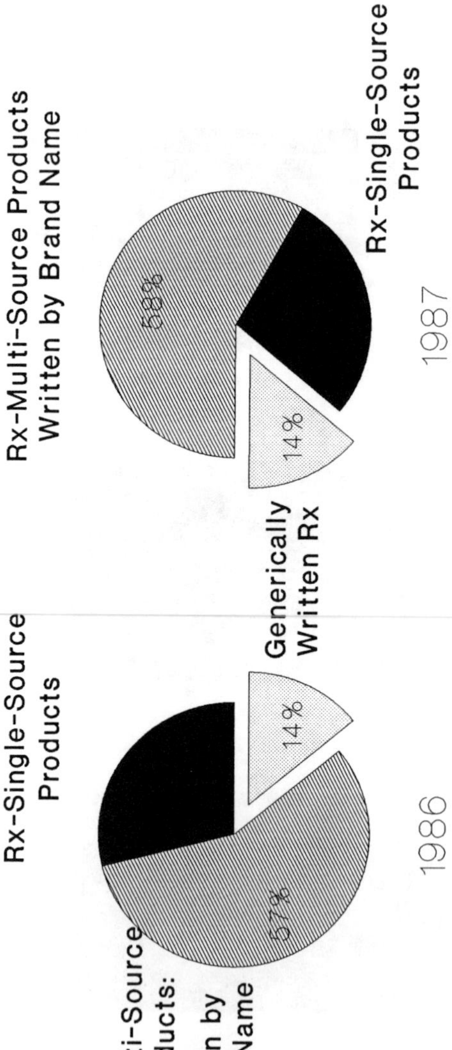

Source: Year-in-Review, 1987
IMS America, LTD., 1988.

Order Item ID: 169730609017801

Condition note: OUT OF PRINT. NO PRINT LINE. NO DUST JACKET. INSIDE IS VERY GOOD.

Returning your item:

Go to "Your Account" on Amazon.com, click "Your Orders" and then click the "seller profile" link for this order to get information about the return and refund policies that apply.

Visit https://www.amazon.com/returns to print a return shipping label. Please have your order ID ready.

Thanks for buying on Amazon Marketplace. To provide feedback for the seller please visit www.amazon.com/feedback. To contact the seller, go to Your Orders in Your Account. Click the seller's name under the appropriate product. Then, in the "Further Information" section, click "Contact the Seller."

Ship To:

AMZ Order -APTP - 1033840-1-0764
Main Address
800 Avondale Ave
1033840-1-0764
Grandview Heights, OH 43212

Buyer PO #: 1033840-1-0764

Order ID: 113-3781371-4994612

Thank you for buying from uniquebooksplus on Amazon Marketplace.

Shipping Address:	Order Date:	Mon, Sep 14, 2026
AMZ Order -APTP	Shipping Service:	Standard
Main Address	Buyer Name:	CollegeBooksDirect
800 Avondale Ave	Seller Name:	uniquebooksplus
1033840-1-0764		
Grandview Heights, OH		
43212		

Quantity	Product Details
1	**Pharmaceutical Chartbook [Hardcover] [1990] Hartzema, Abraham G.; Peretto, Eleanor; Hirsch, Jan D.** **SKU:** EWB*J 10/9/2017 11734 1CG/.25[NPL,OOP]

Decline in the Percentages of Total New and Refill Prescriptions of the Top 200 Drugs, 1980 - 1987.

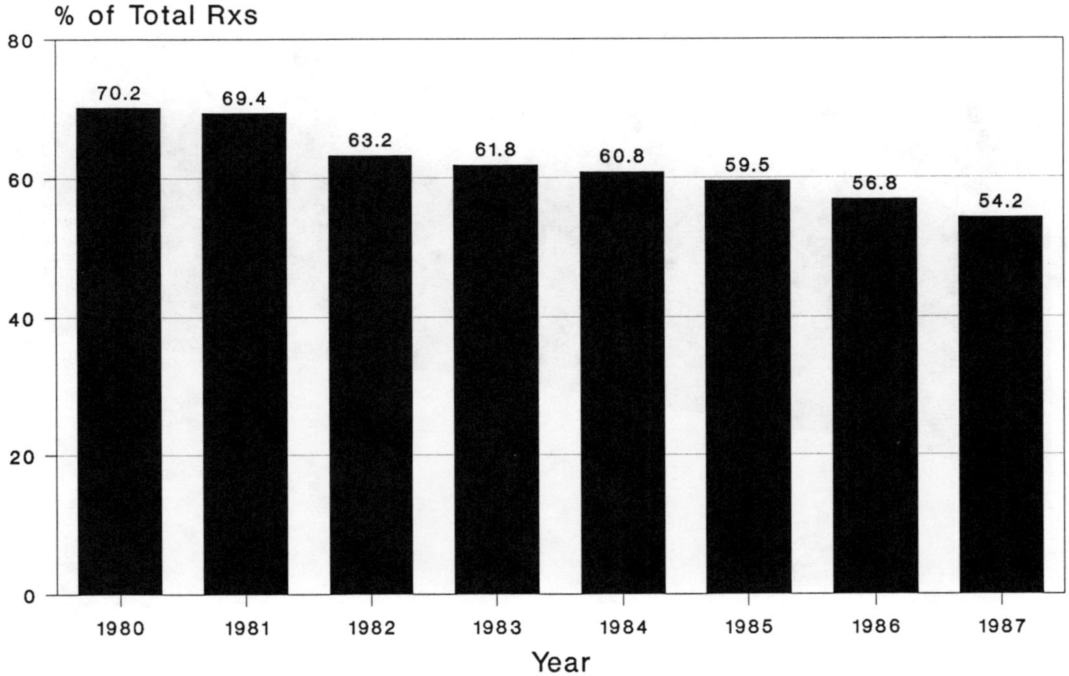

Source: Pharmacy Times, April 1988

Percent of Prescriptions Filled by Chains

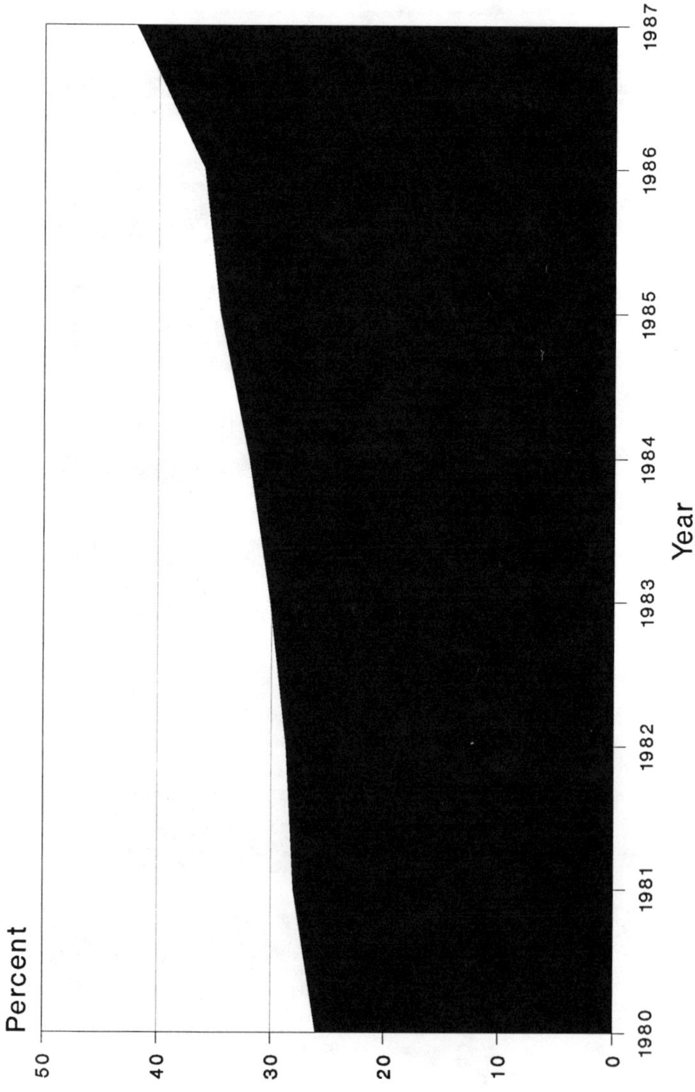

Source: National Association of Chain Drug Stores, Inc. 1987

U.S. Prescription Volume 1977-1987

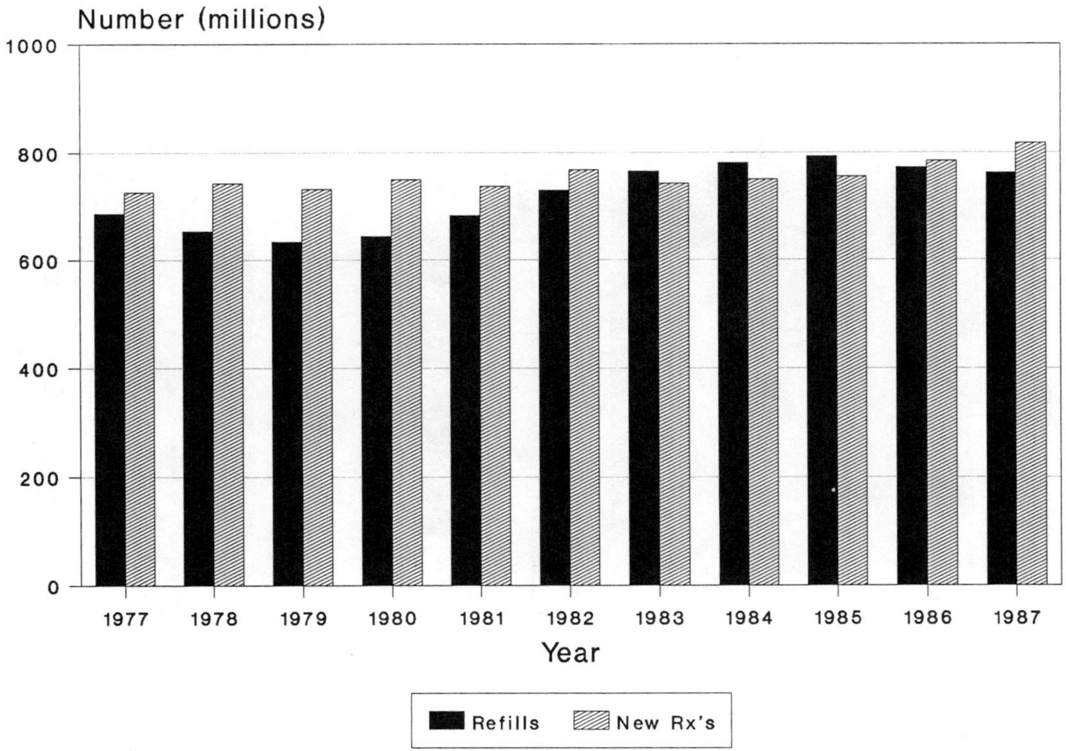

Source: National Prescription Audit, IMS America, LTD, 1988.

New Prescription Volume: Product Source

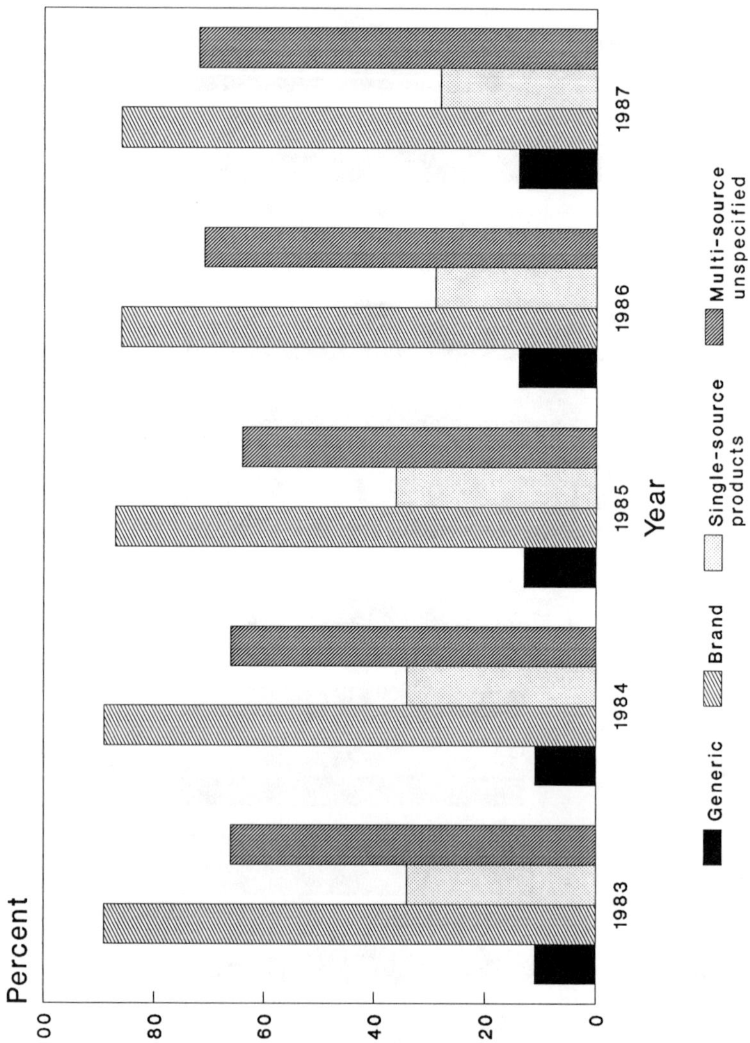

Source: Year-in-Review, 1987
IMS America, LTD., 1988.

Top 25 Prescription Drugs- New and Refill Rxs Dispensed by Drugstores (1987)

Rank 1987	Rank 1986	Drug Product	(% Change) Rxs Dispensed	Manufacturer
1	1	Dyazide	-12	SK&F
2	2	Amoxil	-10	Beecham
3	4	Lanoxin	- 1	Burroughs
4	12	Xanax	14	Upjohn
5	6	Tagamet	-11	SK&F
6	5	Tylenol w/Codeine	-14	McNeil
7	3	Inderal	-25	Ayerst
8	10	Tenormin	- 5	ICI Pharma
9	22	Zantac	23	Glaxo
10	15	Premarin	3	Ayerst
11	17	Ortho-Novum	-24	Ortho
12	16	Synthroid	- 3	Flint
13	9	Lasix	- 8	Hoechst-Roussel
14	19	Naprosyn	7	Syntex
15	13	Darvocet-N	- 8	Lilly
16	11	Motrin	-20	Upjohn
17	32	Cardizem	26	Marion
18	27	Ceclor	25	Lilly
19	8	Valium	-26	Roche
20	60	Seldane	38	Merrell Dow
21	17	Theo-Dur	- 8	Key
22	31	Halcion	12	Upjohn
23	41	Capoten	25	Squibb
24	18	Lopressor	- 8	Geigy
25	26	Procardia	- 4	Pfizer

Source: Pharmaceutical Data Services: Drug Topics, March 7, 1988.

Top 25 Prescription Drugs
New Rxs Dispensed in Drugstores
(1987)

Rank 1987	Rank 1986	Drug Product	Manufacturer
1	1	Amoxil	Beecham
2	2	Tylenol w/Codeine	McNeil
3	7	Ceclor	Lilly
4	12	Xanax	Upjohn
5	3	Keflex	Dista
6	6	Dyazide	SK&F
7	8	Darvocet-N	Lilly
8	13	Monistat	Ortho
9	11	Lanoxin	Burroughs Wellcome
10	16	Naprosyn	Syntex
11	10	Tagamet	SK&F
12	5	Valium	Roche
13	52	Seldane	Merrell Dow
14	21	Zantac	Glaxo
15	9	Motrin	Upjohn
16	152	Trimox	Squibb
17	23	Halcion	Upjohn
18	4	E.E.S.	Abbott
19	15	E-Mycin	Upjohn
20	36	Augmentin	Beecham
21	17	EryC	Parke-Davis
22	20	Premarin	Ayerst
23	48	Veetids	Squibb
24	18	Lasix	Roechst-Roussel
25	26	Synthroid	Flint

Source: Pharmaceutical Data Services, Drug Topics, March 7, 1988.

Top Ten Retail Drugs: 1987-1988

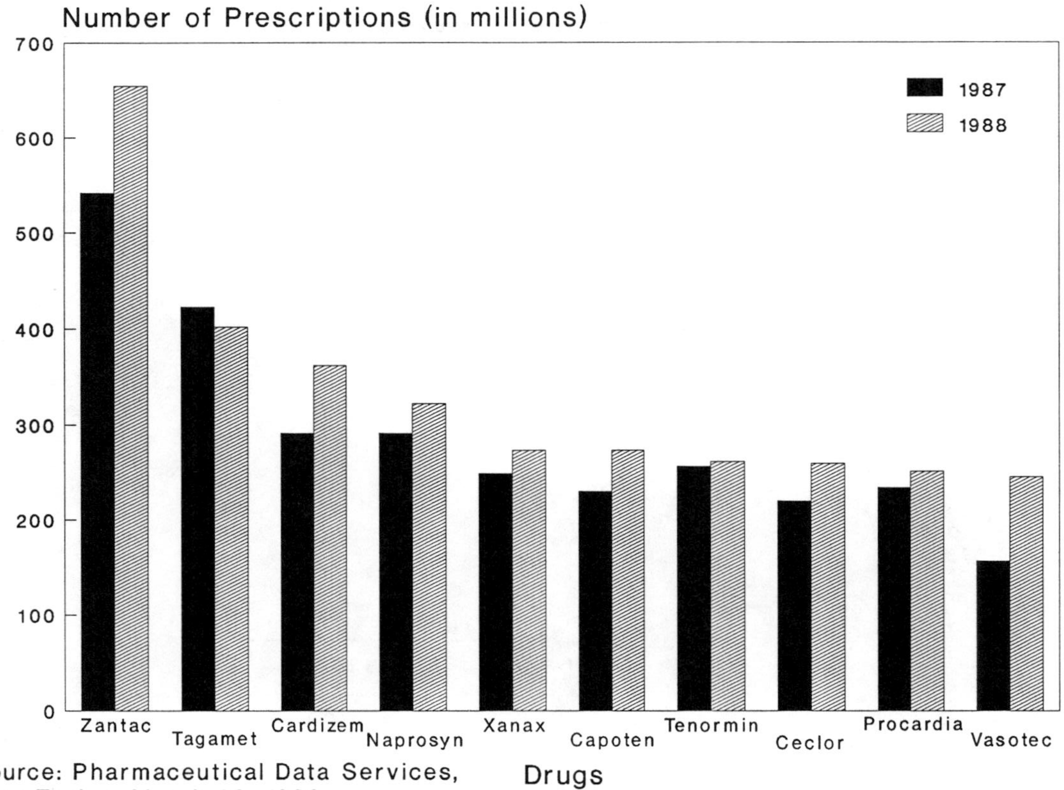

Source: Pharmaceutical Data Services, Drug Topics, March 20, 1989.

1988's Biggest Gainers

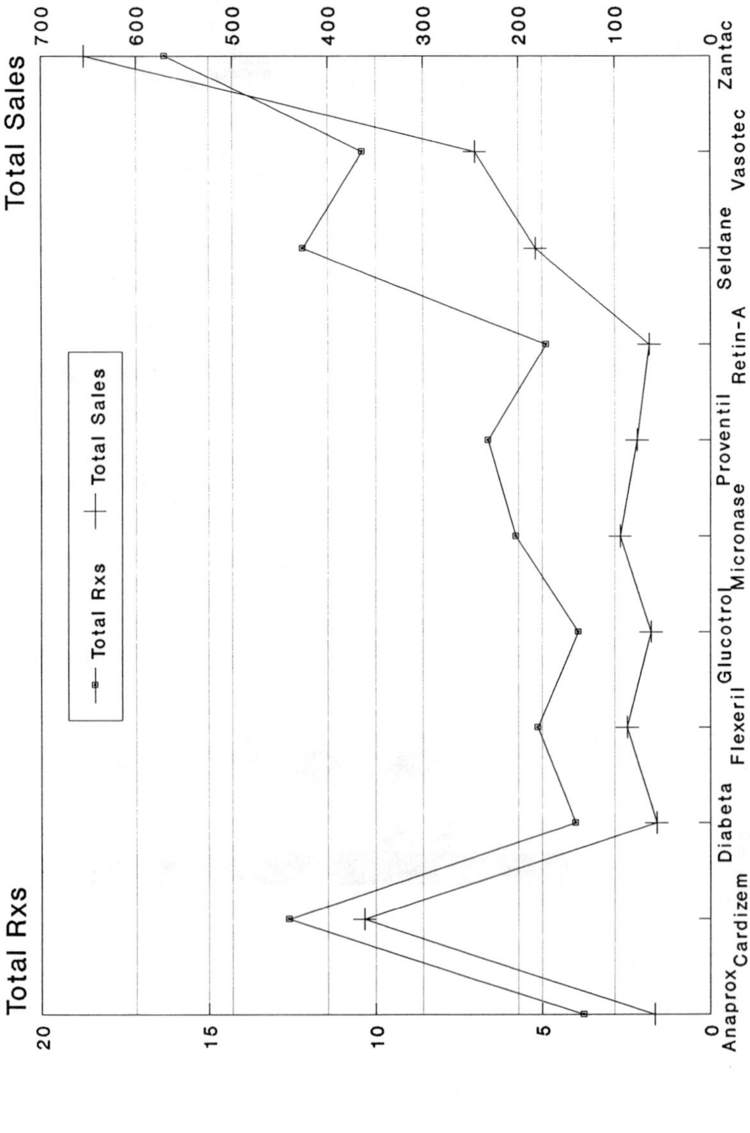

Source: Pharmaceutical Data Services;
Drug Topics, March 20, 1989.

Ranking of the Leading Products 1986 and 1987

Drug	1986	1987
Amoxil	3	1
Dyazide	1	2
Lanoxin	2	3
Xanax	7	4
Tagamet	6	5
Tylenol w/Codeine	4	6
Zantac	16	7
Inderal LA	5	8
Tenormin	11	9
Premarin	12	10

Source: Year in Review 1987, IMS America Ltd, 1988

Ranking of the Leading Products for Hospitals 1986 and 1987

Drug	1986	1987
Mefoxin	1	1
Zantac	7	2
Vancocin	2	3
Rocephin	11	4
Ancef	3	5
Cleocin Phos.	4	6
Claforan	8	7
Forane	13	8
Platinol	10	9
Cefobid	5	10

Source: Year in Review 1987, IMS America Ltd, 1988

The Top Ten Therapeutic Classes Worldwide (1987)

Hospital Sector	Pharmacy Sector
Cephalosporins	Antirheumatic Non-steroid
Anti-peptic Ulcerants	Anti-peptic Ulcerants
I.V. Solutions	Cephalosporins
Blood Products	Cerebral & Peripheral Vasotherapy
Broad Spectrum Penicillins	Beta-blockers
Anti-metabolics	Calcium Antagonists
Cytostatic Immunodilators	Non-narcotic Analgesics
Sera & Gamma Globulin	Diuretics
Neuroleptics	Tranquillisers
Cerebral & Peripheral Vasotherapy	Blood Spectrum Penicillins

Source: Glaxo, Scrip Yearbook, 1988.

1988 New Product Launches U.S. Retail Market

Brand Name	1988 Sales (000 omitted)	No. of Months on Market
Prozac (Dista) Antidepressant	$75,993	12
Voltaren (Geigy) Antiarthritic	40,922	4
Ceftin (Allen & Hanbury's) Antibiotic	35,319	10
Zestril (Stuart) Antihypertensives	13,282	12
Prinivil (MSD) Antihypertensives	12,129	12
Axid (Lilly) Antiulcer	11,108	8
Rogaine (Upjohn)	7,943	3

Pharmaceutical Data Services; Drug Topics, March 20, 1989.

Use of Psychotropic Drugs: Total U.S. Population

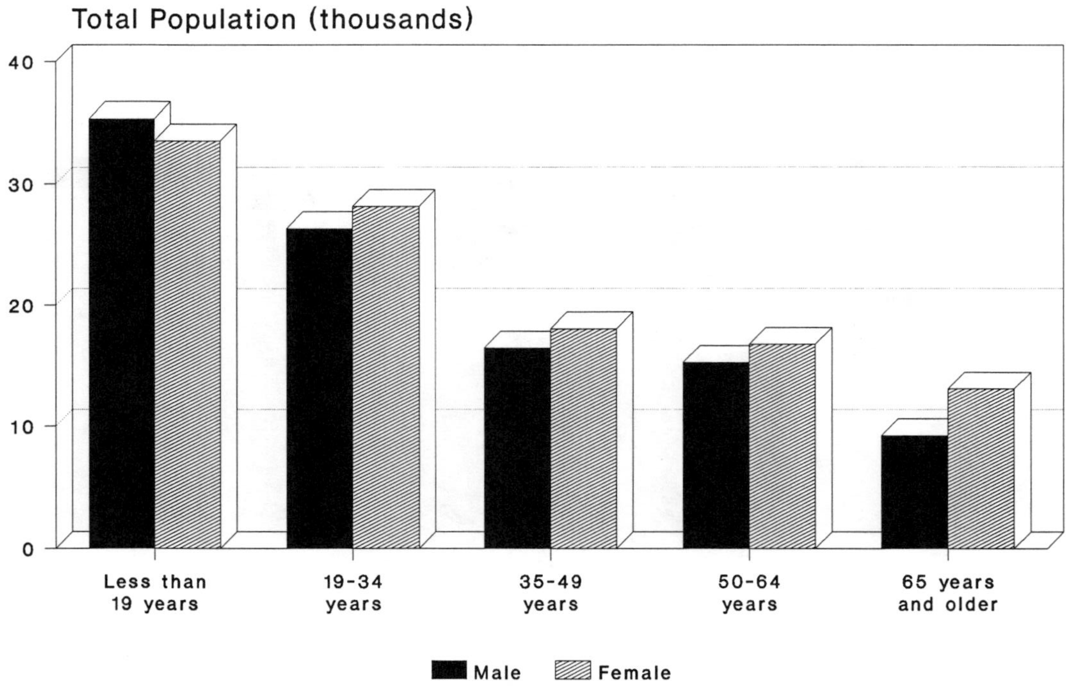

Source: National Center for Health Services, 1983.

Use of Psychotropic Drugs: Persons with at least One Psychotropic Drug Prescription

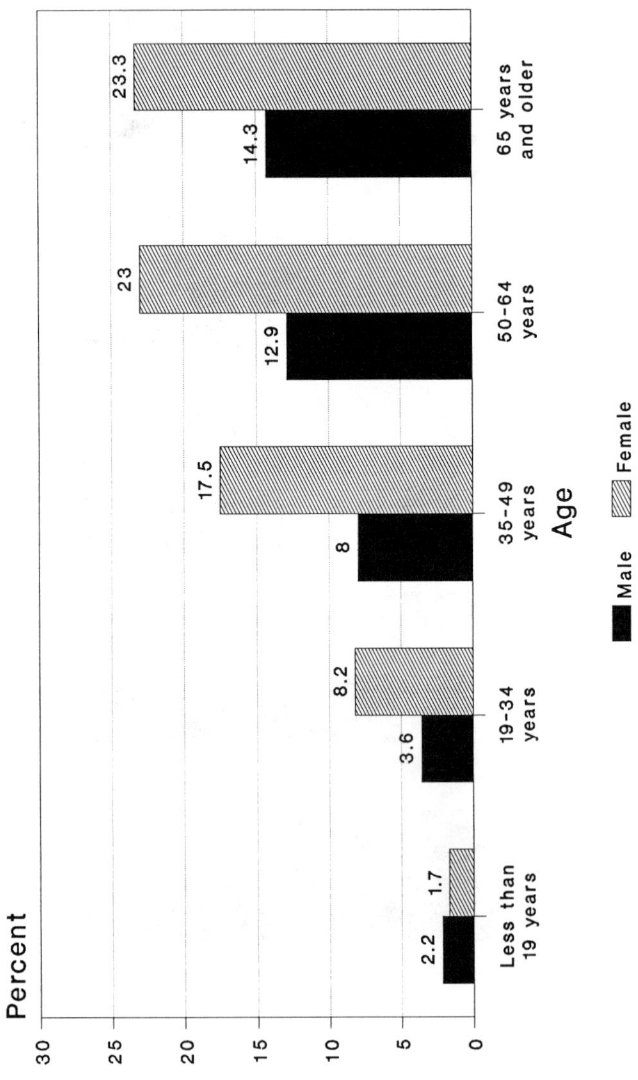

Source: National Center for Health Services Research, 1983.

Use of Psychotropic Drugs: Psychotropic Drugs as Percent of All Prescribed Medicines

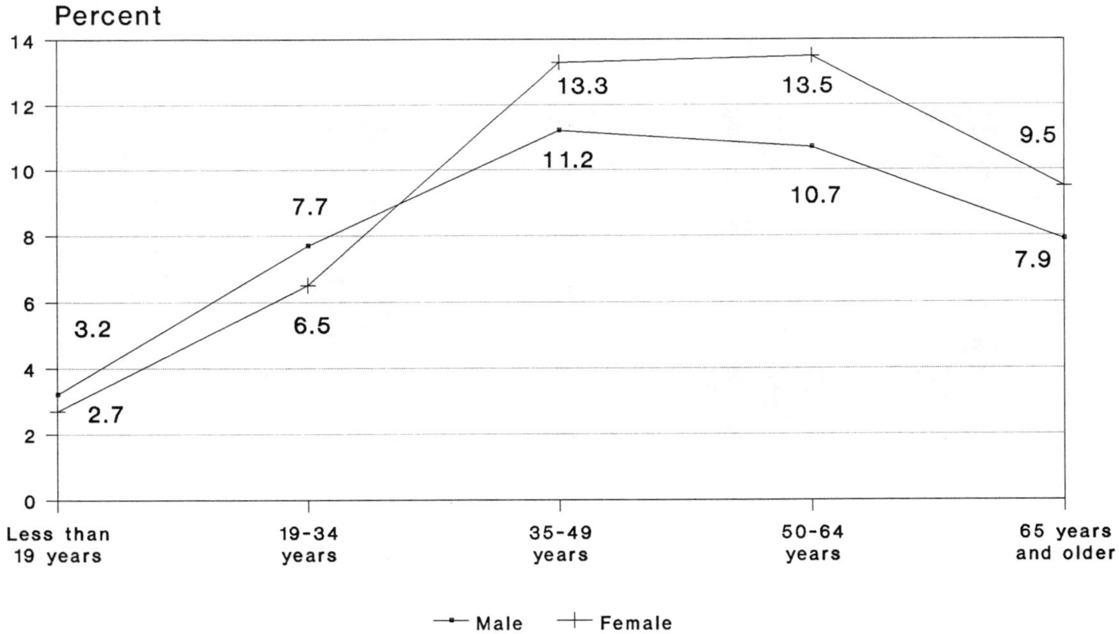

Source: National Center for Health Services Research.

Annual Expenses and Sources of Payment for Psychotropic Drugs: Mean Expense per Person with Expense

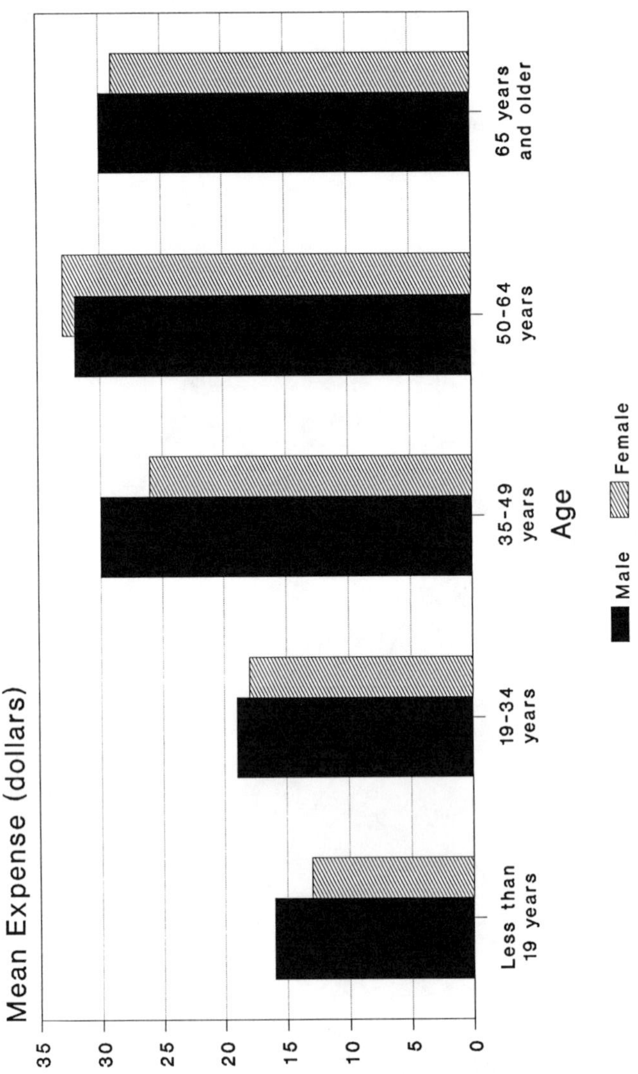

Source: National Center for Health Services Research.

Top Ten Diagnostic Related Groups

DRG Description	Discharges (thousands)
1. Heart failure & shock	323
2. Specific cerebrovascular disorder (transient ischemic attack excluded)	210
3. Angina pectoris	209
4. Simple pneumonia & pleurisy, ›17 yrs, w/complication &/or comorbidity	170
5. Esophagitis, gastroenteritis & misc digestive disorders, ›17 yrs, w/ complication &/or comorbidity	160
6. Major joint & limb reattachment procedures	146
7. Cardiac arrhythmia & conduction disorders w/complication &/or comorbidity	139
8. Nutritional & misc metabolic disorders, ›17 yrs, w/complication &/or comorbidity	136
9. Other factors influencing health status	135
10. Bronchitis & asthma, › 17 yrs, w/complication &/or comorbidity	123

Source: IHS Hospital Pharmacy Data Base , International Health Services, LTD

Ten Most Frequently Performed Surgical Procedures in 1986

Procedure	Numbers (thousands)
Biopsy	1,412
Cesarean section	906
Hysterectomy	644
Repair OB (Birth) laceration	612
Operations on spinal chord & spinal canal	571
Excision of skin lesions	565
Arthroplasty of joints	537
Cholecystectomy	502
Oophorectomy & salpingo-oophorectomy	502
Dilation & curettage of uterus	472

Source: The Division of Health Care Statistics of the National Center for Health Statistics

Use of Prescribed Medicines by Age

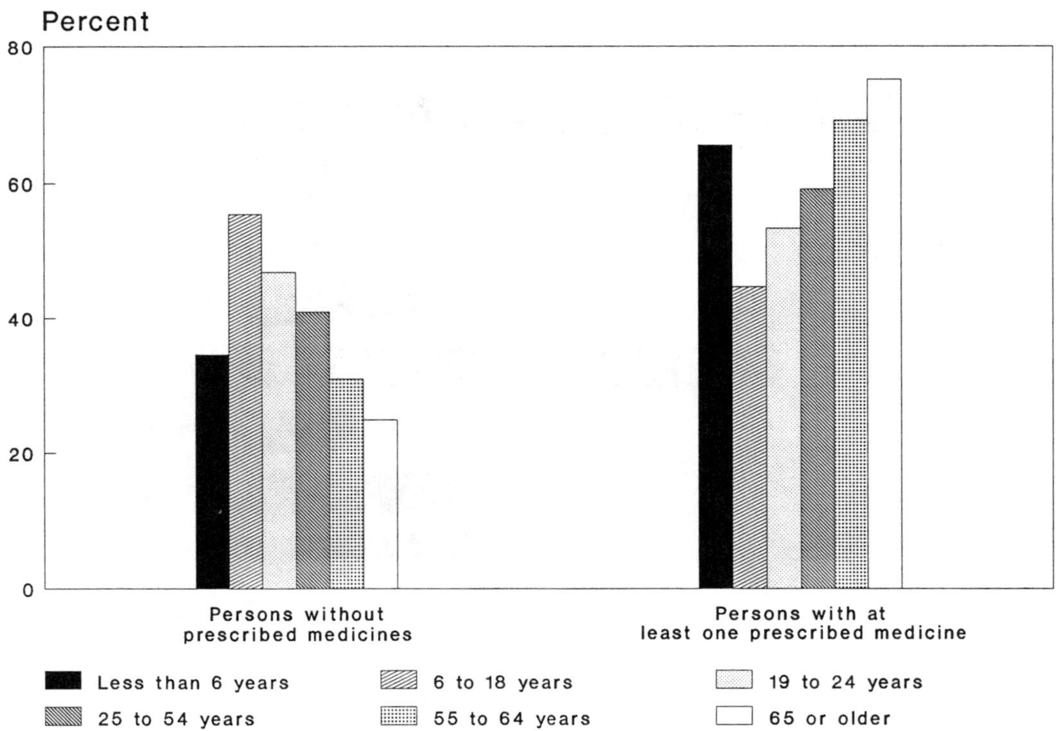

Source: National Center for Health Services Research, 1982.

Average Rate of Adverse Drug Reaction Reports in Nine Major Countries

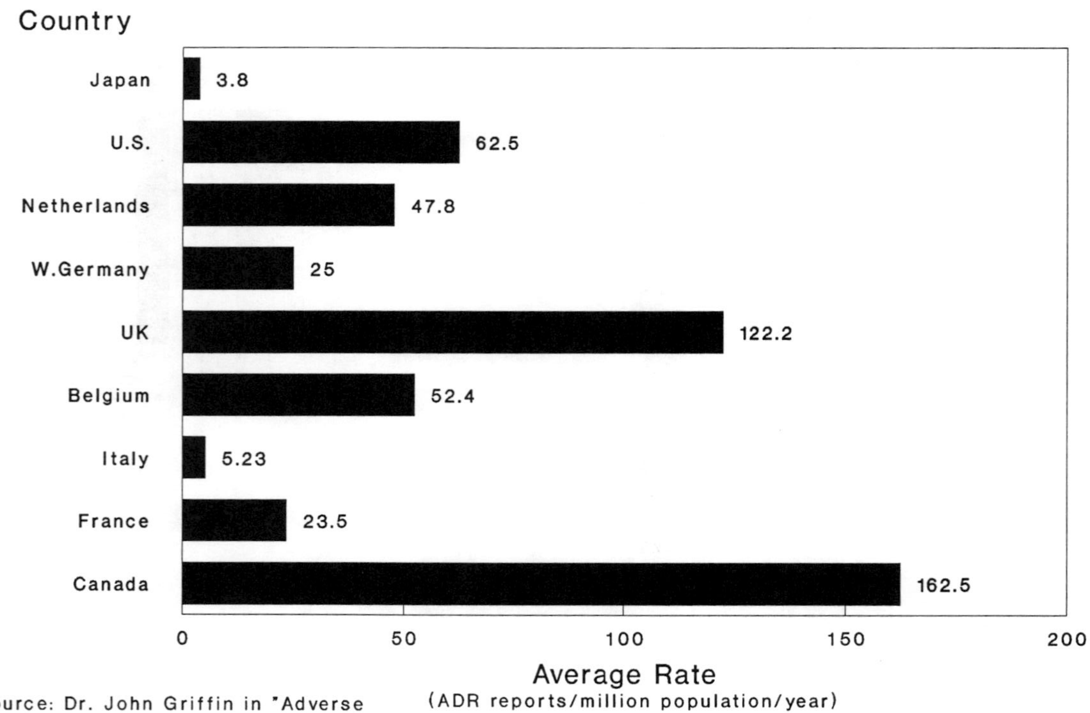

Source: Dr. John Griffin in "Adverse Drug Reactions-the scale and nature of the problem and the way forward"

Patients' Rating of Communication on Medication

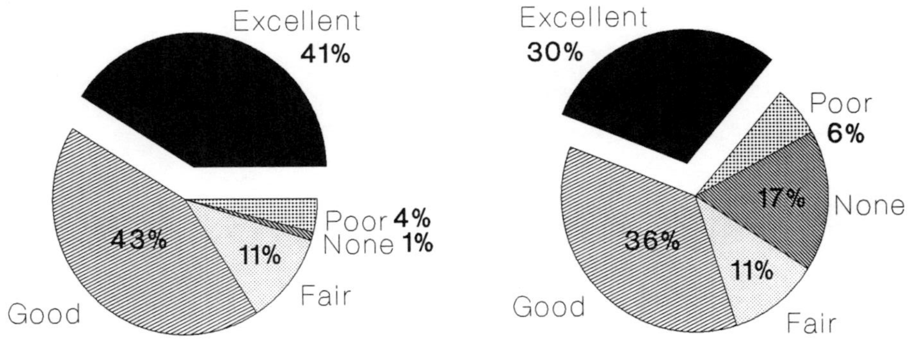

With Physician — With Pharmacist

Source: 1987 Industry Review

Chapter 3

DRUG COST EXPENDITURES

Drug cost expenditures are presented and contrasted with overall expenditure levels. This chapter also includes Consumer Price Index and other indicators.

Expenditures for Total Medical Care in the United States (1950-1987)

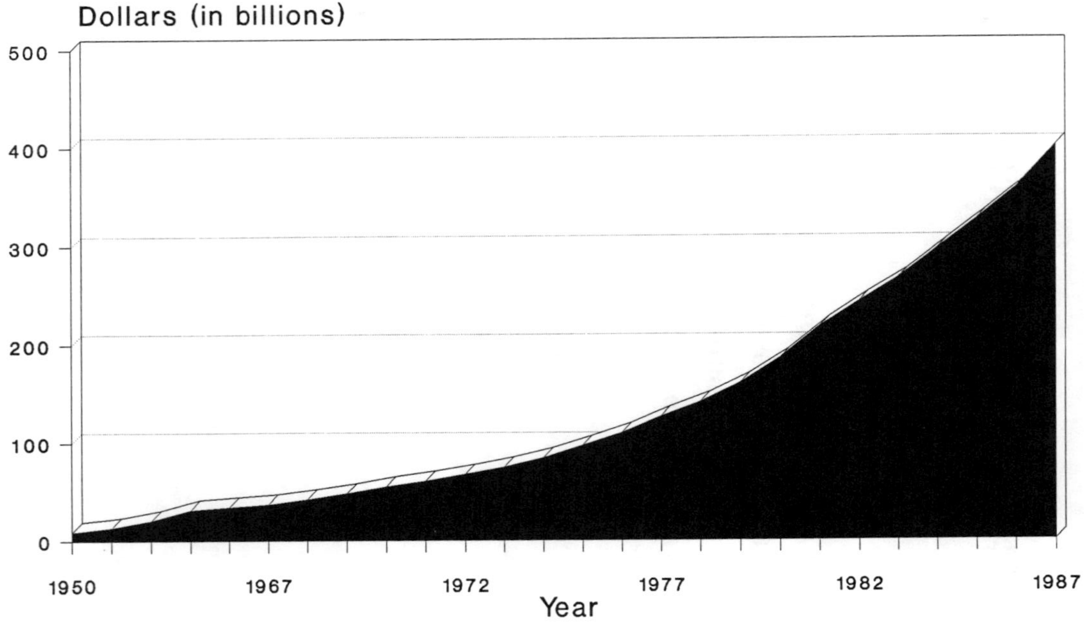

Source: U.S. Department of Commerce, Bureau of Economic Analysis, Survey of Current Business, various issues.

United States Total Health Care Expenditures

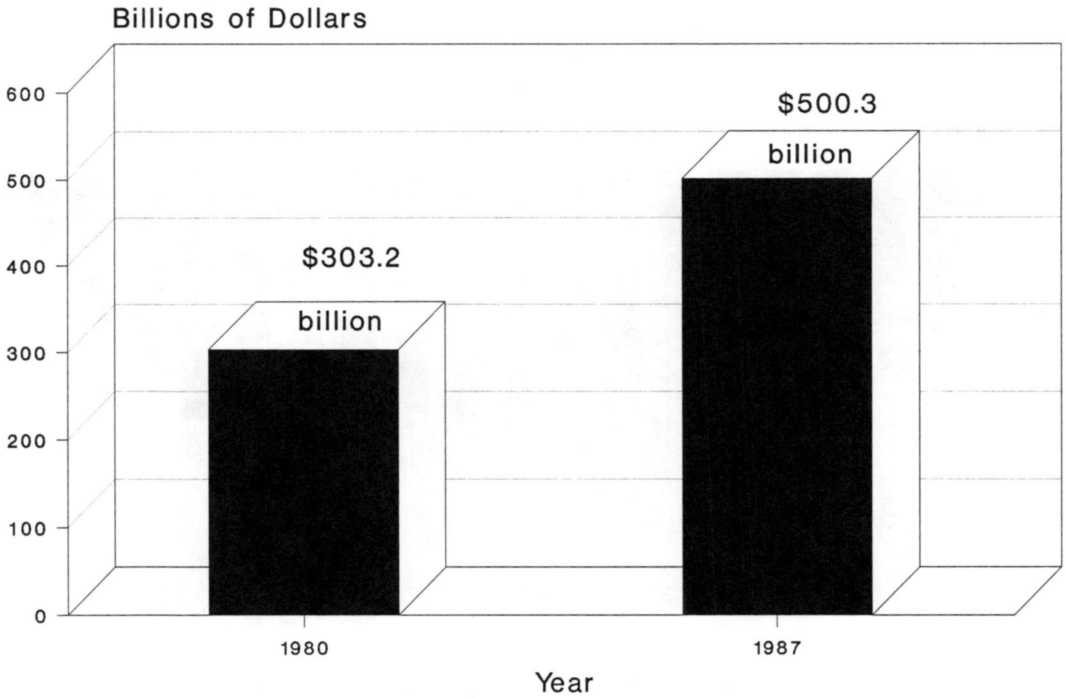

Source: Health Care Finance Administration, Volume 10, No.2, 1989.

Comparison of Annual Growth Rates of Gross National Product and National Health Expenditures, 1970-1987

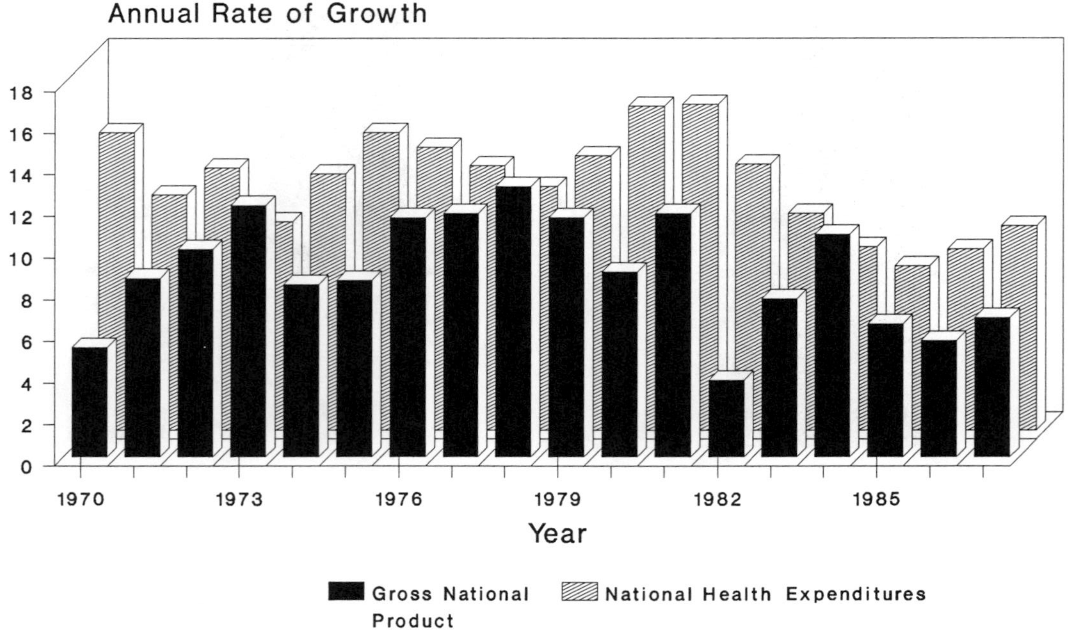

Source: U.S. Department of Health and Human Services, Health Care Financing Administration, 1989.

National Health Expenditures Aggregate
(selected calendar years 1970-1987)

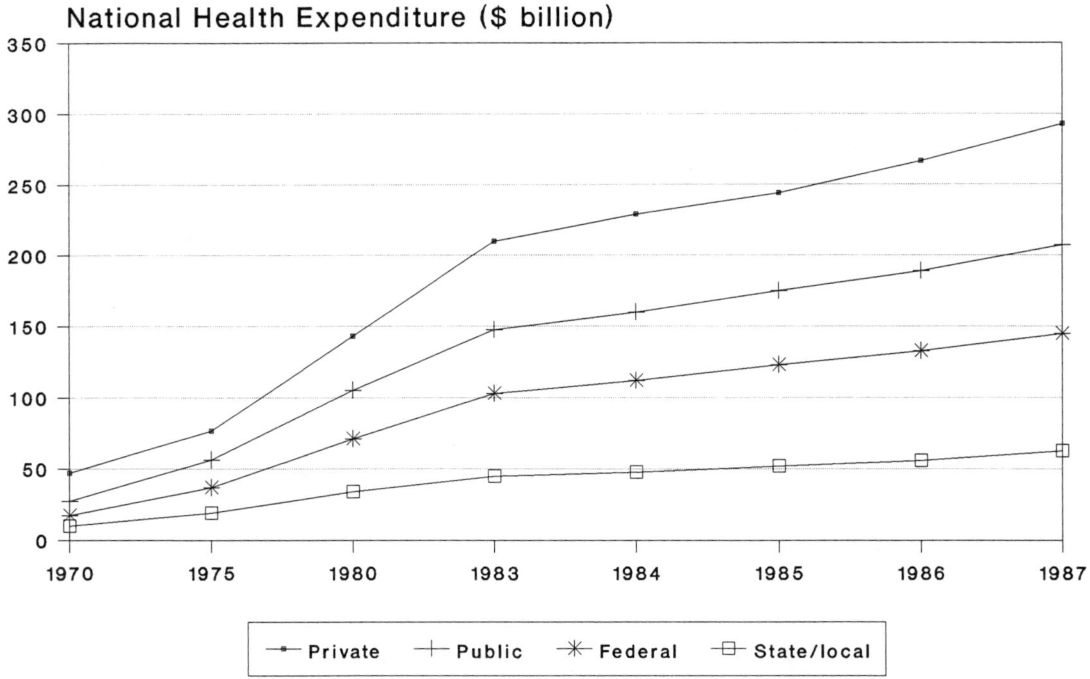

Source: Health Care Financing Administration; Source Book of Health Insurance Data, 1989.

Expenditures for Medical Care in the United States, (1965-1987)

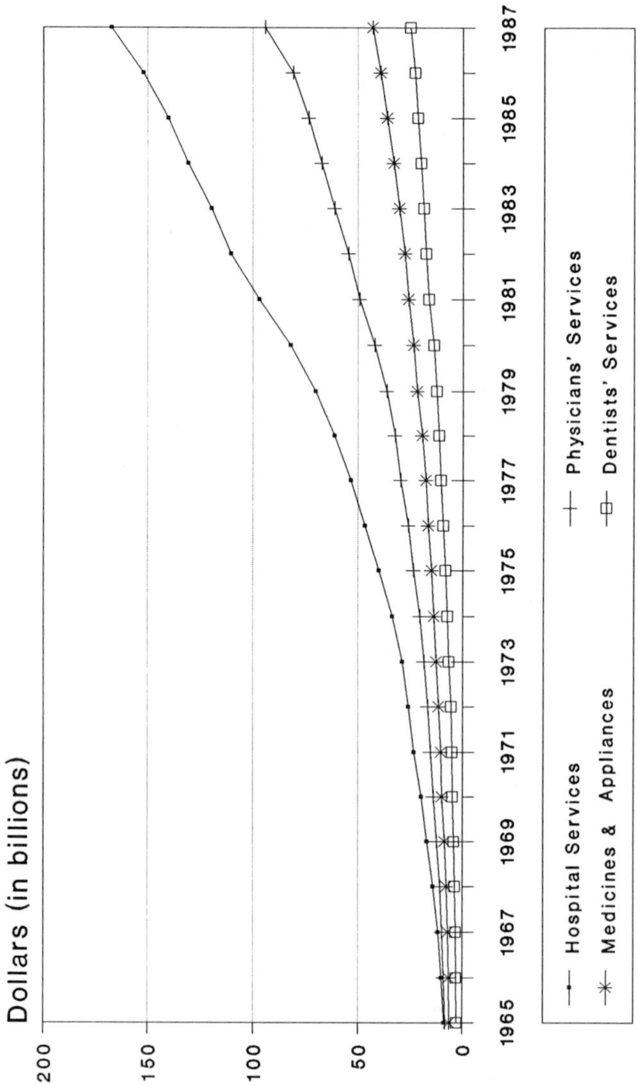

Source: U.S. Department of Commerce, Bureau of Economic Analysis, Survey of Current Business.

Medical Care Price Changes
(1987-1988)

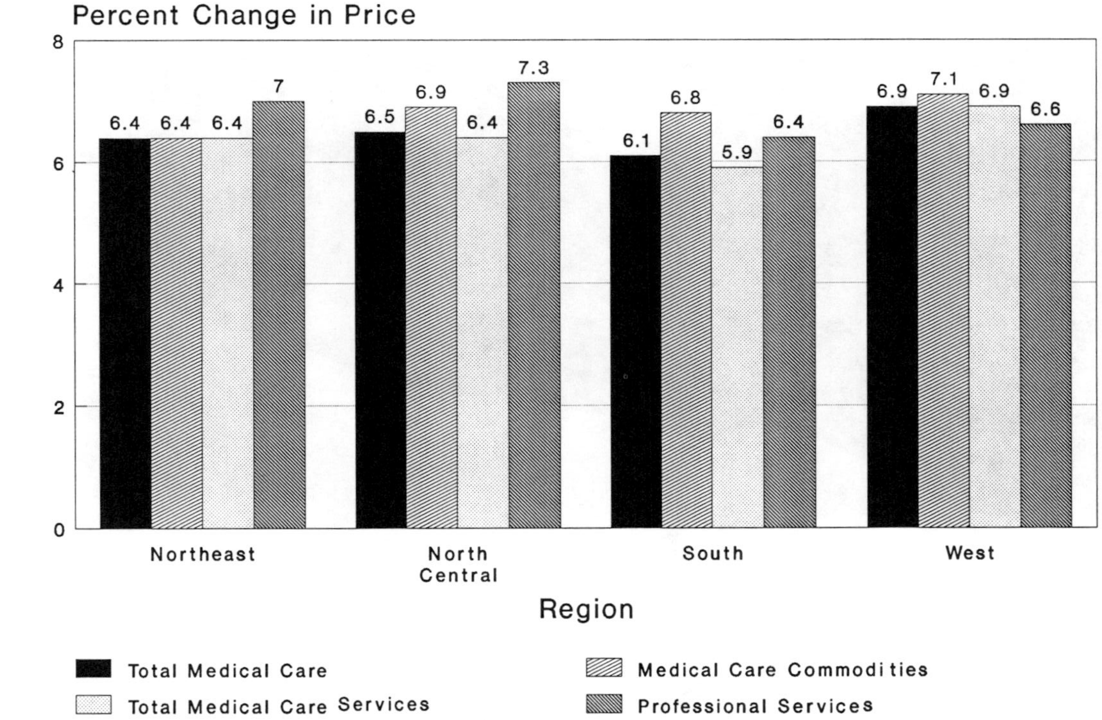

Source: U.S. Bureau of Labor Statistics

National Health Expenditures as a Percent of Gross National Product 1970-1986

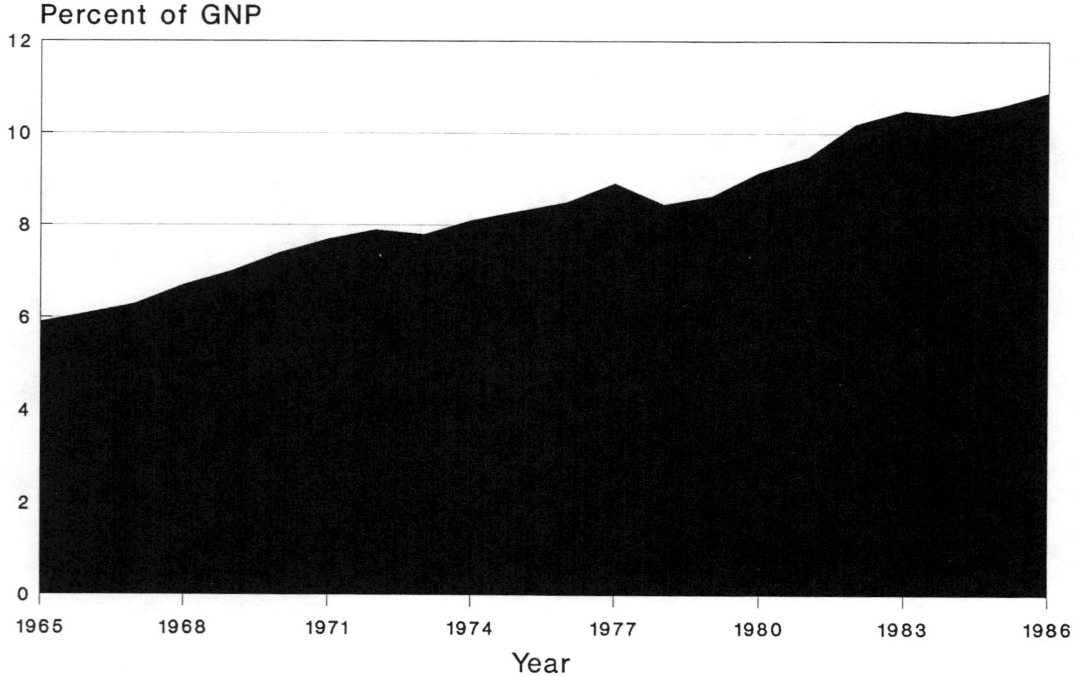

Source: HCFA, Fall 1986

Health Expenditures as Percent of Gross Domestic Product, 1986 (selected countries)

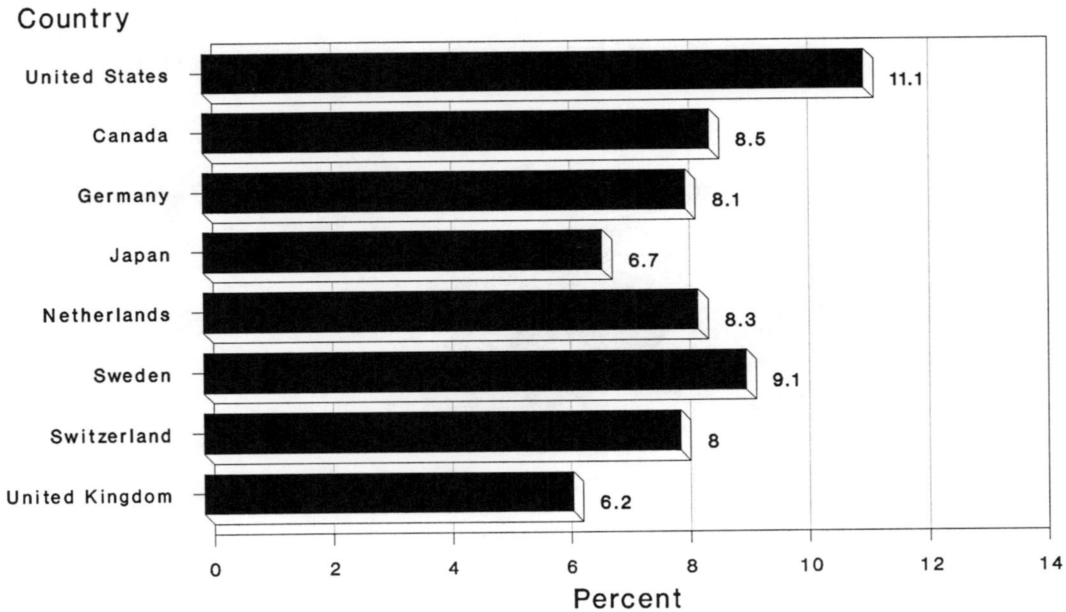

Source: Health Affairs, International Health Care Spending and Utilization Trends, Fall 1988

U.S. Total Health Care Expenditure: How the Bill is Paid

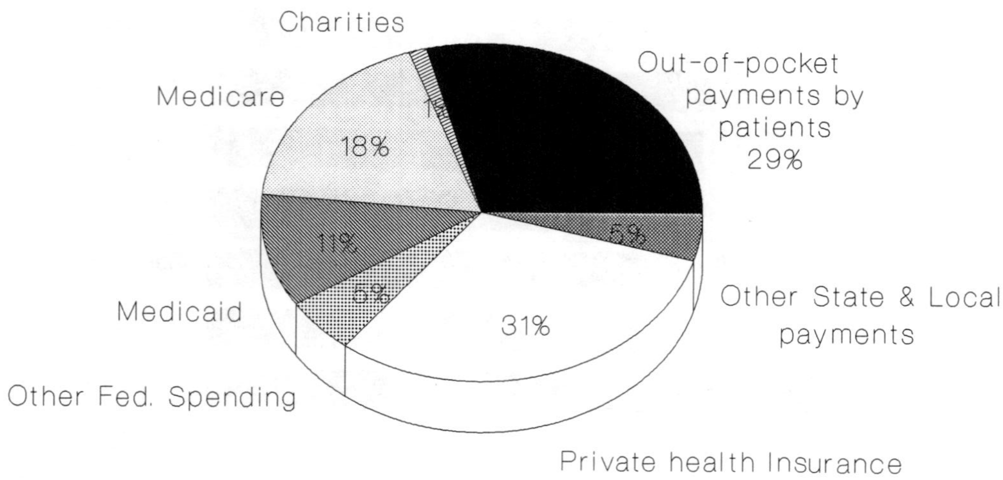

Source: Health Care Finance Administration, 1986.

The Nation's Health Dollar
1986

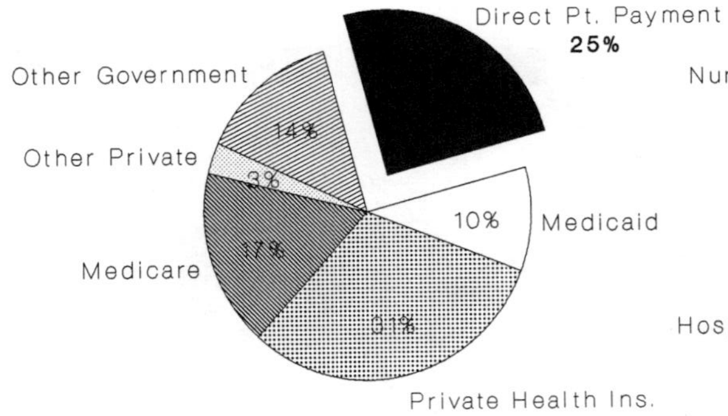

Where It Came From

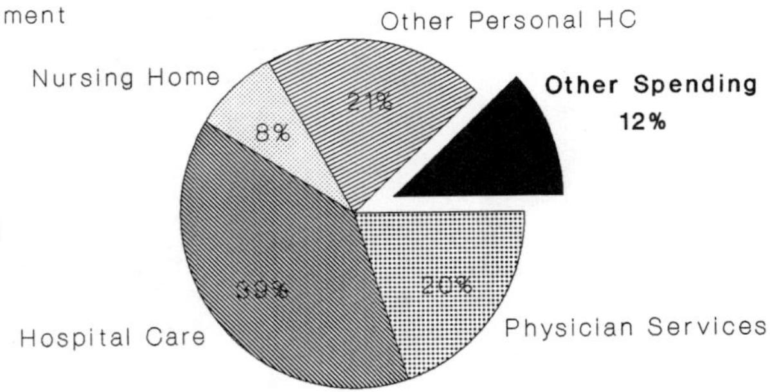

Where It Went

Source: HCFA 1986

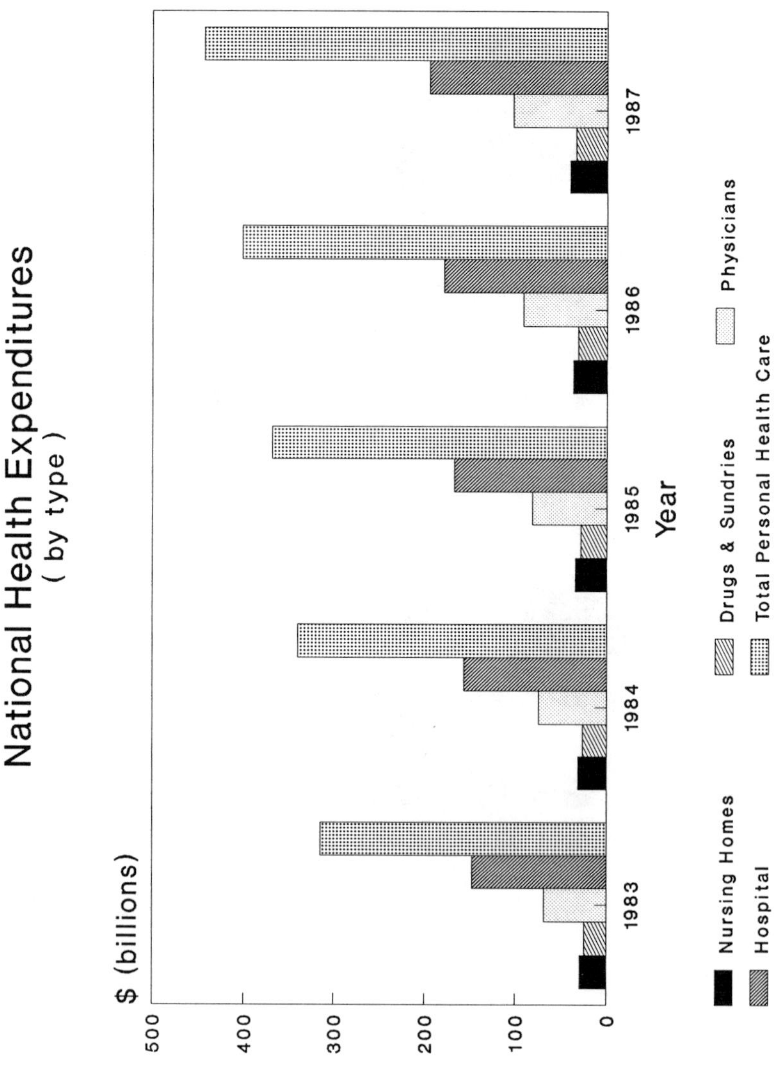

Source: "Health Care Financing Review", Volume 10, No.2, Health Care Financing Administration, 1989.

U.S. Total Health Care Expenditure: Where the Money Goes

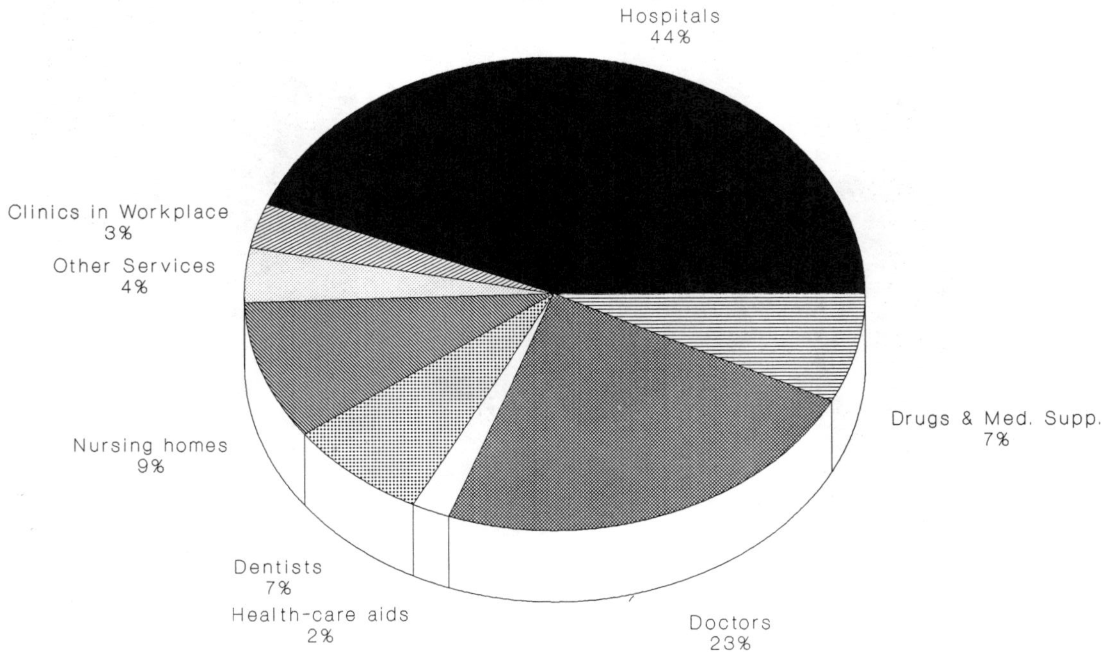

Source: Health Care Finance Administration, 1986.

1986 Health Care Expenditures
(before tax household income)

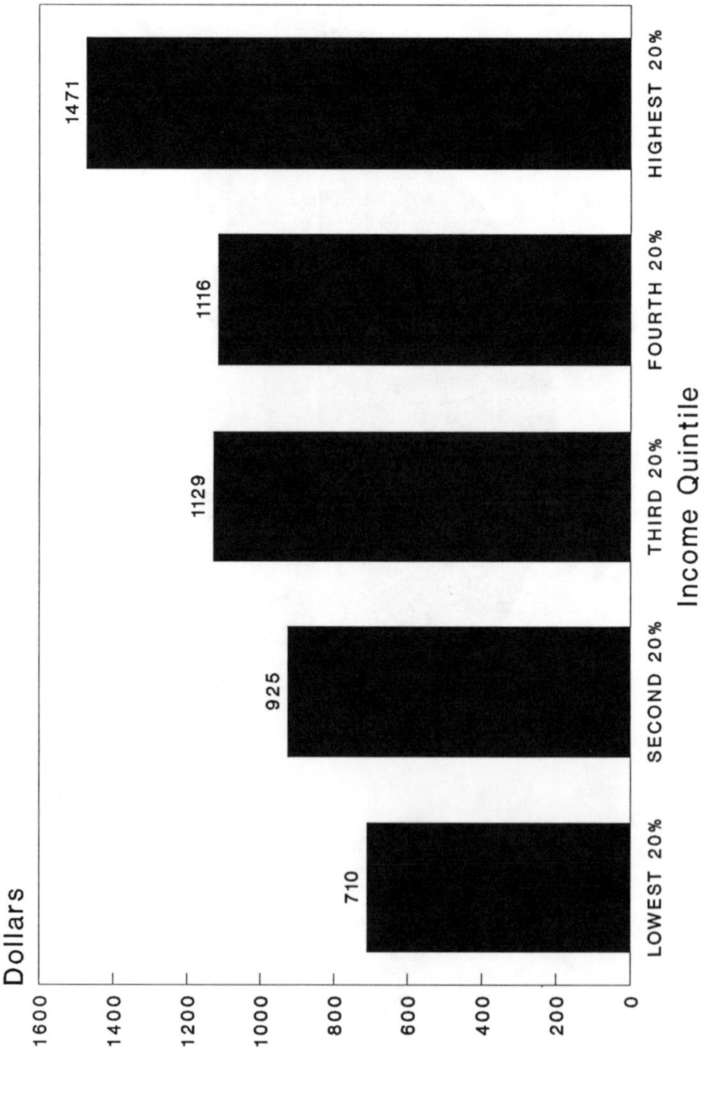

Source: U.S. Bureau of Labor Statistics, 1989 Statistical Abstracts.

Spending on Health Care: A Look at Eight Countries 1986

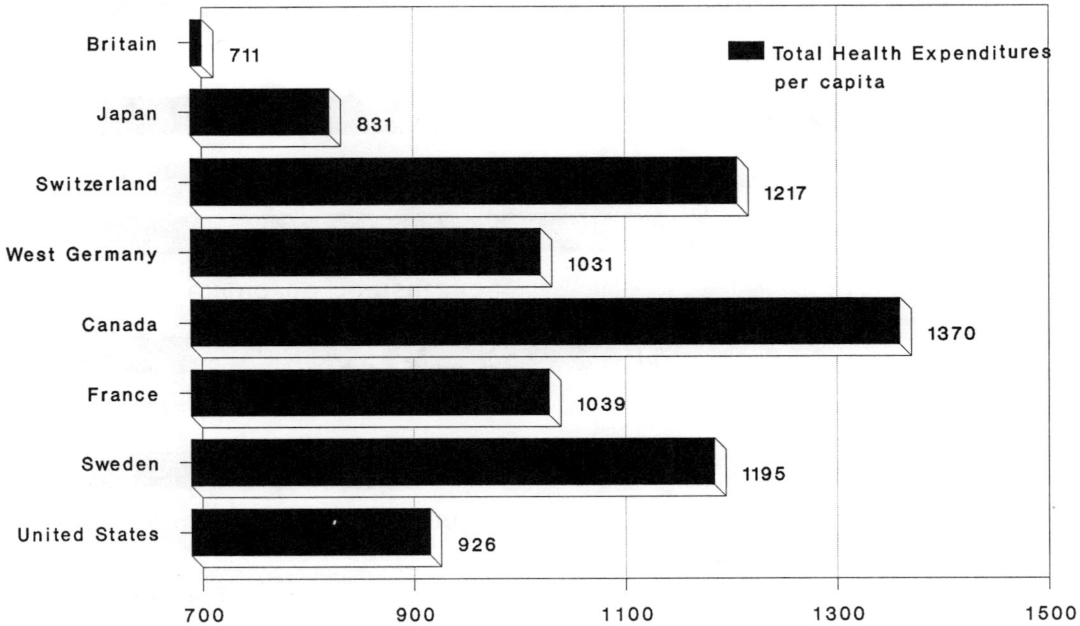

Source: U.S. Department of Health and Human Services, 1986.

Health Care Cost-Containment Measures

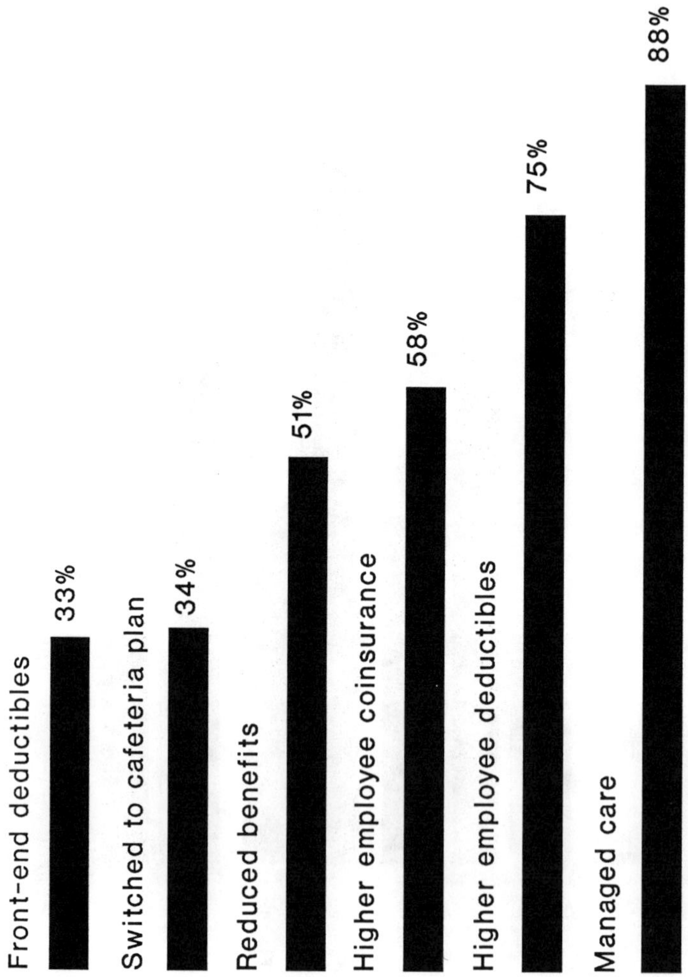

Source: Business Insurance, July 10, 1989. Managed HealthCare, August 14, 1989.

Consumer Price Index for Medical Care Items in the United States. 1967-1988

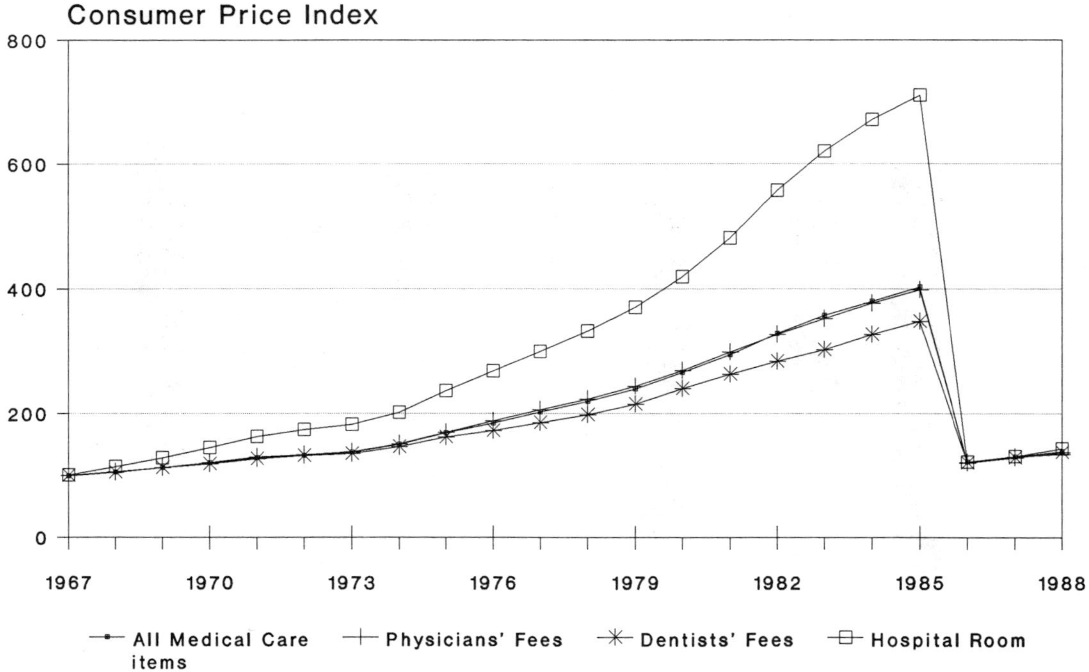

Source: U.S. Department of Labor, Bureau of Labor Statistics, CPI Detailed Report, various issues.

All Urban Consumers

Trends in Pharmaceuticals

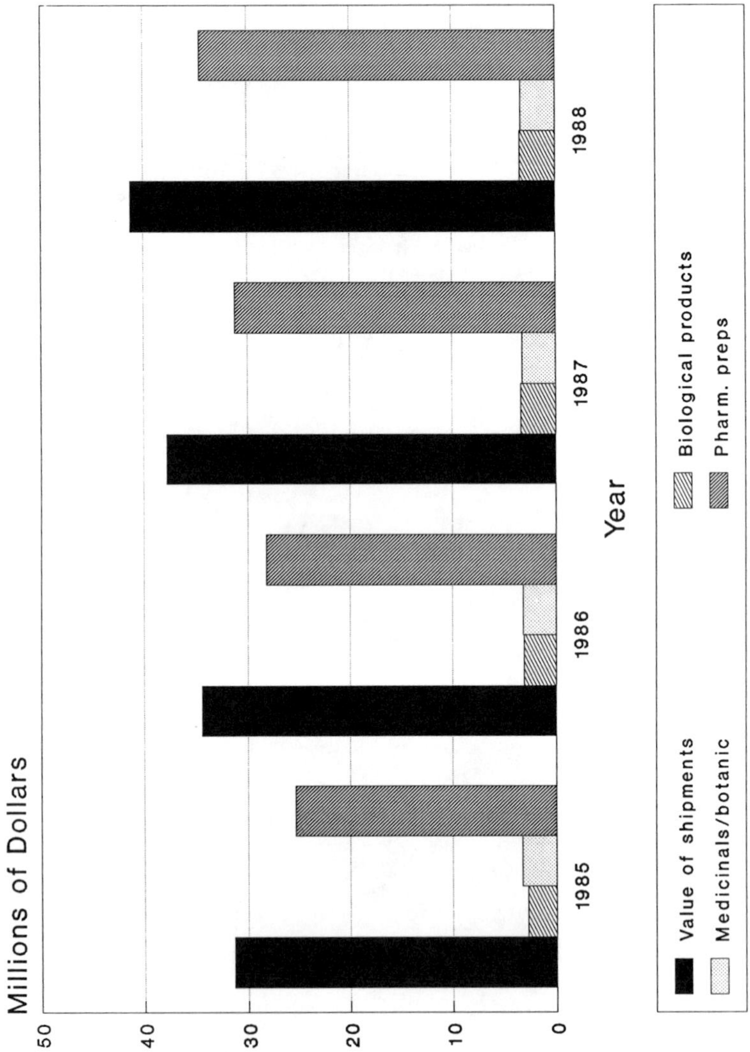

Source: U.S. Department of Commerce, Bureau of Census.

Consumer Price Index for Drugs and Prescriptions in the United States, 1967-1988

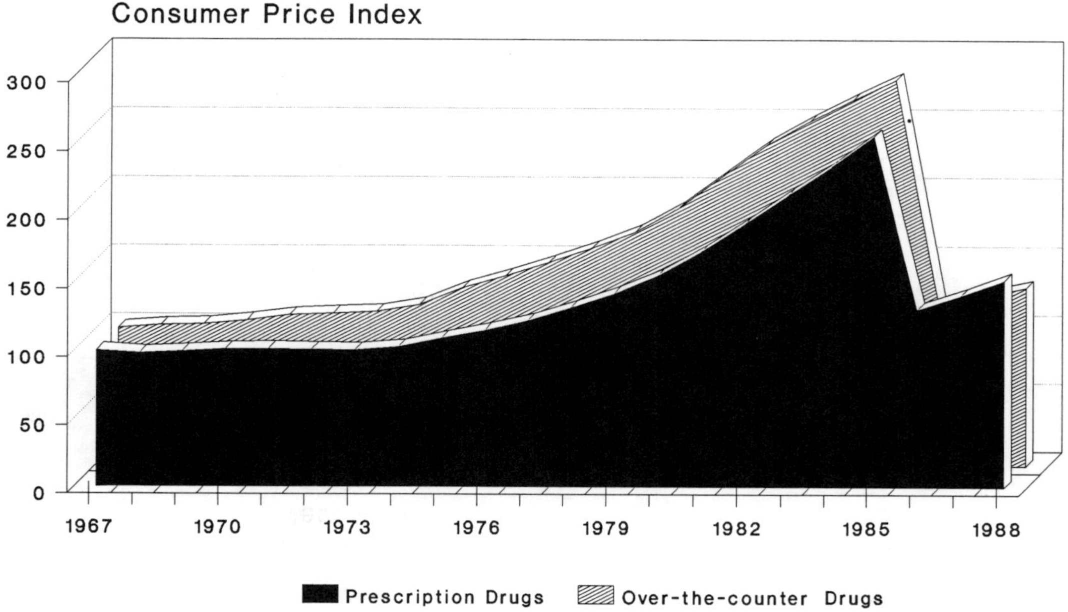

Source: U.S. Department of Labor, Bureau of Labor Statistics, CPI Detailed Report, Various issues.

All Urban Consumers

Per Capita Expenditure on Medicines by Country (1986)

Country	Per Capita Spend ($)
Japan	166.04
West Germany	136.32
France	127.63
Belgium	114.38
Italy	109.05
United States	109.00
Austria	98.24
Sweden	73.47
Netherlands	57.03
United Kingdom	50.75
Spain	50.70
Portugal	41.80
Australia	36.00
Argentina	31.00
South Korea	20.00
South Africa	13.00
Brazil	11.96
Mexico	9.00
Turkey	8.70

Source: Abifarma, Scrip 1264/21, Scrip Yearbook, 1

International Drug Price Comparison
Weighted Average Retail Price
Per Brand Drug, 1987

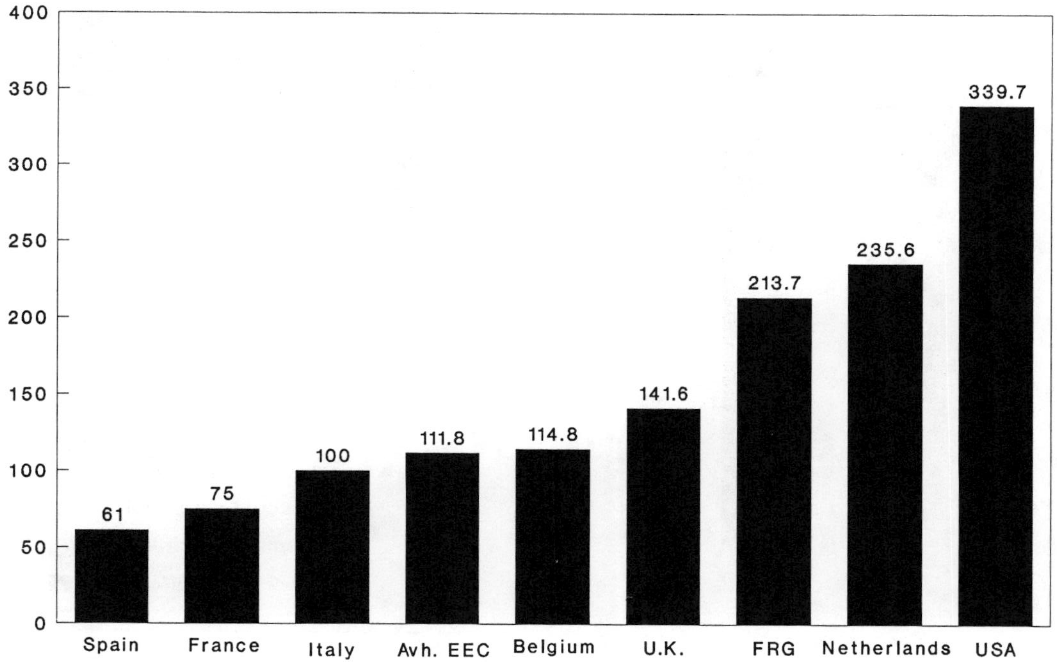

Source: Italian Pharmacutical
Manufacturers Association, 1988

Range of Market Prices Paid for Brand Name Prescription Drugs, Spring 1989

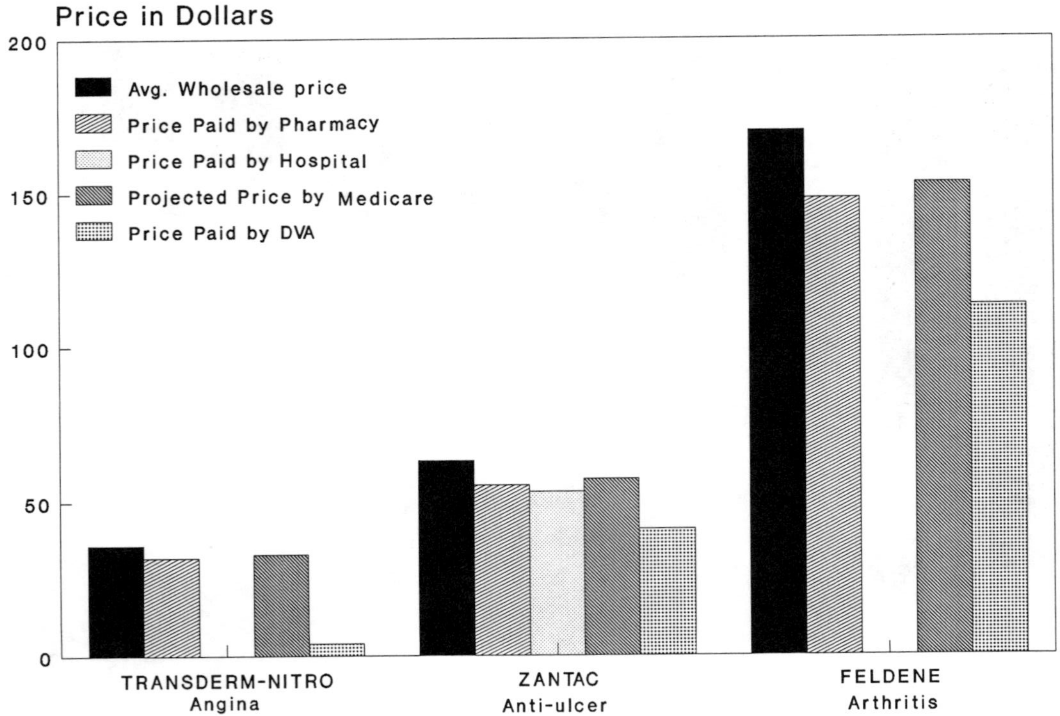

Source: U.S. Senate Special Committee on Aging, 1989.

Pharmaceutical Preparations- Producer Price Indexes

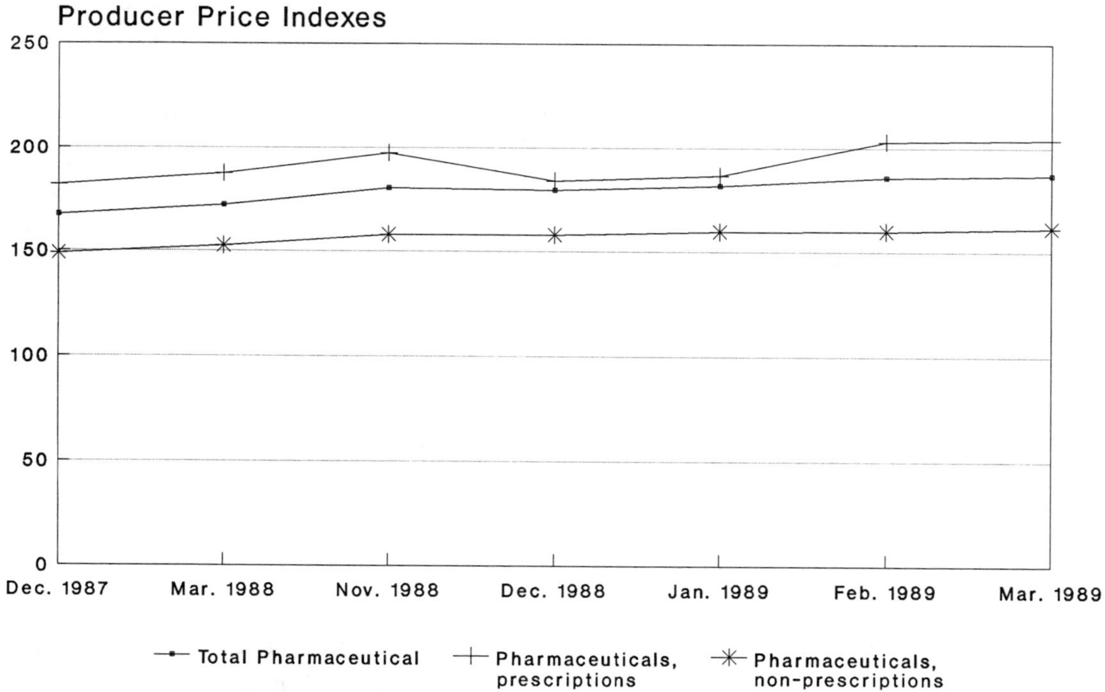

Sources: Bureau of Labor Statistics, Producer Price Indexes Data for March 1989, Table 5, & earlier periods.

Pharmaceutical Preparations-Producer Price Indexes

(comparison of selected OTC categories)

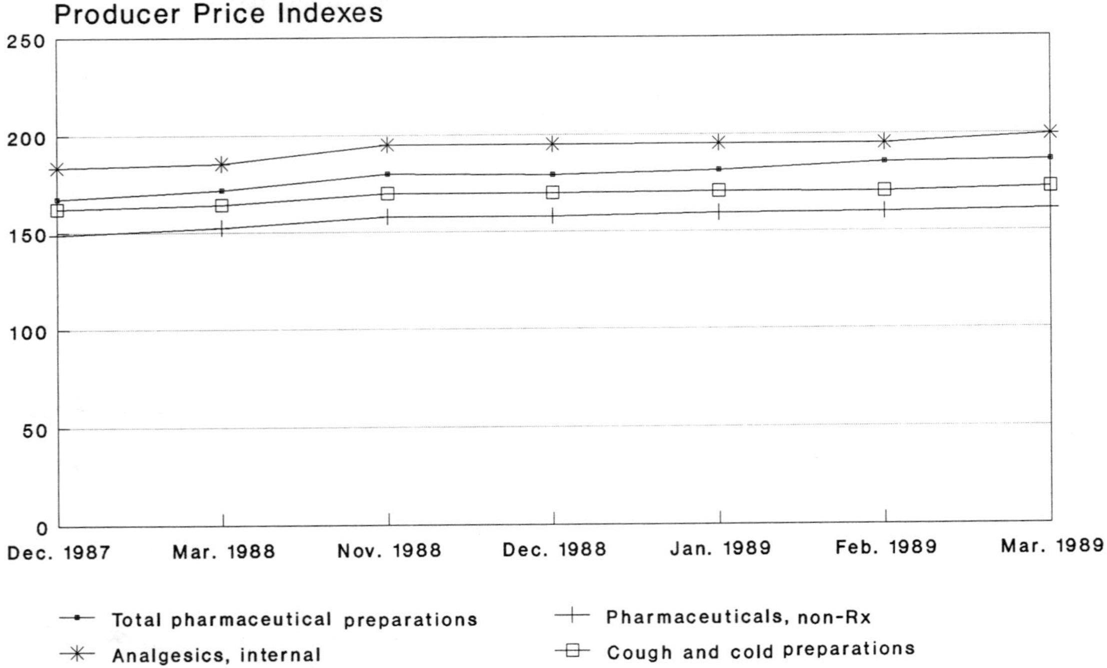

Bureau of Labor Statistics, Producer Price Indexes Data for March 1989, Table 5, and earlier periods.

Pharmaceutical Preparations-
Producer Price Indexes

(comparison of selected therapeutic categories)

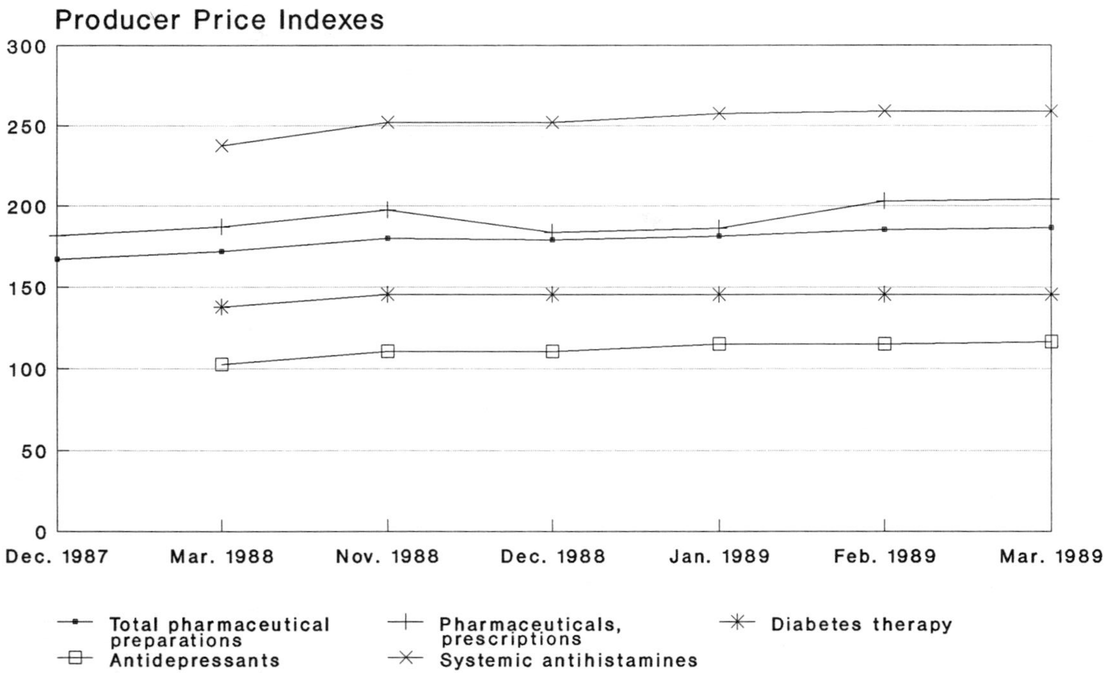

Bureau of Labor Statistics, Producer Price Indexes Data for March 1989, Table 5, and earlier periods.

Pharmaceutical Preparations-Producer Price Indexes

(comparison of selected prescription drugs)

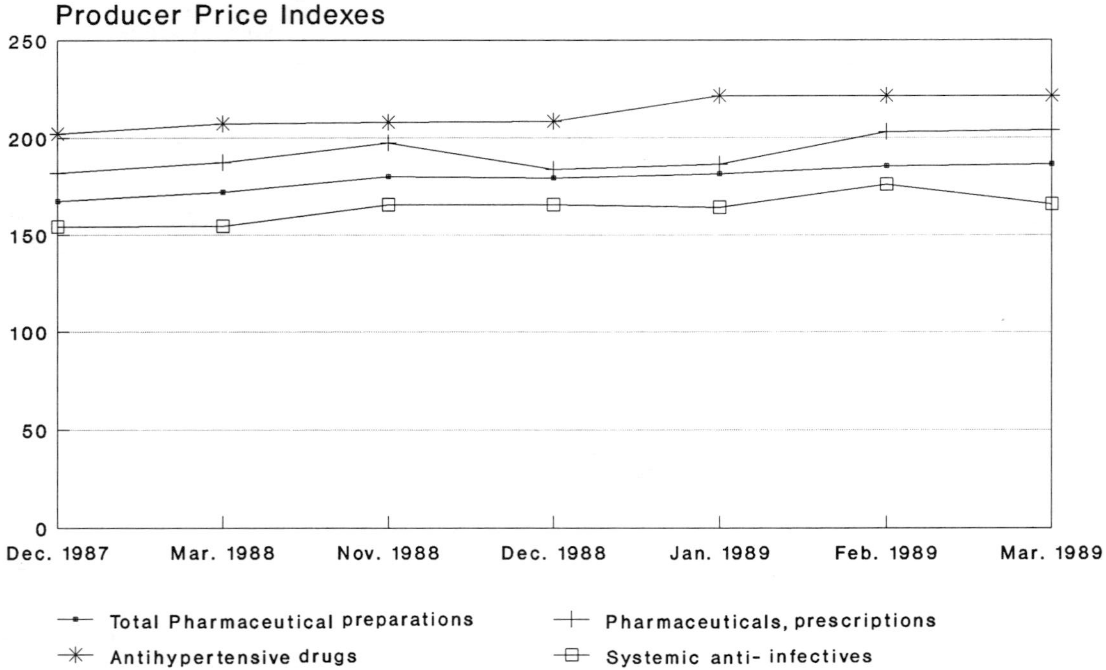

Bureau of Labor Statistics, Producer Price Indexes Data for March 1989, Table 5, and earlier periods.

Annual Percent Change in the Consumer Price Index for Urban Consumers

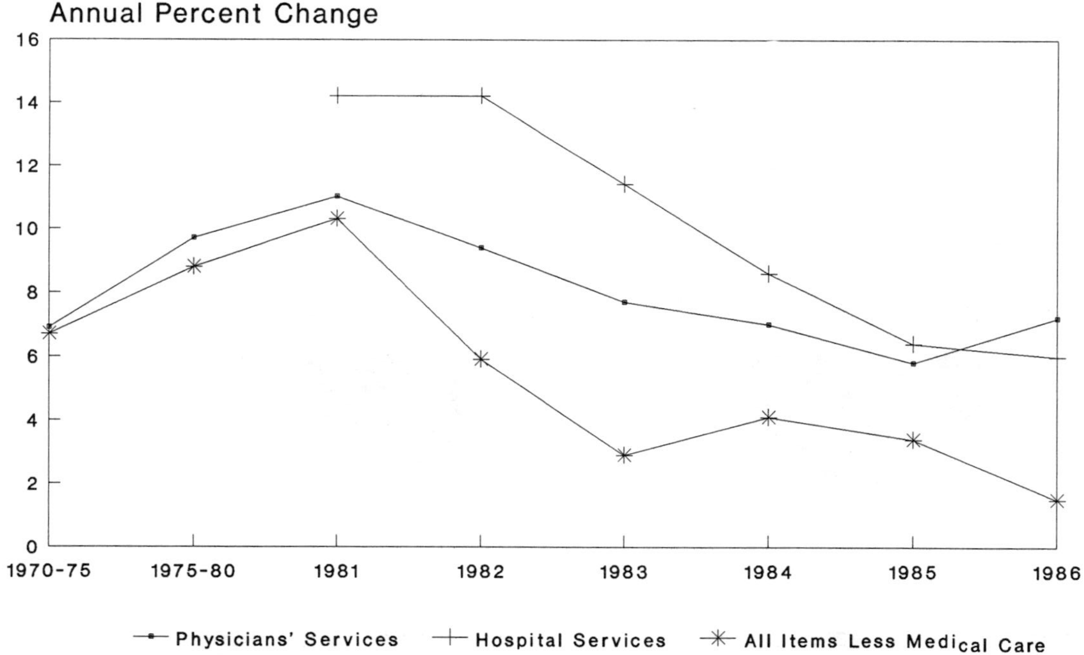

Source: Bureau of Labor Statistics: Detailed CPI Report. Washington. U.S. Printing Office, 1986 and 1987.

Antiulcer Products-Total Sales in Retail Market

1987

Total sales: $1.1 billion

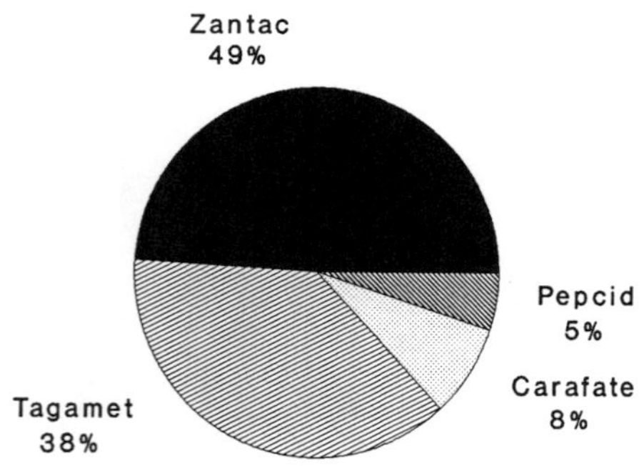

1988

Total sales: $1.3 billion

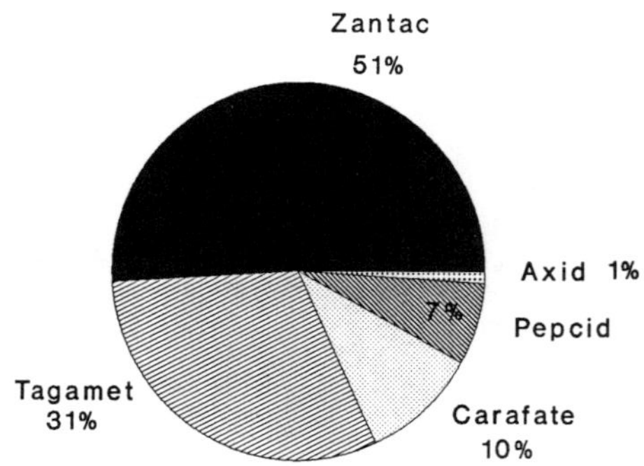

Source: Pharmaceutical Data Services:
Drug Topics, March 20, 1989.

Antiulcer Products:
Number of Total Prescriptions

1987

Total Rxs: 34 million

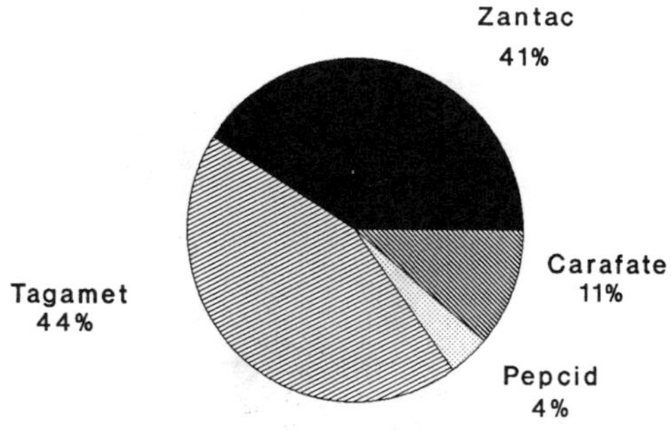

1988

Total Rxs: 38 million

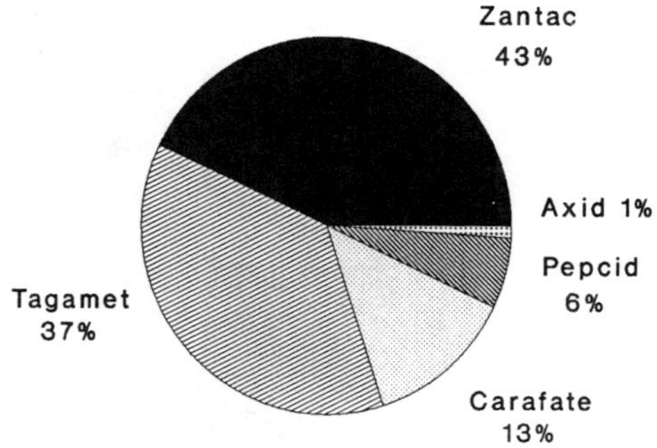

Source: Pharmaceutical Data Services:
Drug Topics, March 20, 1989.

Antiarthritic Drug Retail Sales

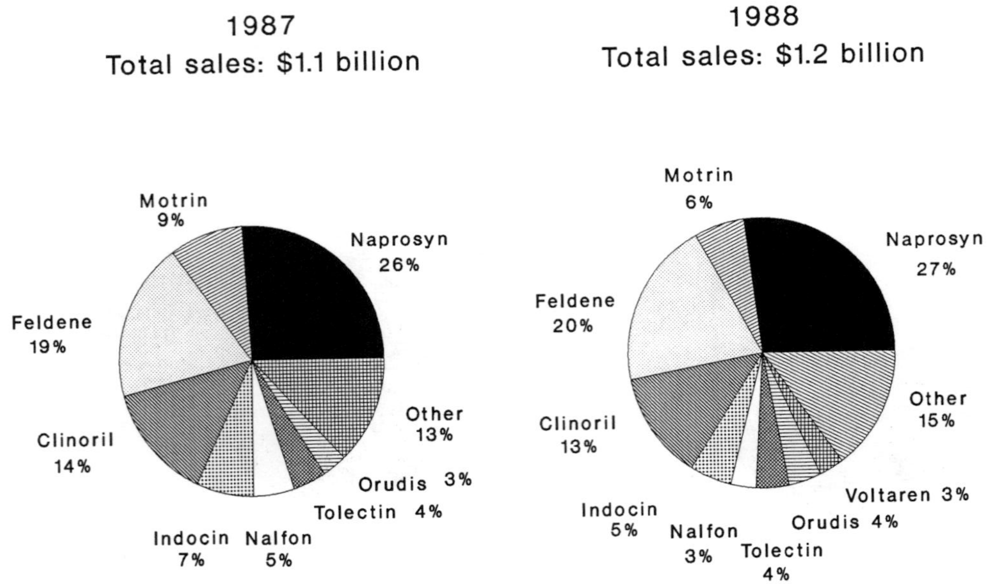

Source: Pharmaceutical Data Services:
Drug Topics, March 20, 1989.

ACE Inhibitors-Retail Market

1987
Total Rxs: 17.8 million

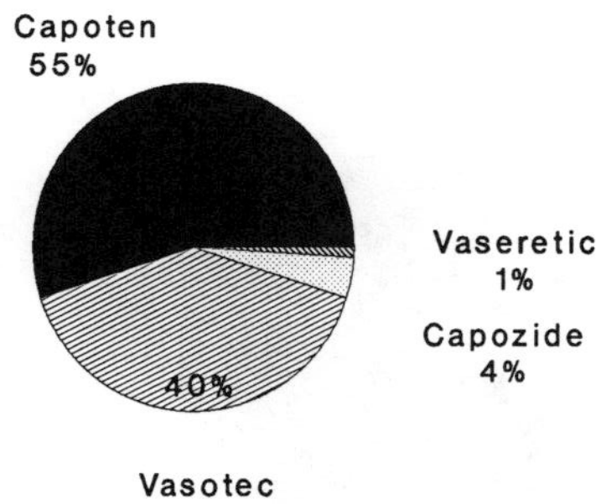

1988
Total Rxs: 24.6 million

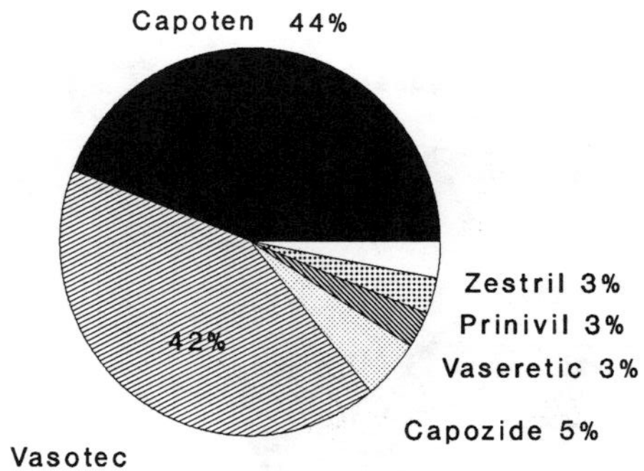

Source: Pharmaceutical Data Services:
Drug Topics, March 20. 1989.

*ACE= Angiotension I-Converting Enzyme.

ACE Inhibitors-Retail Market

1987
Total sales: $405 million

1988
Total sales: $587 million

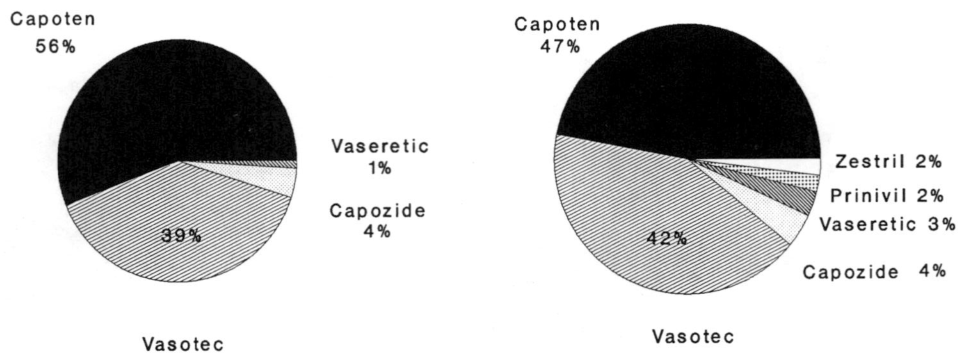

Source: Pharmaceutical Data Service:
Drug Topics, March 20, 1989.

*ACE= Angiotension I-Converting Enzyme

Oral Calcium Channel Blockers: Retail Market

1987
Total sales: $680 million

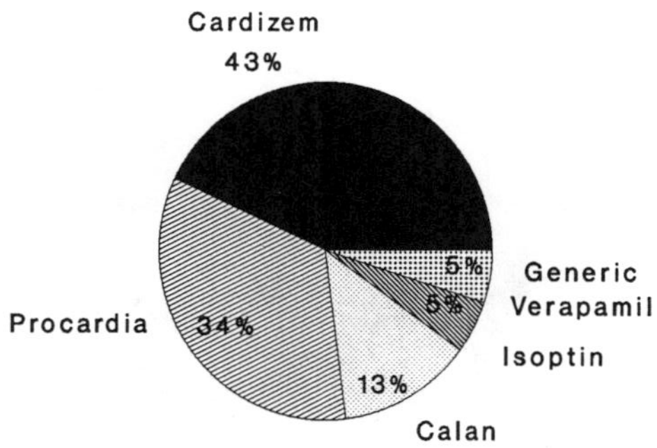

1988
Total sales: $860 million

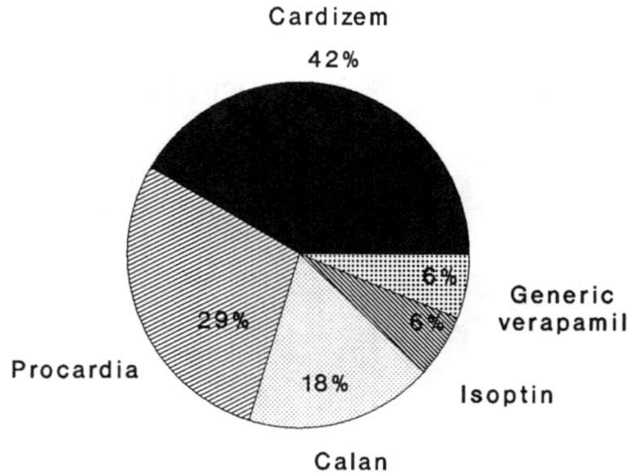

Source: Pharmaceutical Data Services:
Drug Topics, March 20, 1989.

Total Retail Sales: Cardiovascular Drugs

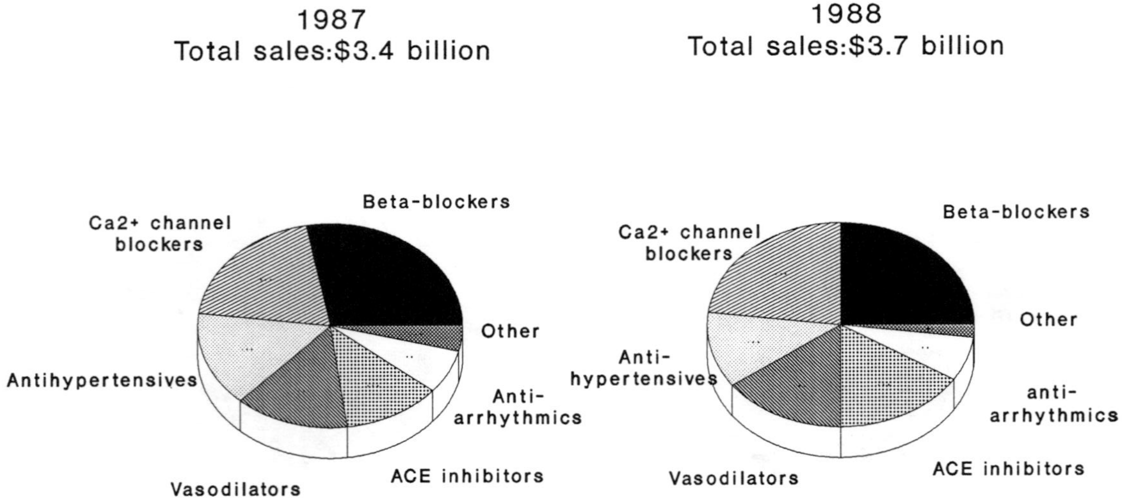

Source: Pharmaceutical Data Services: Drug Topics, March 20, 1989.

Antilipemics-Retail Market

1987
Total sales: $180 million

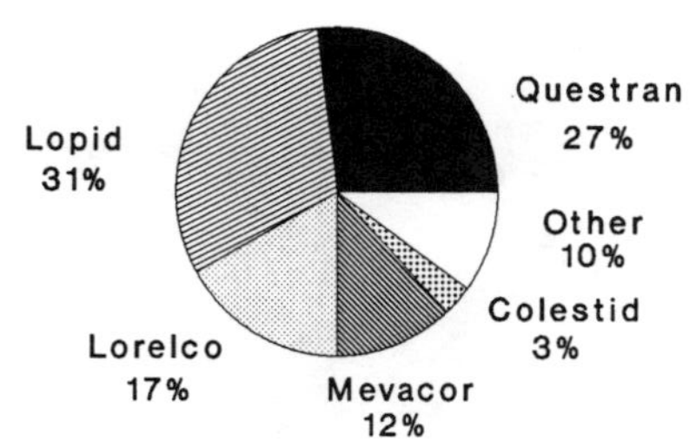

1988
Total sales: $374 million

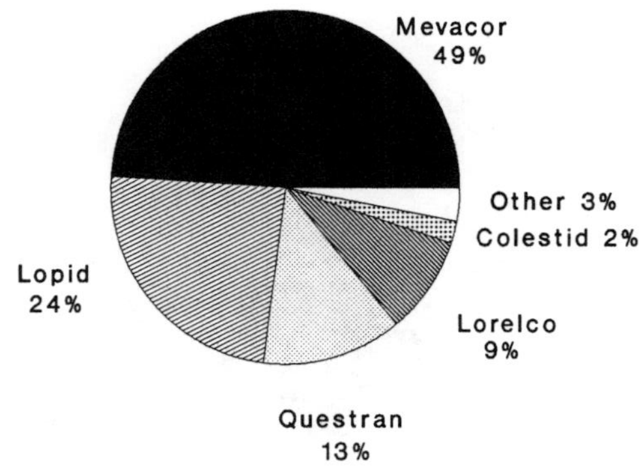

Source: Pharmaceutical Data Services:
Drug Topics, March 20, 1989.

Antilipemics-Total Prescriptions

1987
Total Rxs: 6.4 million

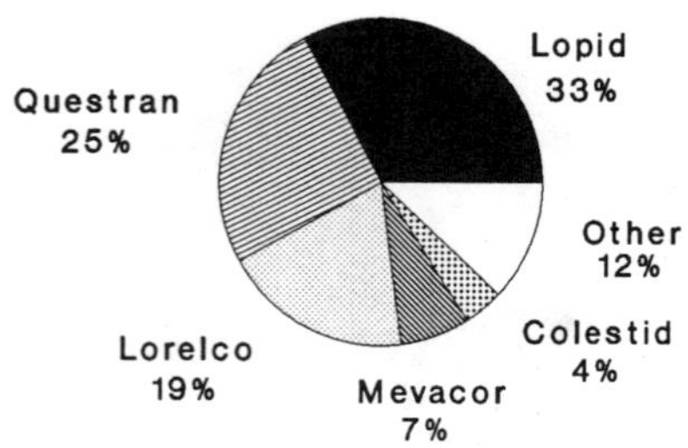

1988
Total Rxs: 11.4 million

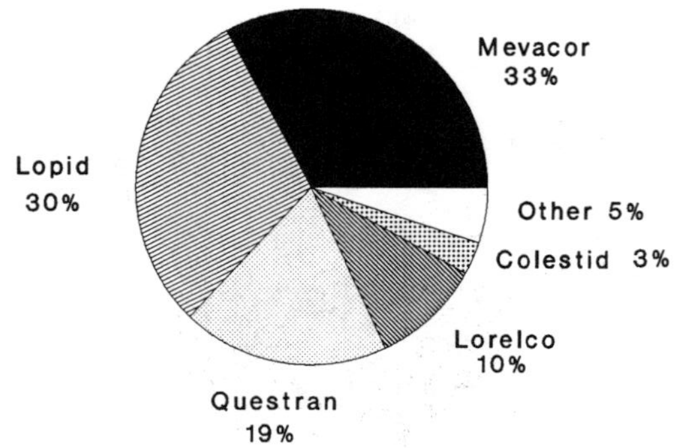

Source: Pharmaceutical Data Services:
Drug Topics, March 20, 1989.

Consumer Price Index for Drugs and Prescriptions in the United States, 1967-1988

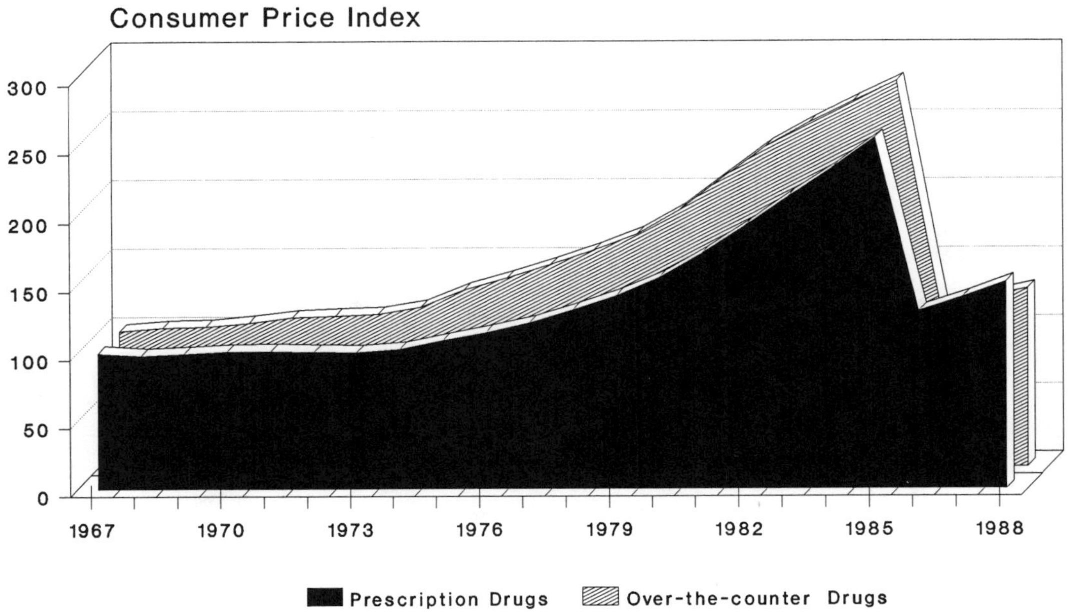

Source: U.S. Department of Labor, Bureau of Labor Statistics, CPI Detailed Report, Various issues.

All Urban Consumers

Chapter 4

THIRD PART COVERAGE, REIMBURSEMENT, AND FINANCING

This chapter provides information on drug reimbursement, financing, out-of-pocket payments, third party payments, private insurance, Medicaid, and Medicare

Sources of Prescription Payment

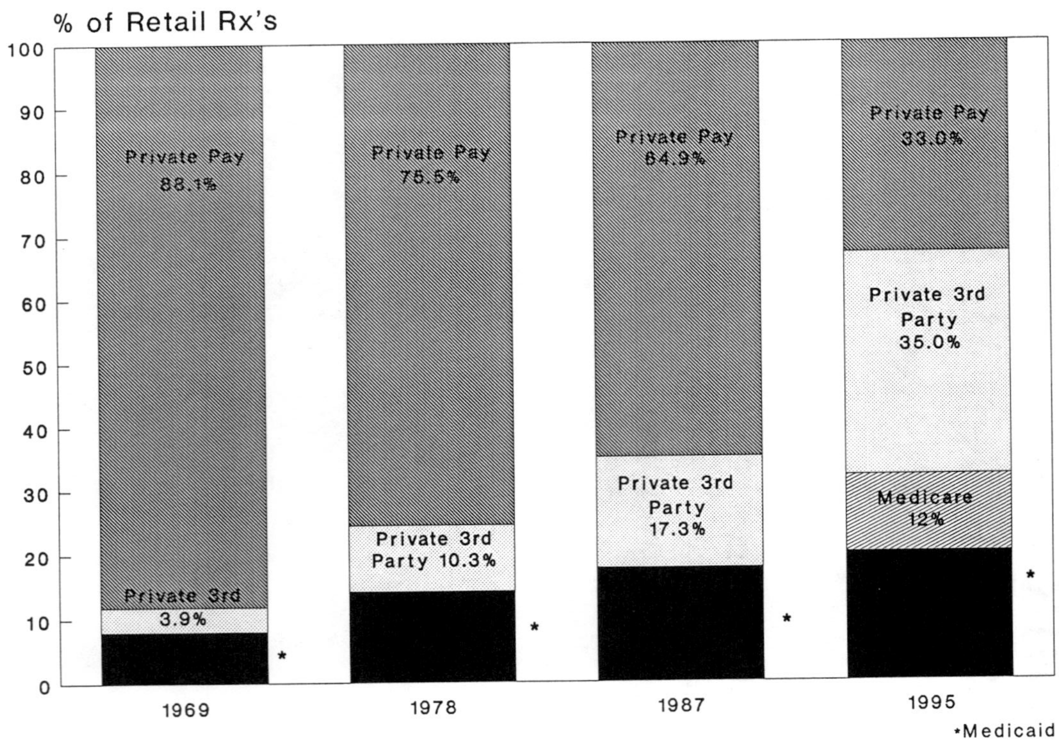

Schondelmeyer, Stephen W., "Trends with Third Parties and Manages Health Care: A Pharmacy Perspective," In proceedings of The Changing Health Care Environment:: Its Impact on Pharmacy and the Pharmaceutical Industry, 1987, p.32.

Third-Party Prescriptions: 1987

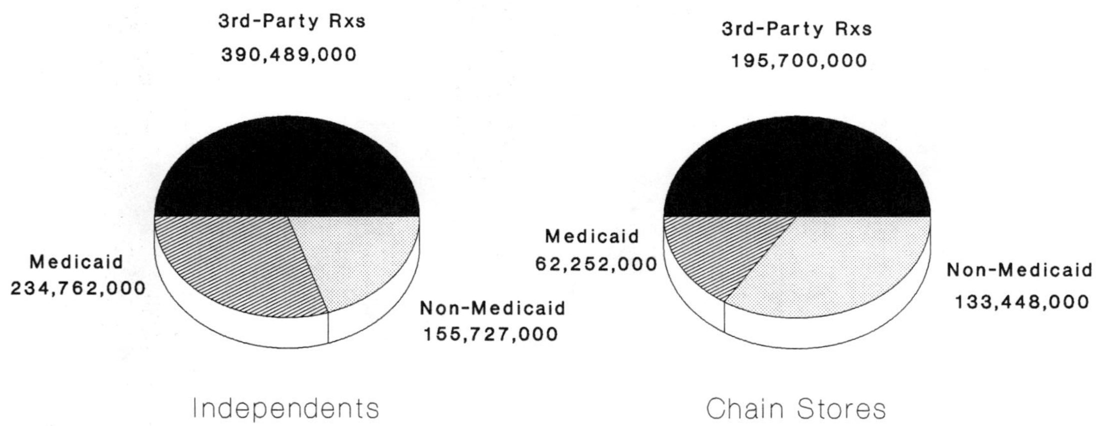

Source: American Druggist, May 1988

Third-Party Prescription Ratios- 1987

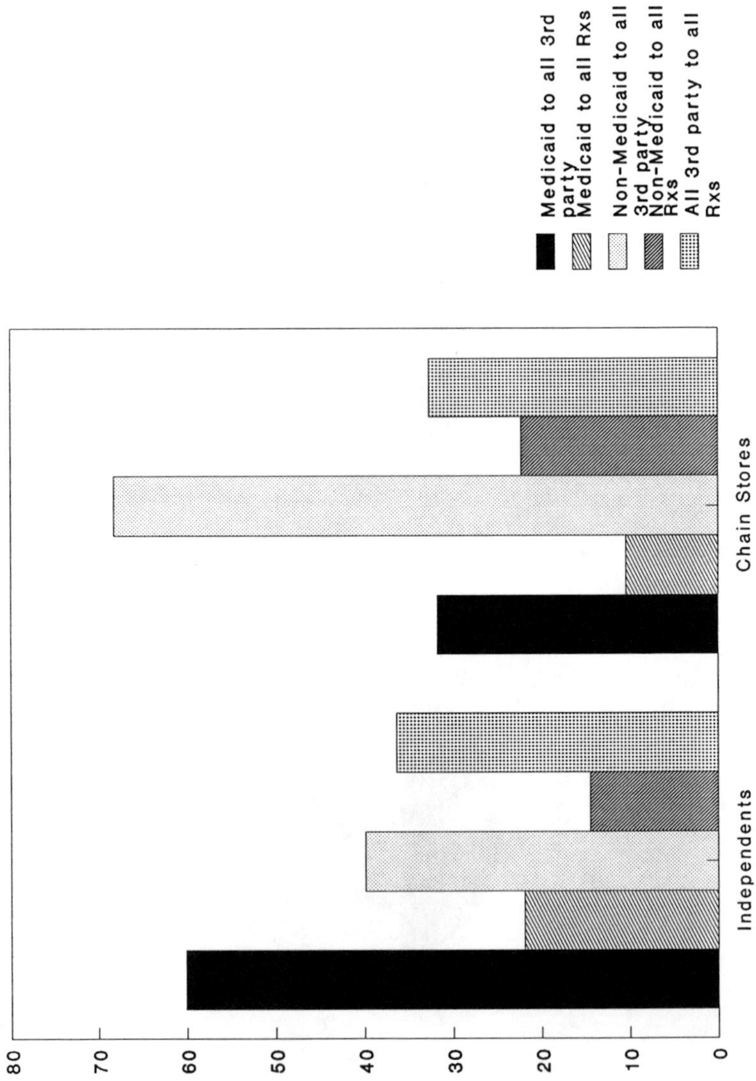

Source: American Druggist, May 1988

Drug Distribution to Members by Third Parties

Means of Distribution	Total HMOs	Staff	Group	IPA	Network	Hybrid	PPO
Contracted pharmacies	87%	64%	77%	93%	93%	89%	77%
In-house pharmacy	24%	79%	56%	2%	25%	42%	11%
Mail	<1%	0	0	<1%	0	0	0
No answer	6%	2%	4%	7%	6%	2%	17%
Total*	117%	145%	137%	102%	124%	133%	105%
Survey base	(455)	(47)	(57)	(243)	(53)	(55)	(47)

*Total exceed 100% because many plans distribute drugs via in-house pharmacies as well as through contracts with community pharmacies.

Source: American Medical Census Corporation ; HMO/PPO Trends, Vol.1, No.1, March/April 1988.

Percentage Distribution of U.S. Ethical Pharmaceutical Sales by Class of Customer

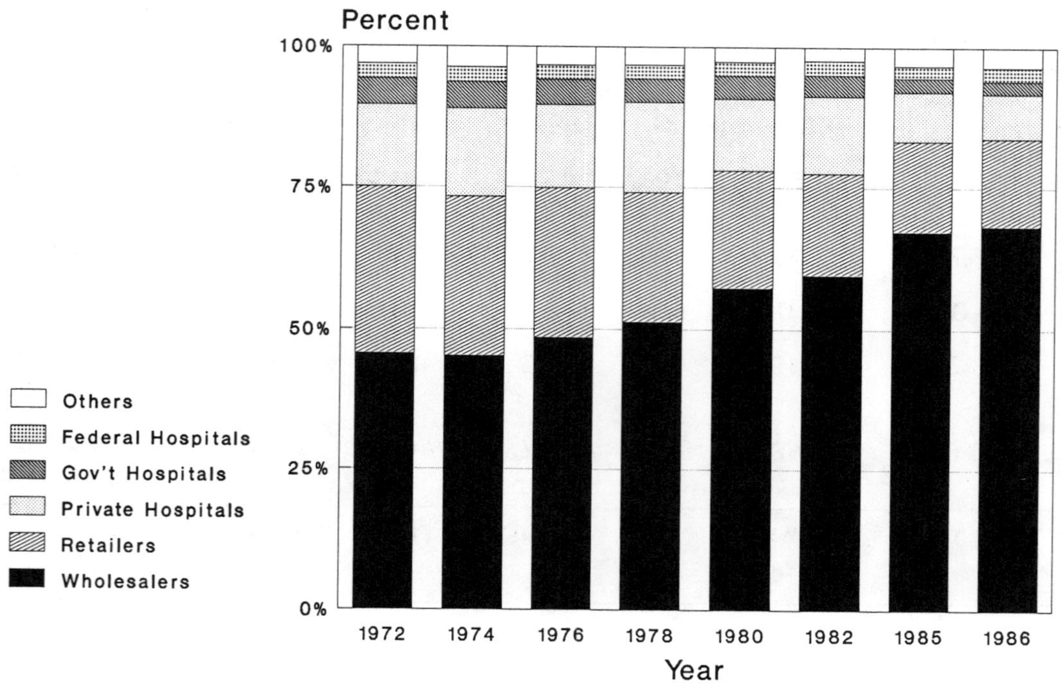

Source: PMA Annual Survey, 1988.

Health Insurance Coverage Status: 1985

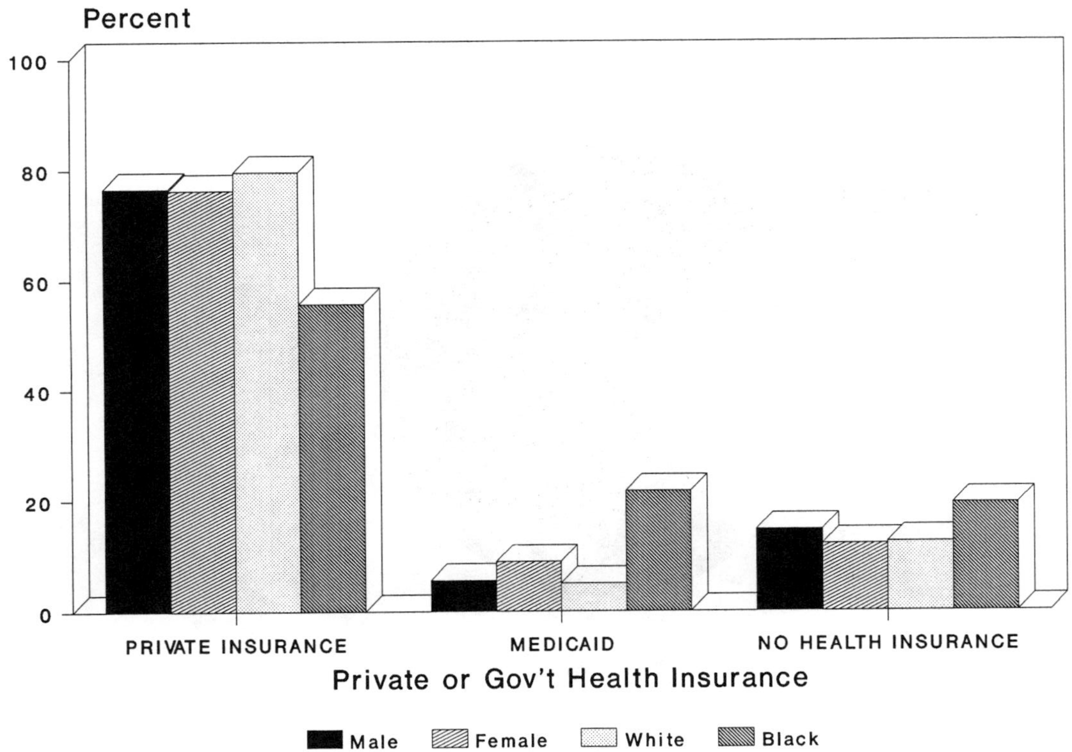

Source: U.S. Bureau of the Census, 1986.

National Health Insurance Coverage Rates 1987

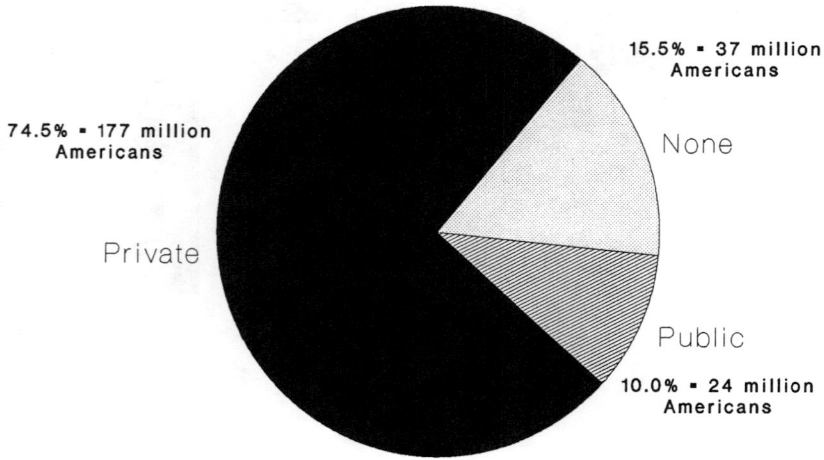

Source: A Profile of Uninsured Americans
(National Medical Expenditure Survey
Research Findings 1, DHHS Publication No. (PHS) 89-3443)

Dollar Outlay by Employers for Employee Insurance Coverage: 1987

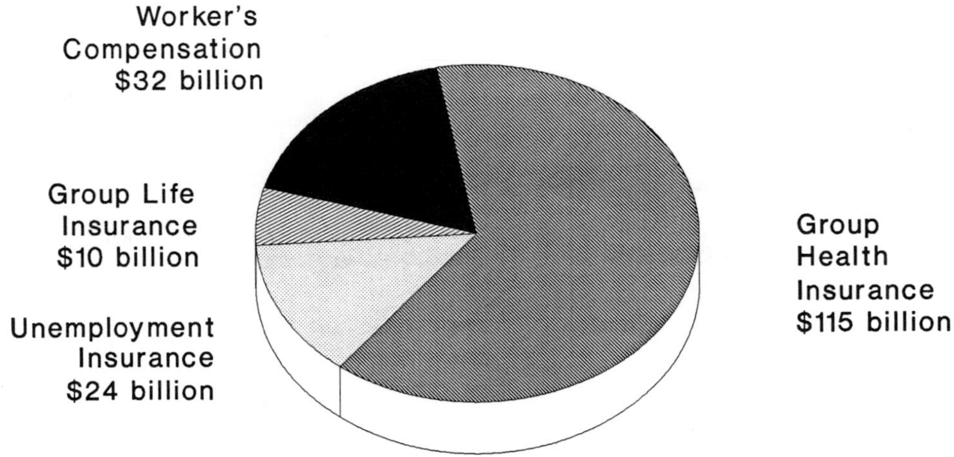

Source: U.S. Department of Commerce, Survey of Current Business, Bureau of Economic Analysis: Source Book of Health Insurance Data, 1989

Major Health Care Service Provider Companies

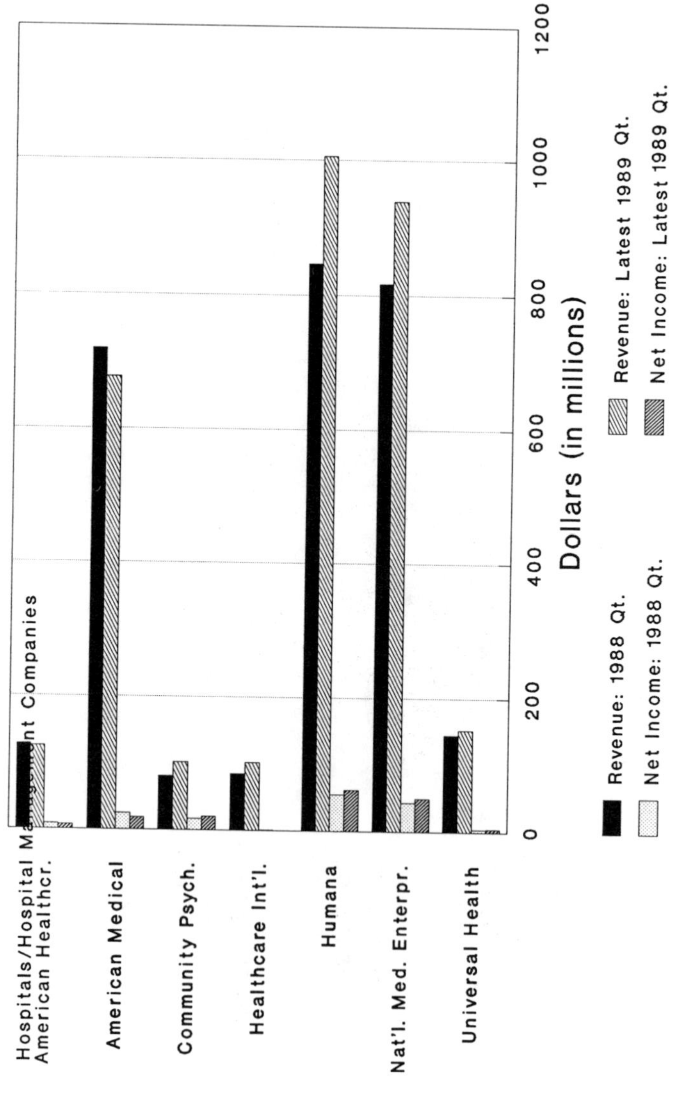

Source: Health Commerce Line, Issue 5, 1989.

Growth in Life Insurance Companies' Pension Reserves in the U.S.

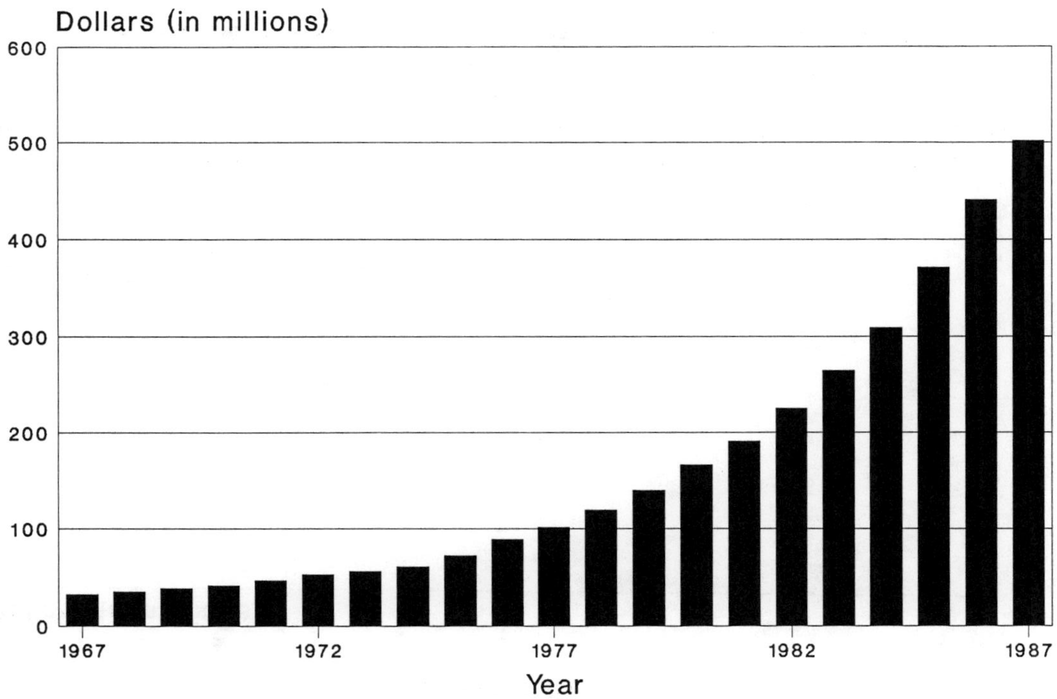

Source: Compiled by the American Council of Life Insurance.

Health Insurance Claims Payments in the United States, (1978-1987)

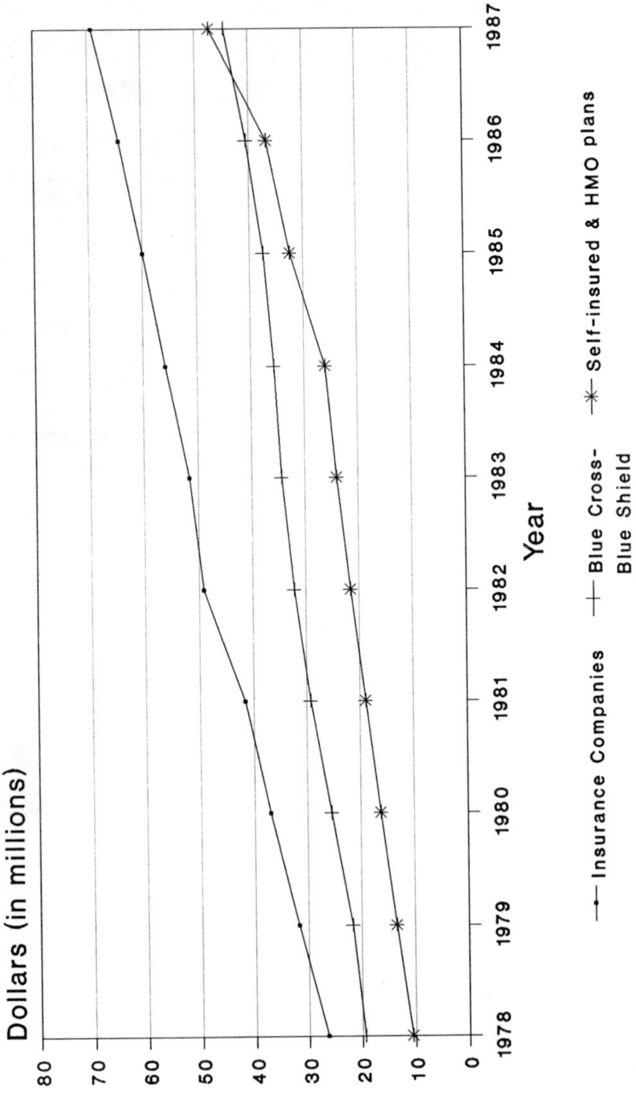

Source: Health Insurance Association of America: Source Book of Health Insurance Data, 1989.

Ratio of Insurance Premiums to Disposable Personal Income

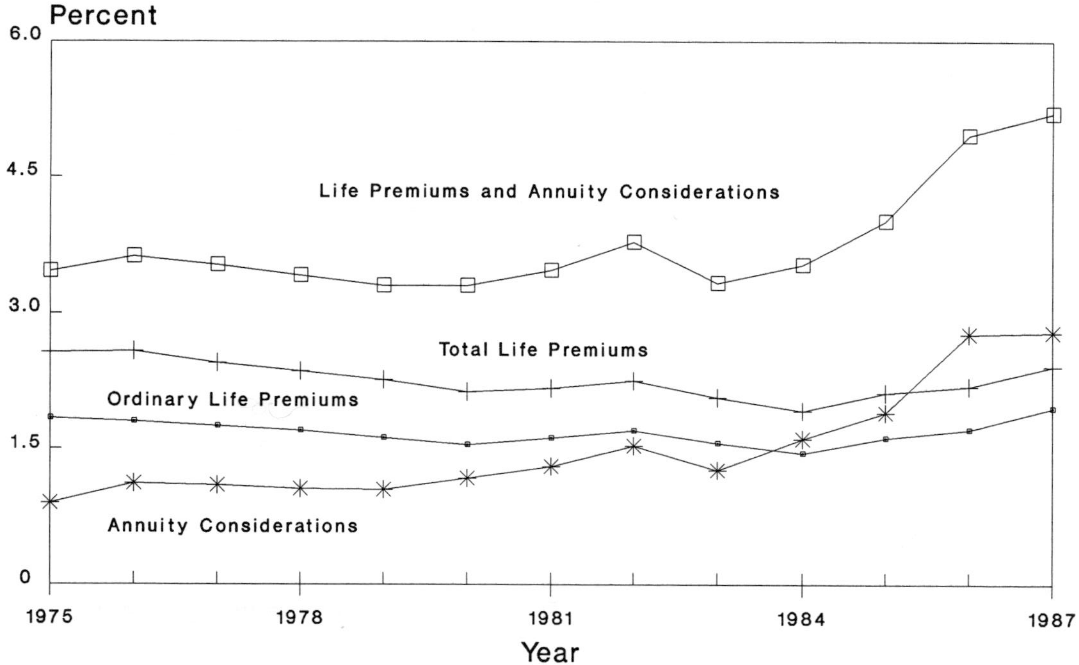

Source: U.S. Department of Commerce, Spectator Year Book and American Council of Life Insurance, 1989.

Life Insurance Policy Value and Disposable Personal Income per Household in the United States

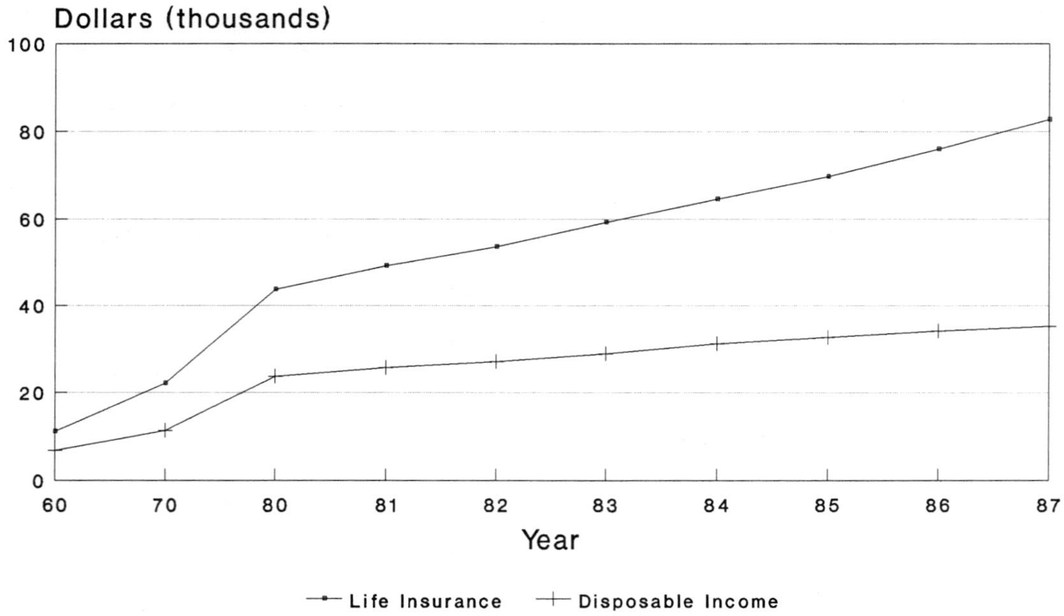

Source: Spectator Year Book, American Council of Life Insurance, Life Insurance Marketing and Research Association, U.S. Bureau of the Census and U.S. Department of Commerce, 1989.

Average Size Life Insurance Policy in Force in the United States

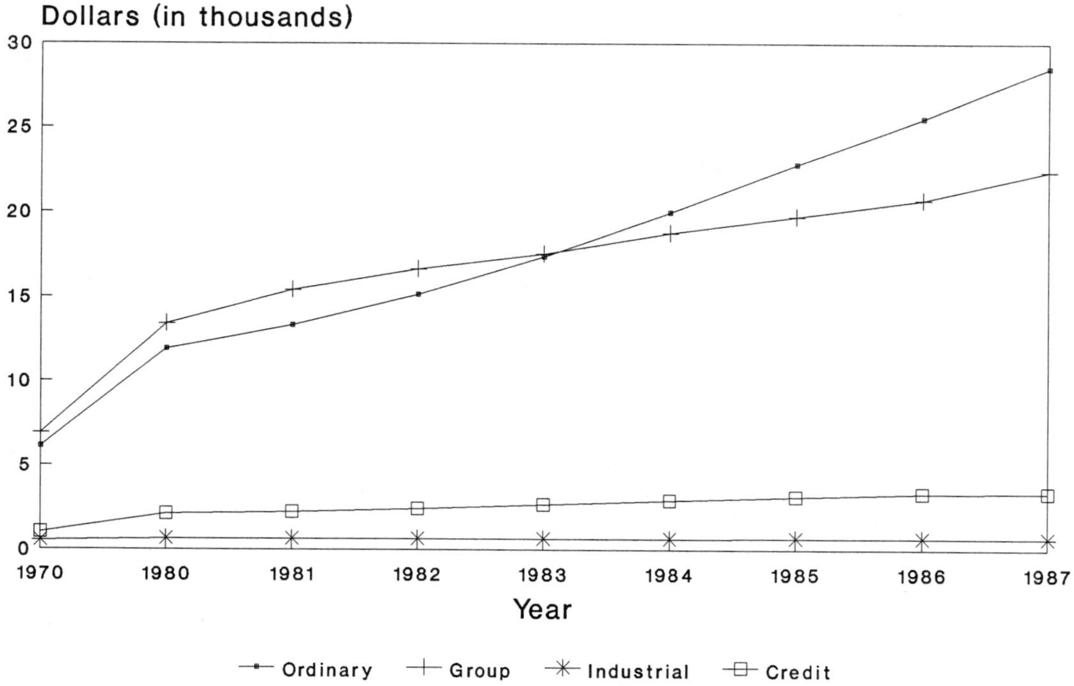

Source: Spectator Year Book and American Council of Life Insurance, 1989.

Percent Change in Average Total Professional and Liability Insurance Expenses of Self-Employed Physicians

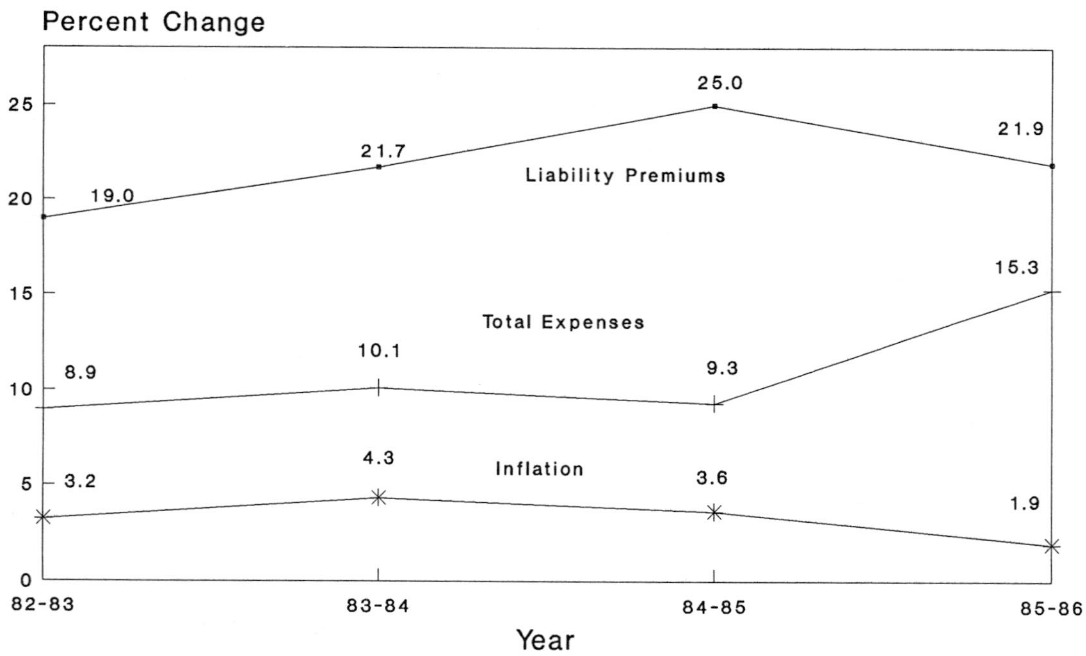

Source: AMA Socioeconomic Monitoring System, 1983-1987 core surveys.

Estimated Health Insurance Premiums to Increase for 1989 Due to:

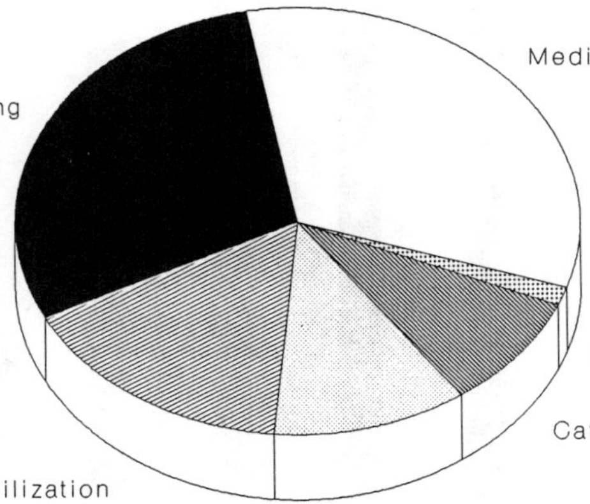

Insurance carriers estimate a 21.5% increase in medical-benefit costs.

Source: Hewitt Associates, 1986.

Medicare Enrollment 1977-1986
(in millions)

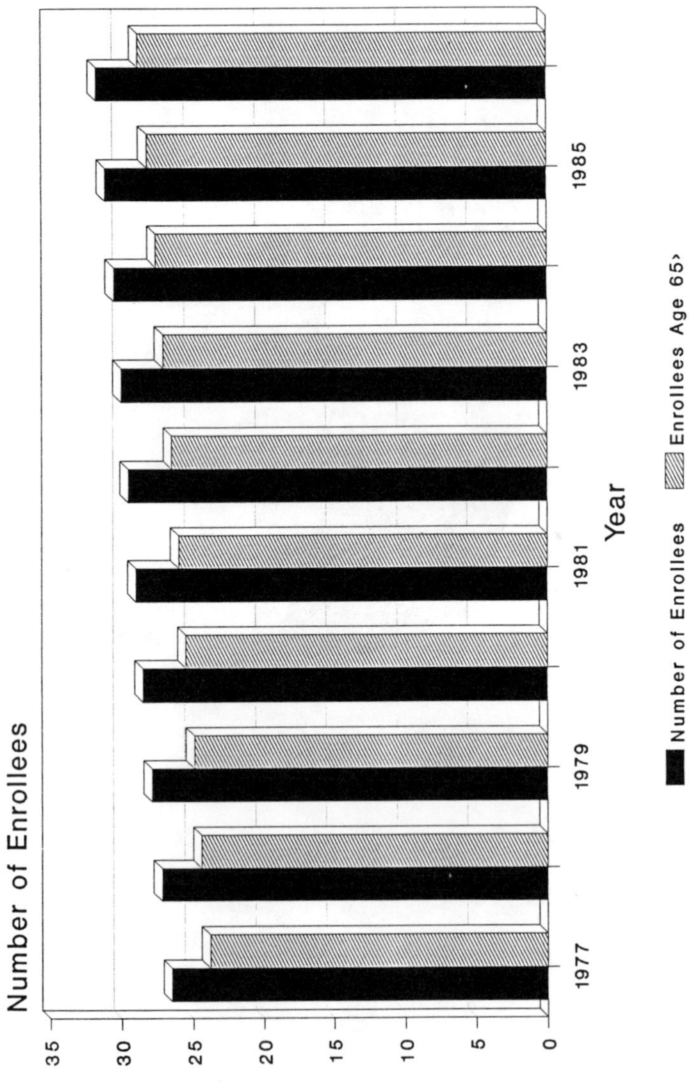

Source: Department of Health and Human Services, 1988.

Distribution of Medicare Enrollees, by Census Region: 1966 and 1987

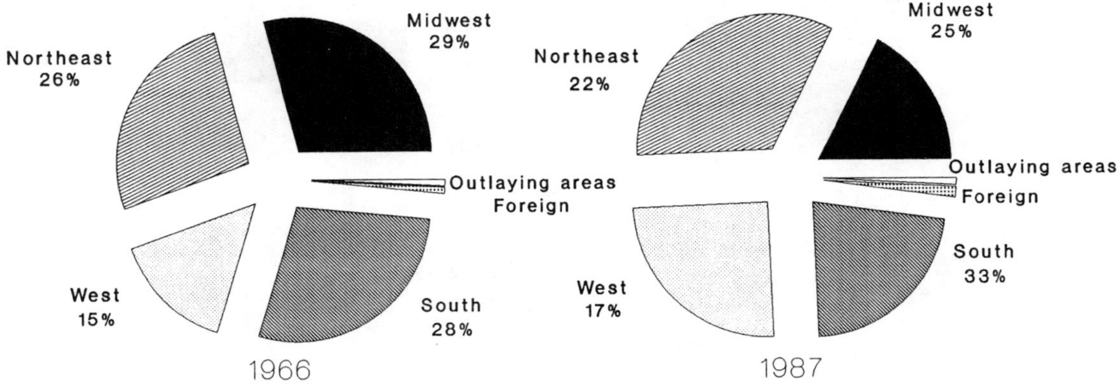

Source: HCFA, Health Care Financing Review, Spring 1989.

Number and Percent Distribution of Medicare Enrollees, 1966 and 1987

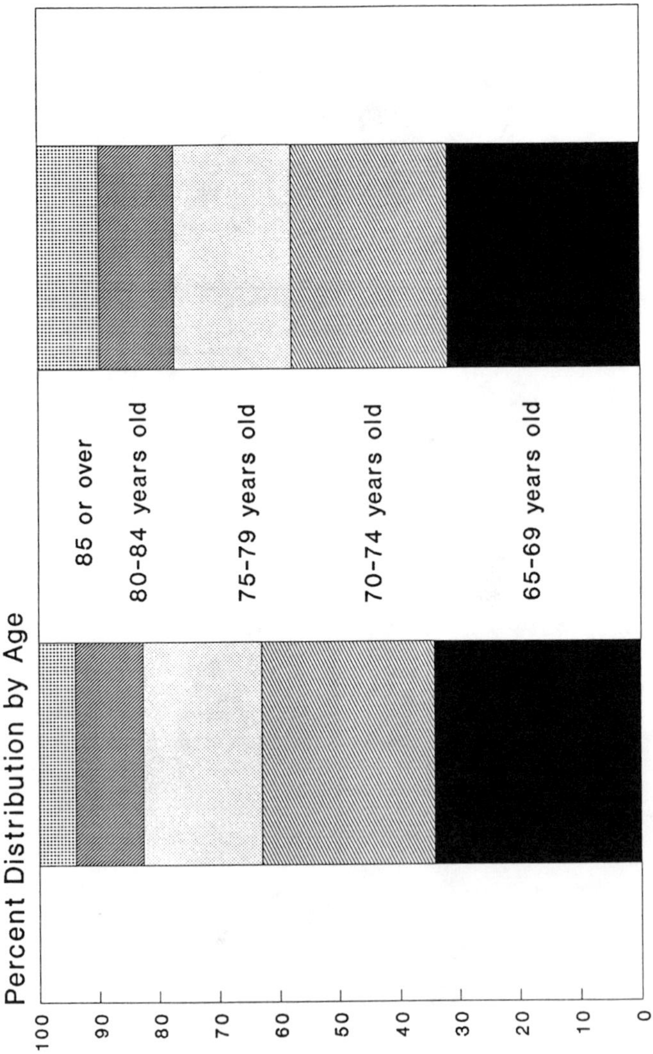

Source: HCFA, Health Care Financing Review, Spring 1989.

Growth of Medicare, Selected Years

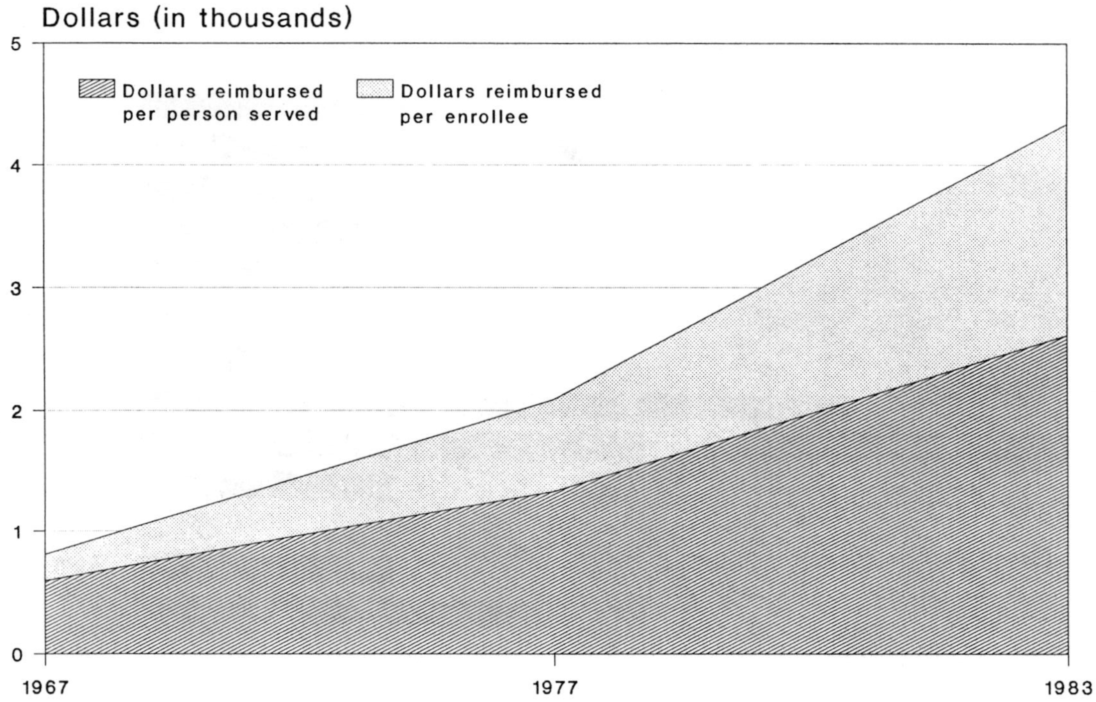

Source: U.S. Department of Health and Human Services, Public Health Service, United States, 1986.

Medicare Physician Services per User
(1986)

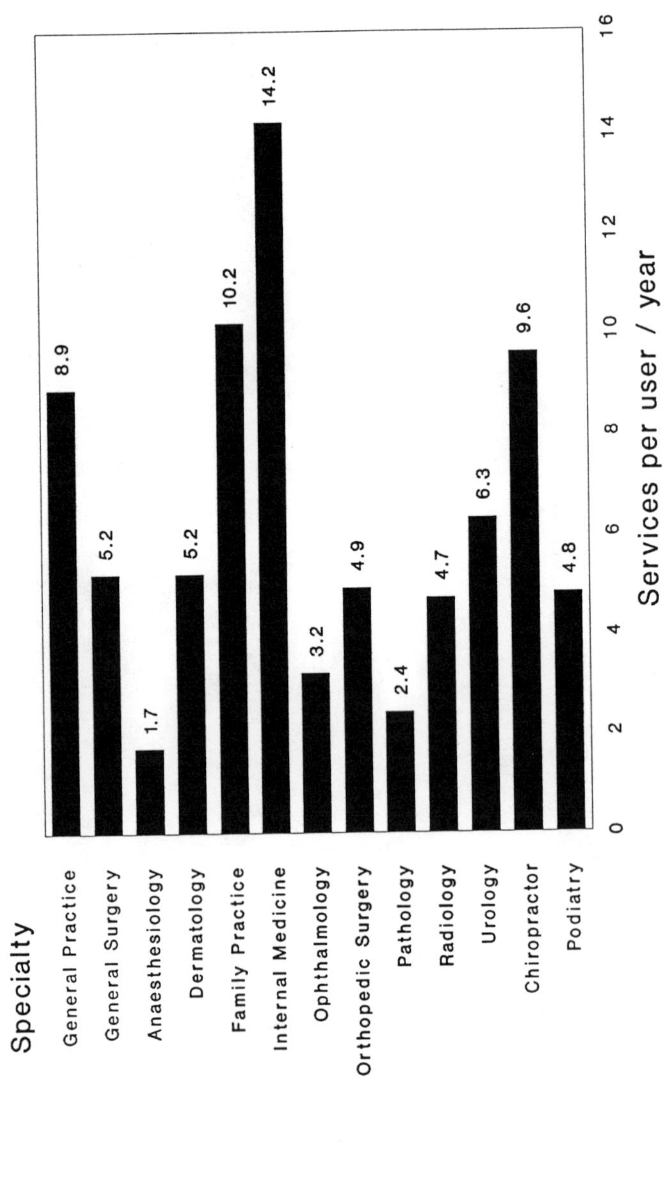

Source: HCFA, Health Care Financing Review, Spring 1989.

Mean Total Medicare and Mean Total Patient Visits Per Week in Selected Specialties 1987

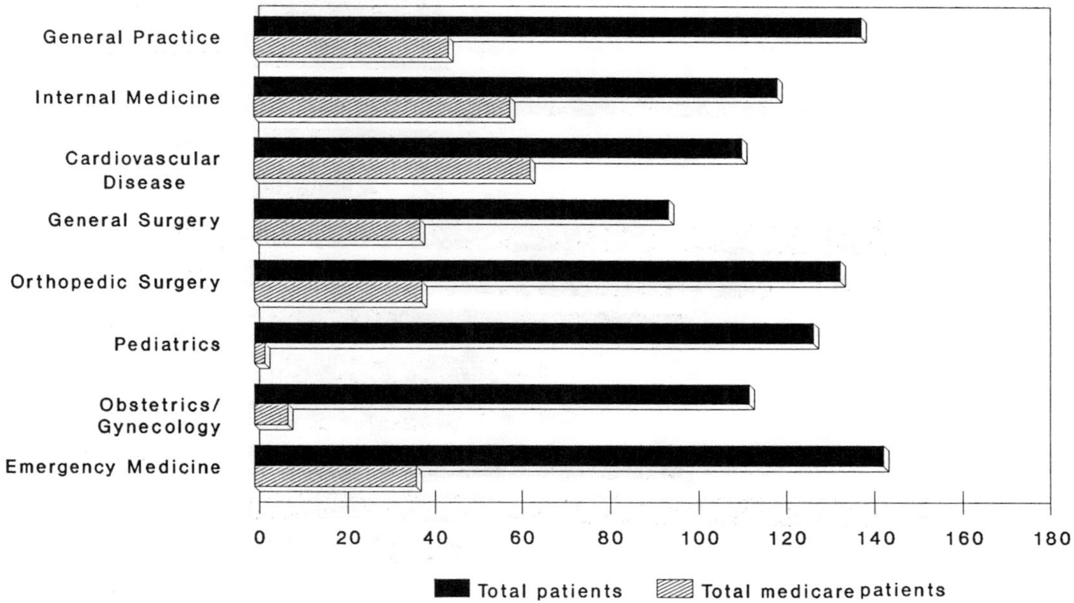

Source: Physician Marketplace Statistics, 1988

Medicare Average Allowed Charge per User
(1986)

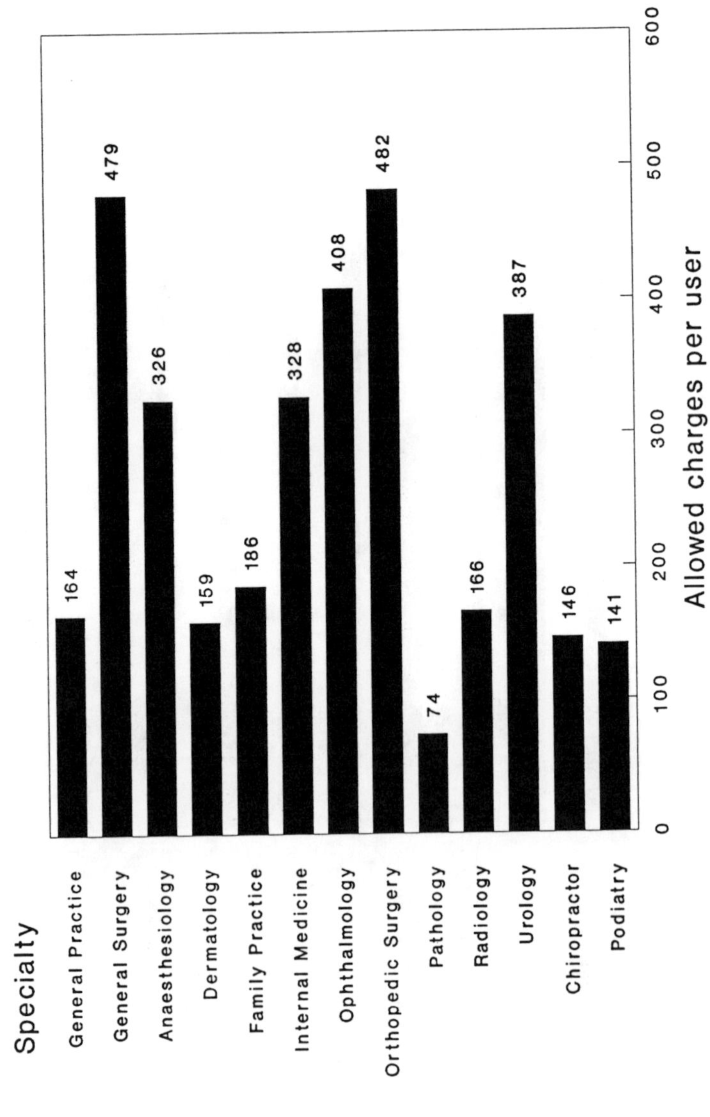

Mean Annual Utilization of Medicare Services

Medicare Service (and utilization unit)	1979 Mean	1979 SD
Home Health Care (visits)	1.38	9.80
Outpatient Hospital (bills)	.99	2.26
Non-Hospital-Based (payment records)	5.75	7.23
Physician (payment records)	5.02	5.93
Surgeon (payment records)	.61	1.26
Supplier (payment records)	.73	2.79
Hospital by MDs (payment records)	.53	1.40
Skilled Nursing Facilities (admissions)	.03	.32
Inpatient Hospital (admissions)	.43	.86

Source:Inquiry, Fall 1987

Mean Annual Reimbursement for Medicare Services
(in dollars)

Medicare Service	1979	
	Mean	SD
Home Health Care	36.68	268.80
Outpatient	54.83	417.20
Non-Hospital-Based	356.88	690.86
Physician	329.29	647.10
Surgeon	119.83	361.27
Supplier	27.37	141.31
Hospital	10.02	50.77
Skilled Nursing Facility	25.82	268.07
Inpatient Hospital	955.84	2,611.95
Total Medicare Plus PAA	2,244.17	4,443.34

Source: Inquiry, Volume 24, Fall 1987

Annual Expenditures for Noninstitutionalized Medicare Beneficiaries, 1987

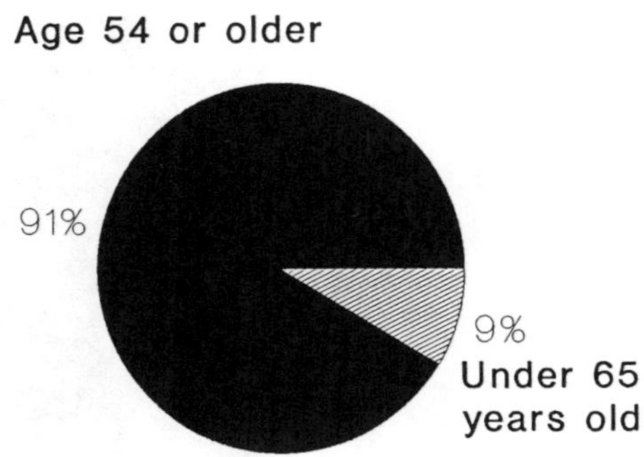

Total Beneficiaries

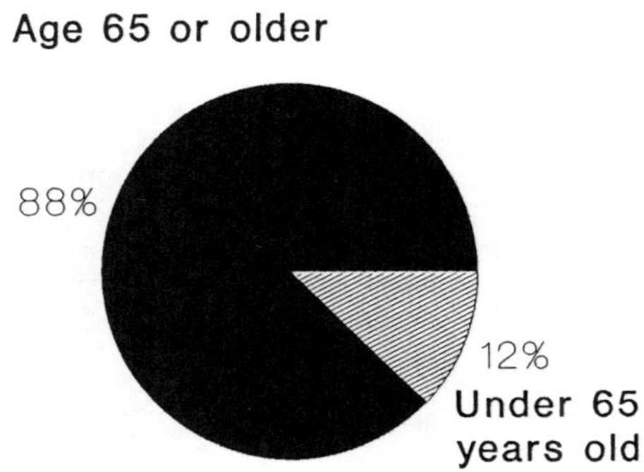

Prescribed Medicines

National Center for Health Services Research & Health Care Technology Assessment, 1987.

Annual Prescription Drug Expenditures for Noninstitutionalized Medicare Beneficiaries, 1987

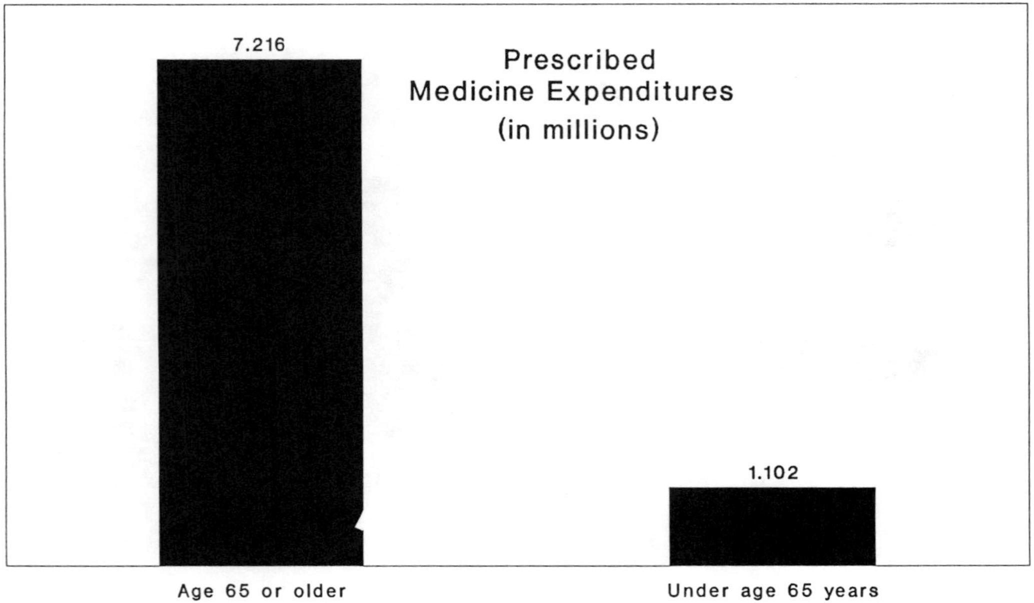

National Center for Health Services Research & Health Care Technology Assessment, 1987.

Prescription Use by Elderly Medicare Beneficiaries, 1980 and 1987

Average charge per prescription

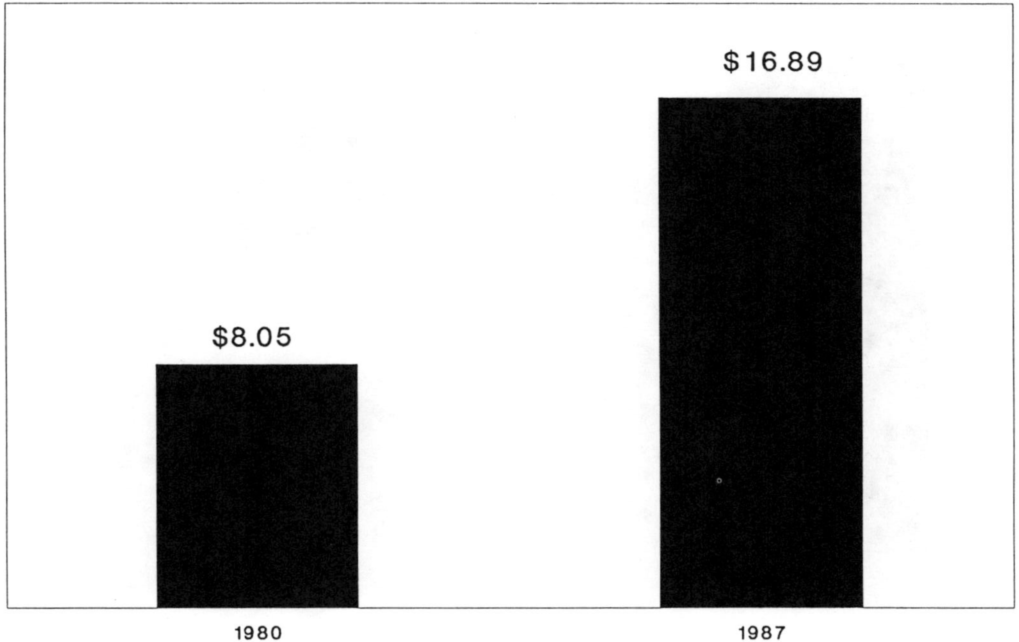

National Medical Expenditure Survey:
Prescribed Medicines : A Summary of Use
& Ependitures by Medicare Beneficiaries, 1988.

Prescription Use by Elderly Medicare Beneficiaries, 1980 and 1987

Average annual prescription expenditures

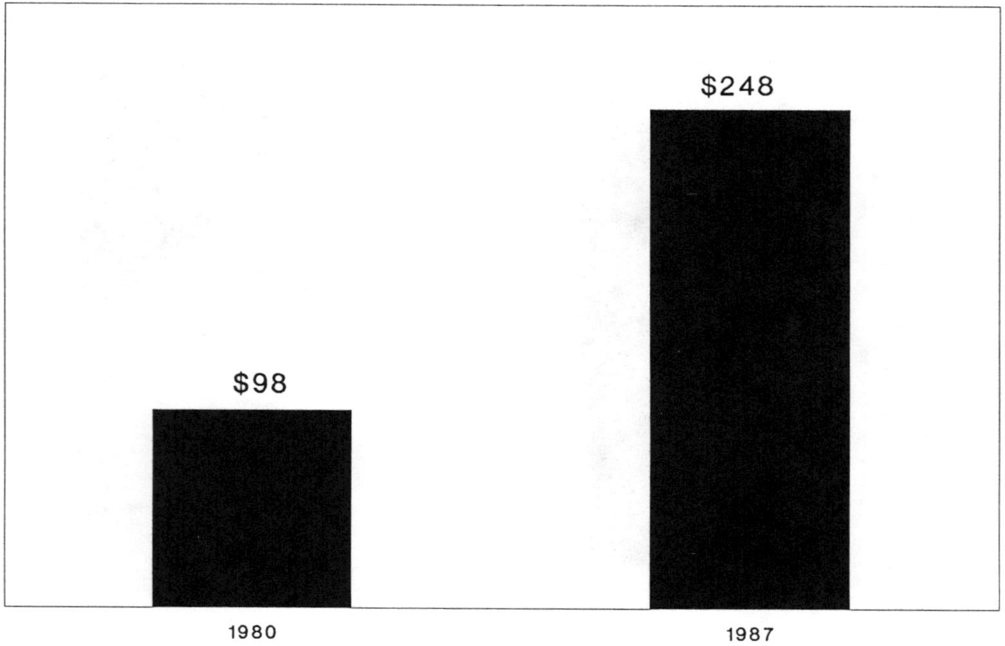

National Medical Expenditure Survey:
Prescribed Medicines: A Summary of Use &
Expenditures by Medicare Beneficiaries

Prescription Use by Elderly
Medicare Beneficiaries, 1980 and 1987

Average annual prescriptions per beneficiary

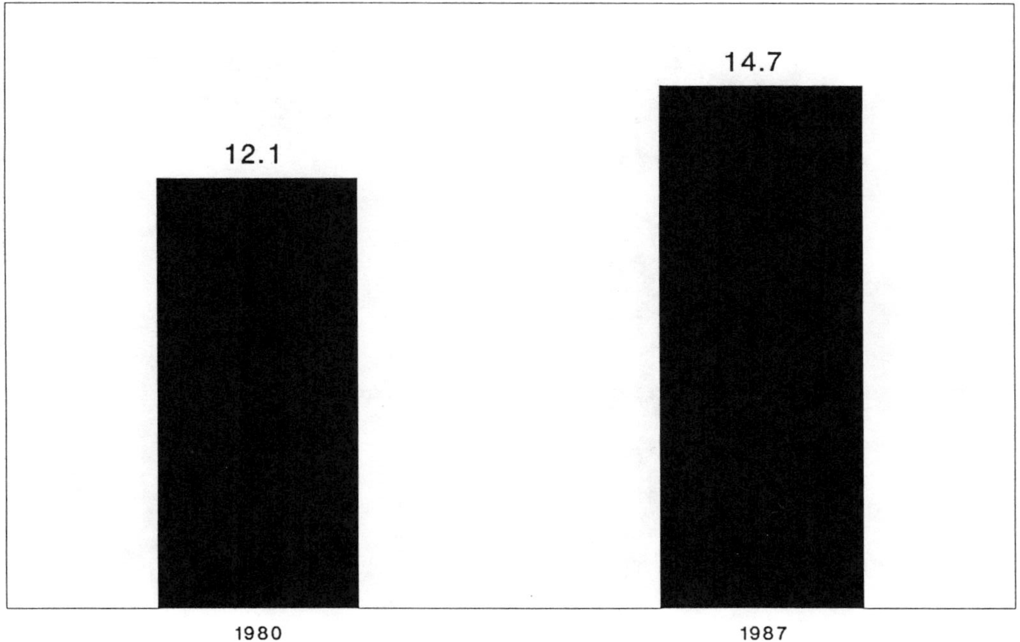

National Medical Expenditure Survey:
Prescribed Medicines : A Summary of Use
& Expenditures by Medicare Beneficiaries

Prescription Use by Elderly Medicare Beneficiaries, 1980 and 1987

Percent with at least one prescription during year

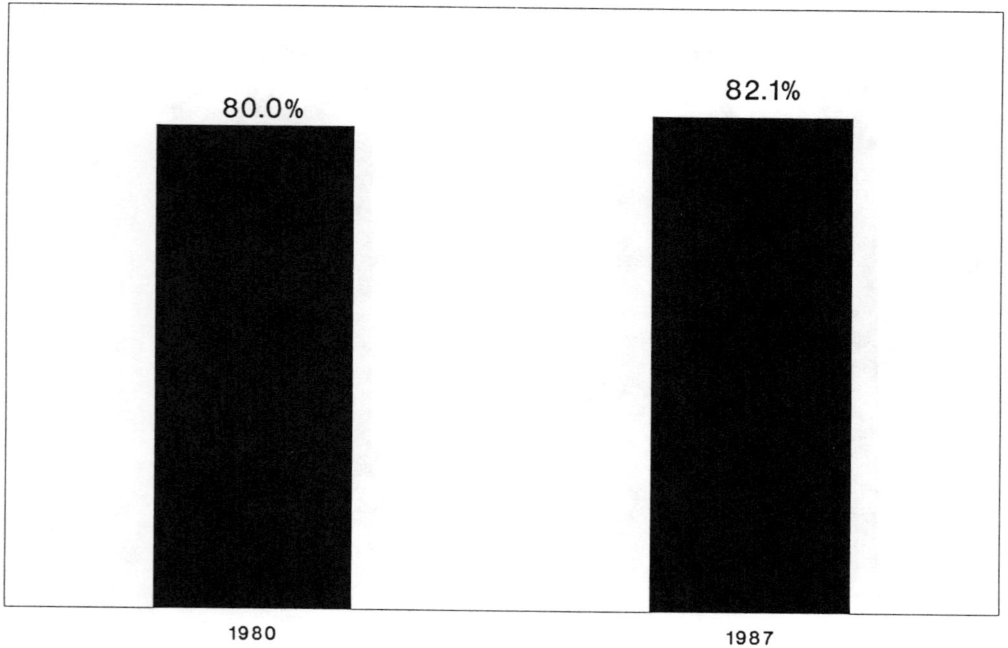

National Medical Expenditure Survey:
Prescribed Medicines: A Summary of Use &
Expenditures by Medicare Beneficiaries, 1989.

Elderly Prescription Drug Use by Medicare Beneficiaries : 1967-1980

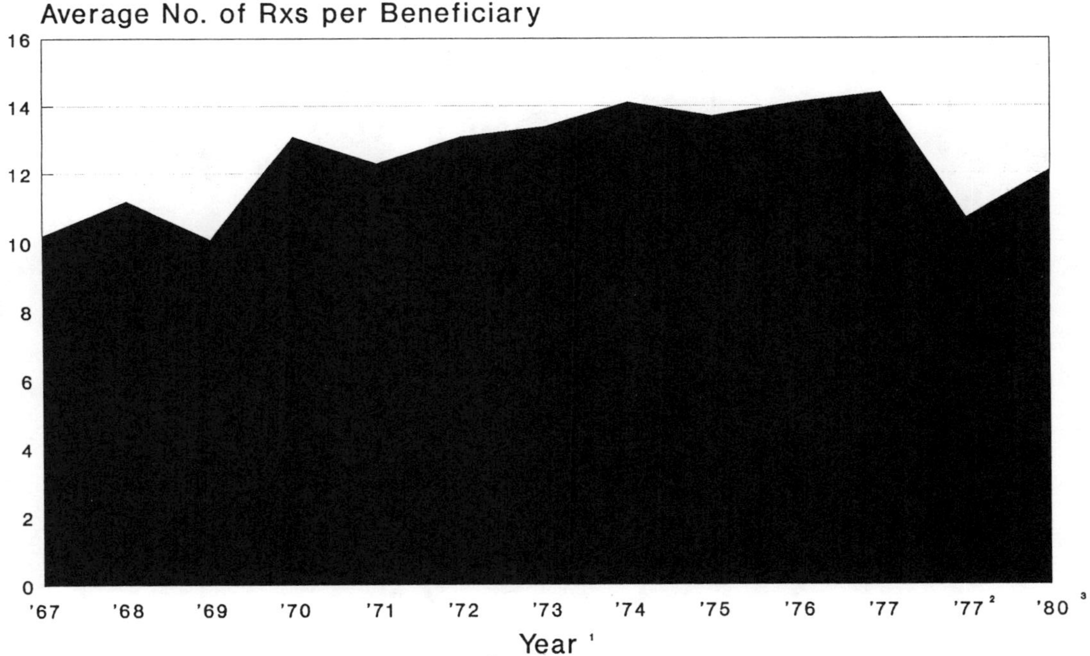

Source: Current Medicare Survey, National Medical Care Expenditure Survey and National Medical Care Utilization, 1983

[1] Data for 1967-77 are from CMS and include institutionalized beneficiaries.

[2] Data are from NMCES, 1977 for all noninstitutionalized persons 65 years of age or over.

[3] Data for 1980 are from NMCUES for noninstitutionalized, aged Medicare beneficiaries.

Medicaid Rx Product Cost as a Percentage of Total Rx Price

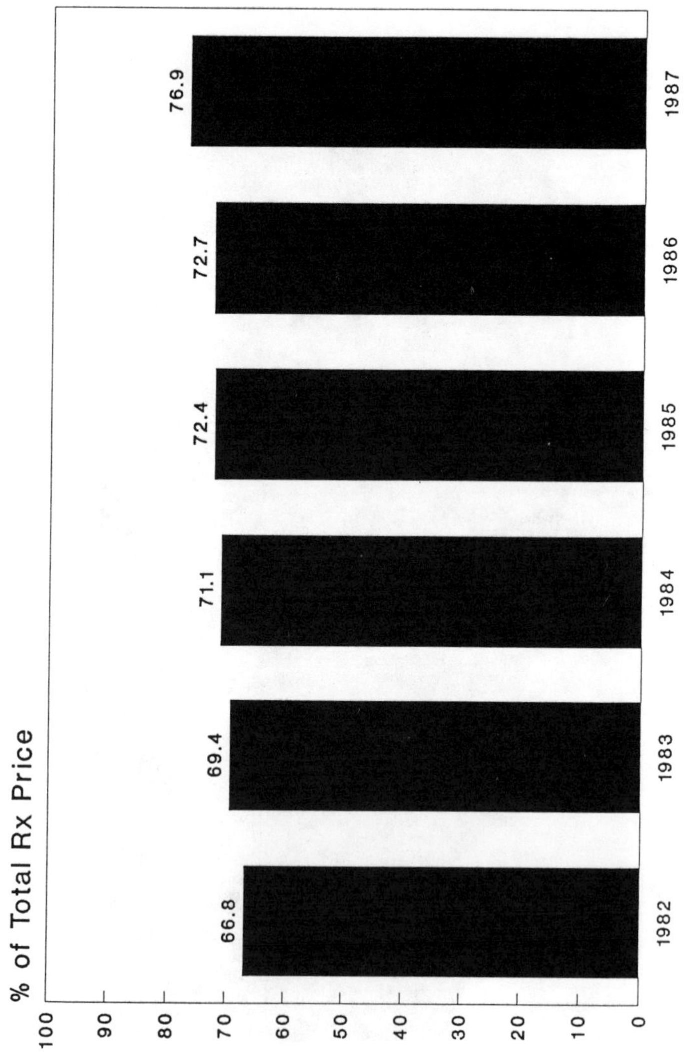

National Pharmaceutical Council,
Pharmaceutical Benefits Under State
Medical Assistance Programs, September 1983 and 1988.

The Impact of Cutting Pharmacy Reimbursement

Medicaid Rx Drug Reimbursement Components

1982-1987

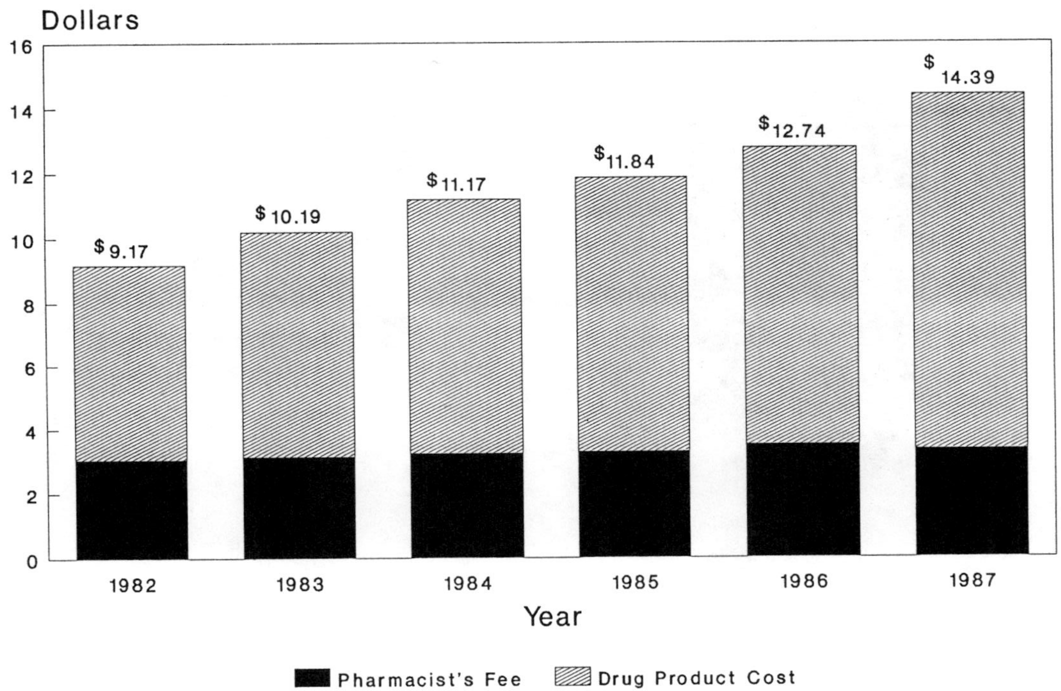

Source: Pharmaceutical Economics Research Center, Purdue University

Labor-Intensive vs. Product-Intensive Industries: Distribution of Expenses

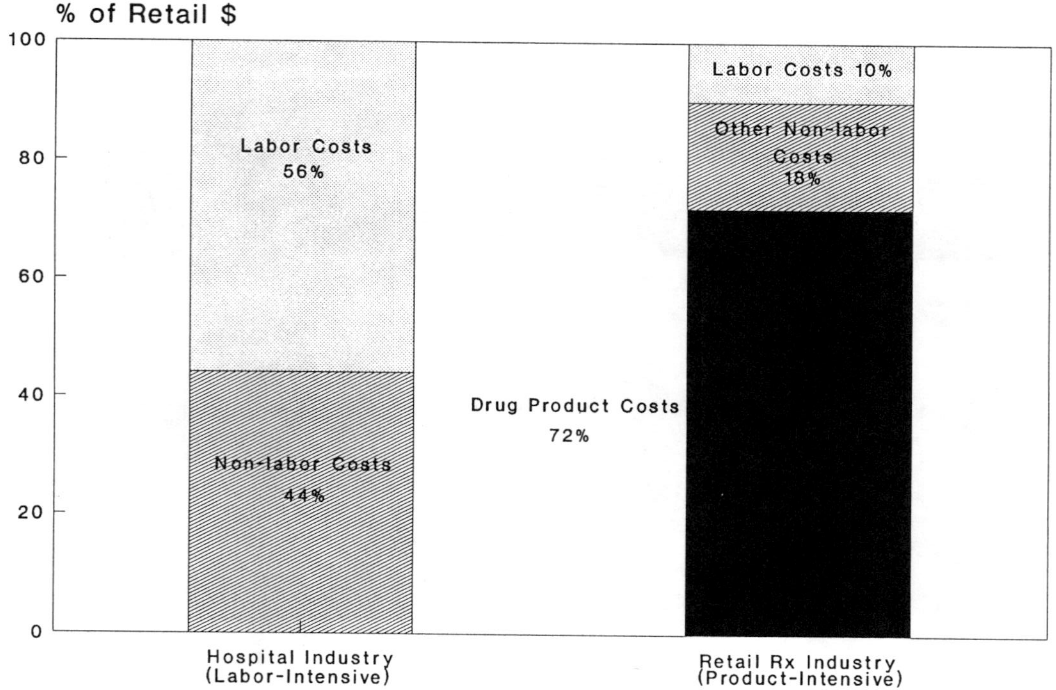

The NACDS-Lilly Digest: 1986 (Indianapolis: Eli Lilly and Company, 1986), p.5.

Pharmacy Fee Increases
(Assume 4% GNP Deflator)

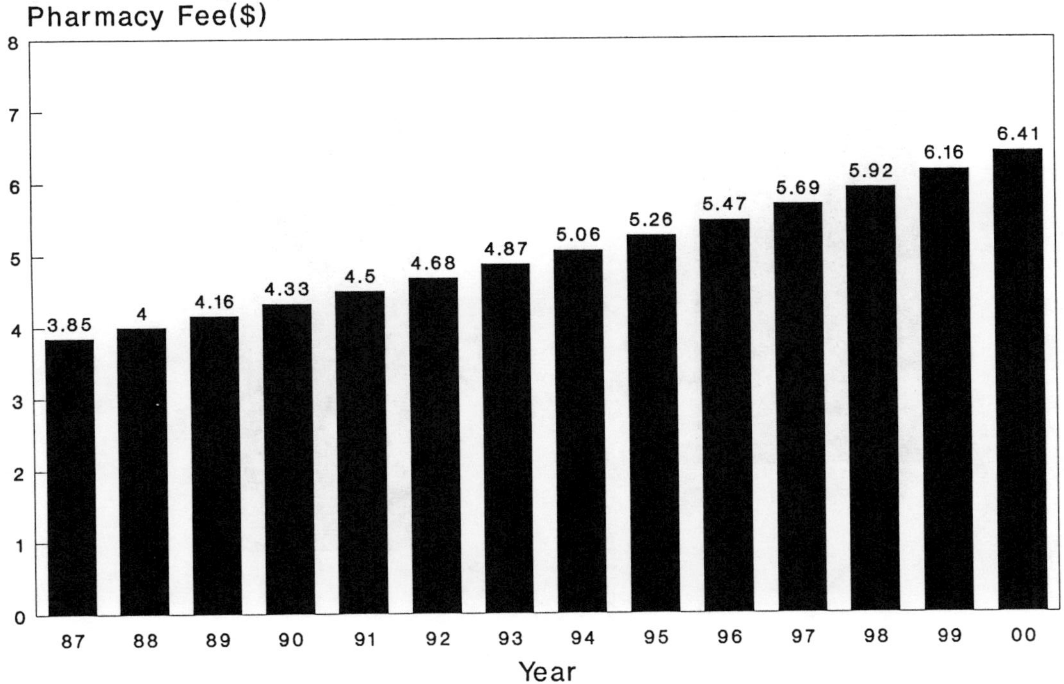

Schondelmeyer, Stephen W., "Demystifying the Pharmacy Component of Medicare," Journal of Research in Pharmaceutical Economics, Volume 1, No.3 (Fall 1989).

Minutes Worked to Pay for an Average Prescription

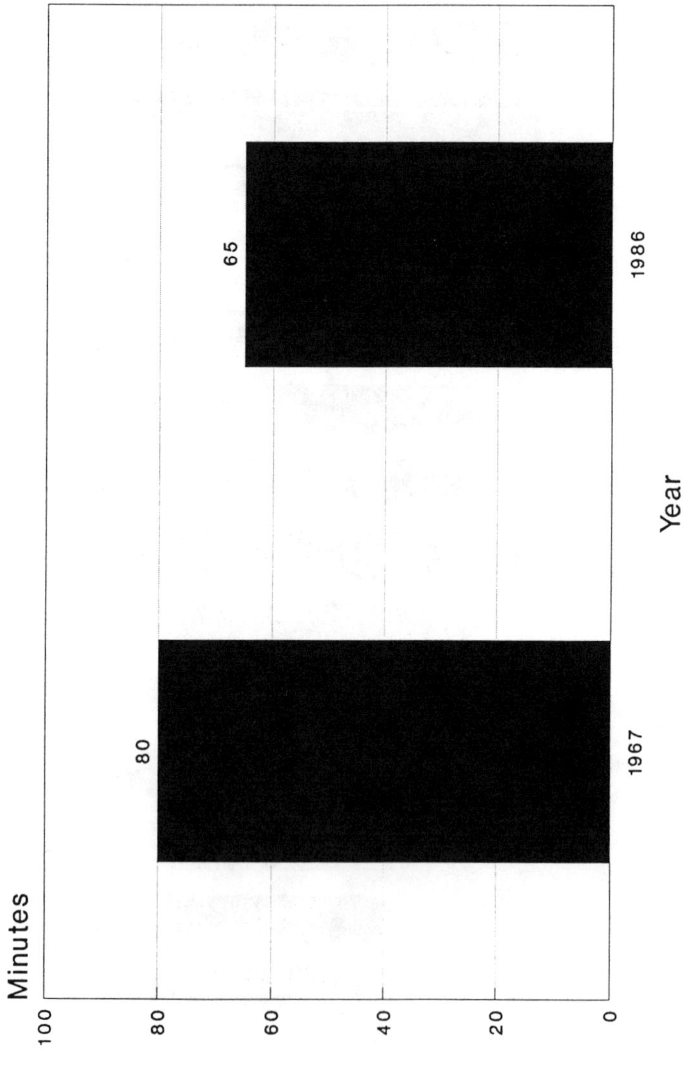

U.S. Department of Commerce, Statistical Abstracts of the United States (Washington DC: U.S. Government Printing Office, 1988)

Predicted Effect of the Catastrophic Drug Insurance Program on Medicare Expenditures

(in billions of dollars)

	1990	1991	1992	1993	Four-Year Total
Outlays					
Benefits	0.1	1.6	3.7	4.3	9.6
Administrative Costs	0.1	0.5	0.7	0.8	2.2
Total	0.2	2.1	4.4	5.1	11.8
Receipts					
Income-Related Premium	0.8	1.8	1.6	2.1	6.3
Flat Premium		0.6	1.0	1.2	2.8
Total	0.8	2.4	2.6	3.3	9.1
Net Effect	-0.7	-0.2	1.8	1.7	2.7

Source: Congressional Budget Office, July 1989

Insurers Step Up Efforts to Reduce Use of Free-Choice Health Plans

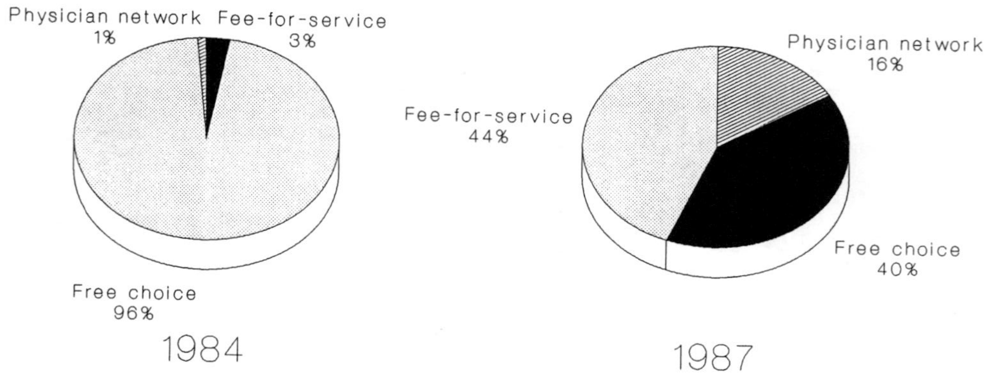

Source: Health Insurance Association Of America, 1988.

Expected Growth of Managed Care

By 1995 it is projected that managed care will cover 76 percent of the population (200 million)

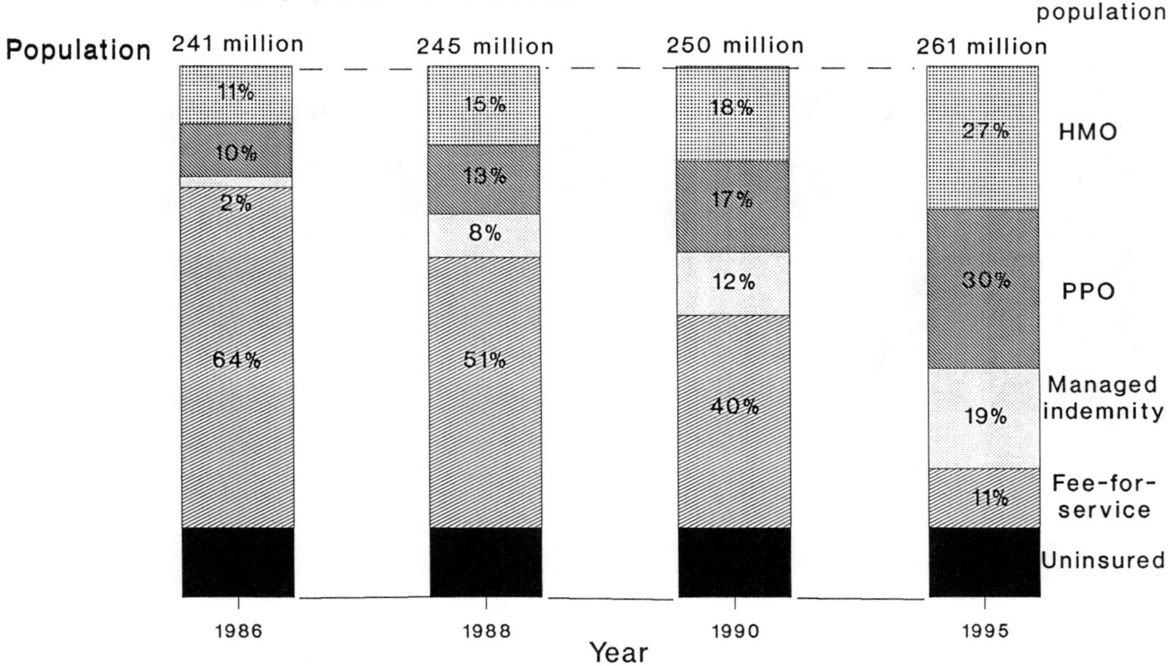

Source: HCFA, Modern Healthcare, Interstudy, The Wilkerson Group. MBSTAT.Medical Benefits. 1988

Total HMO Membership
1978-1987

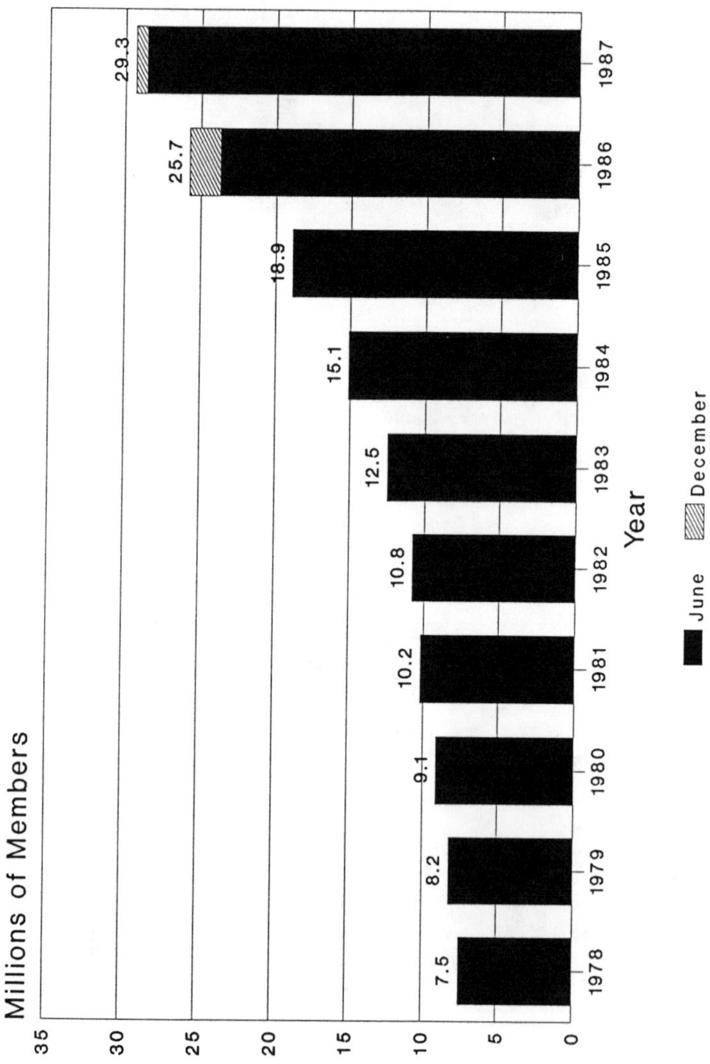

Source: Health Affairs: Summer 1988

Number of HMO Plans
1978-1987

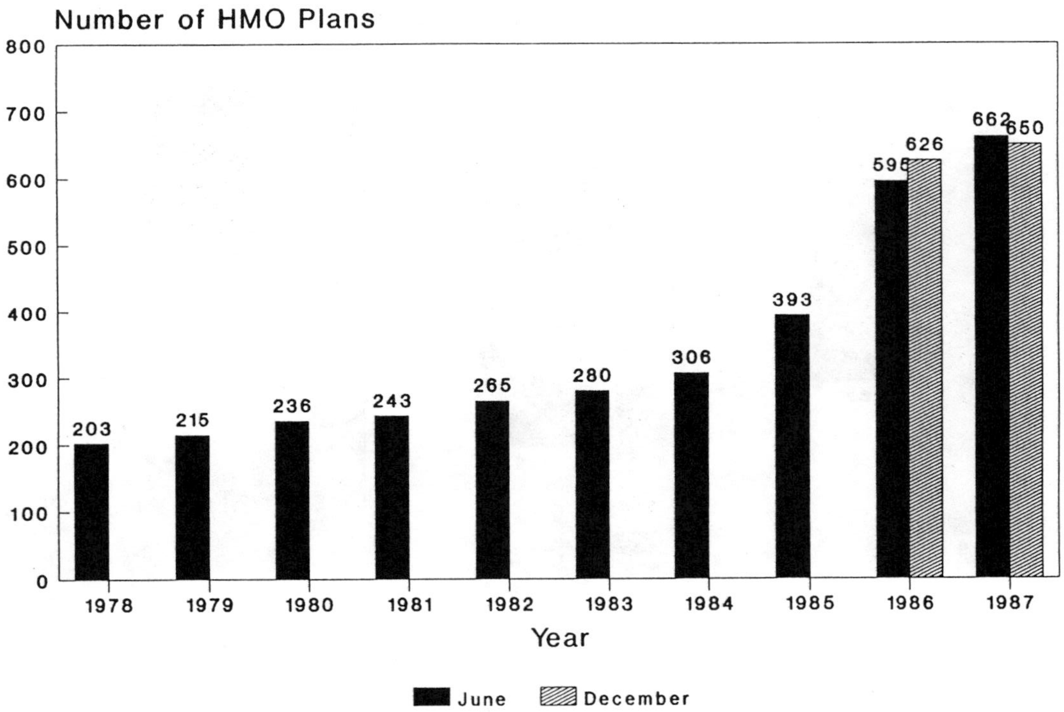

Source: Health Affairs: Summer 1988

Changes in the Total Number of HMOs and PPOs

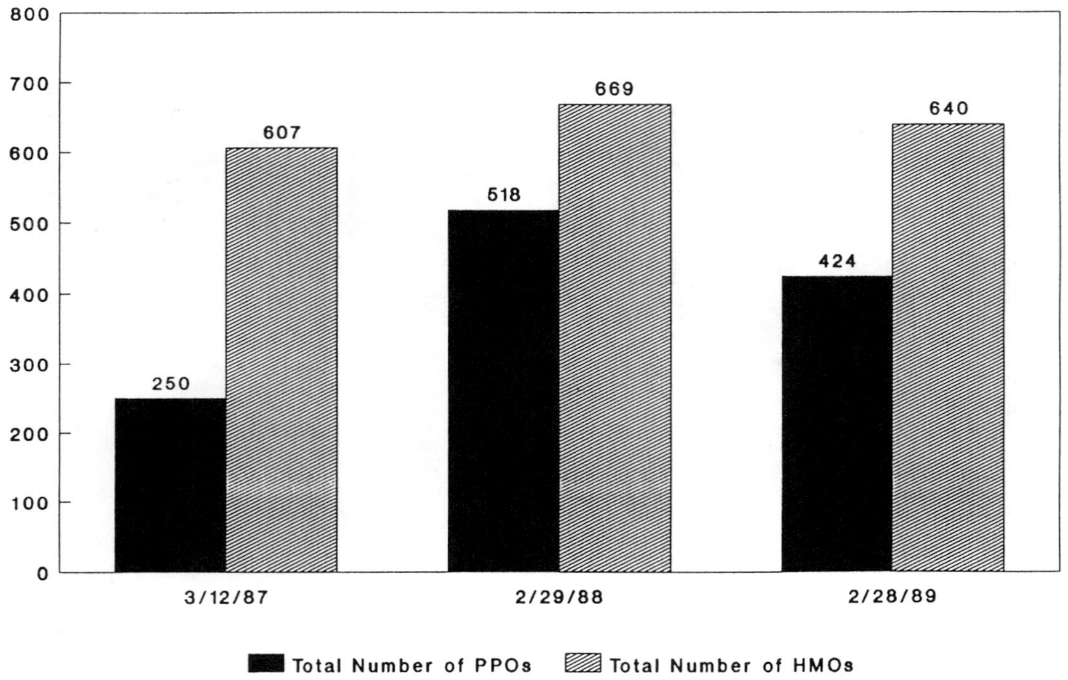

Source: HMO/PPO Census Database Survey, 1989.

Health Maintenance Organizations and Preferred Provider Organizations by Region as of 2/28/89

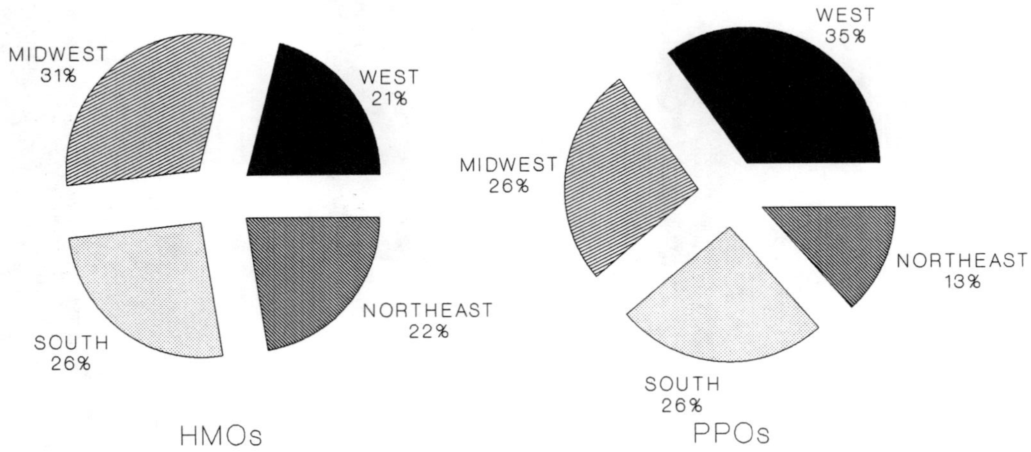

Source: HMO/PPO Census Database Survey, 1989.

New HMO Data:
Counts of HMO Organizations

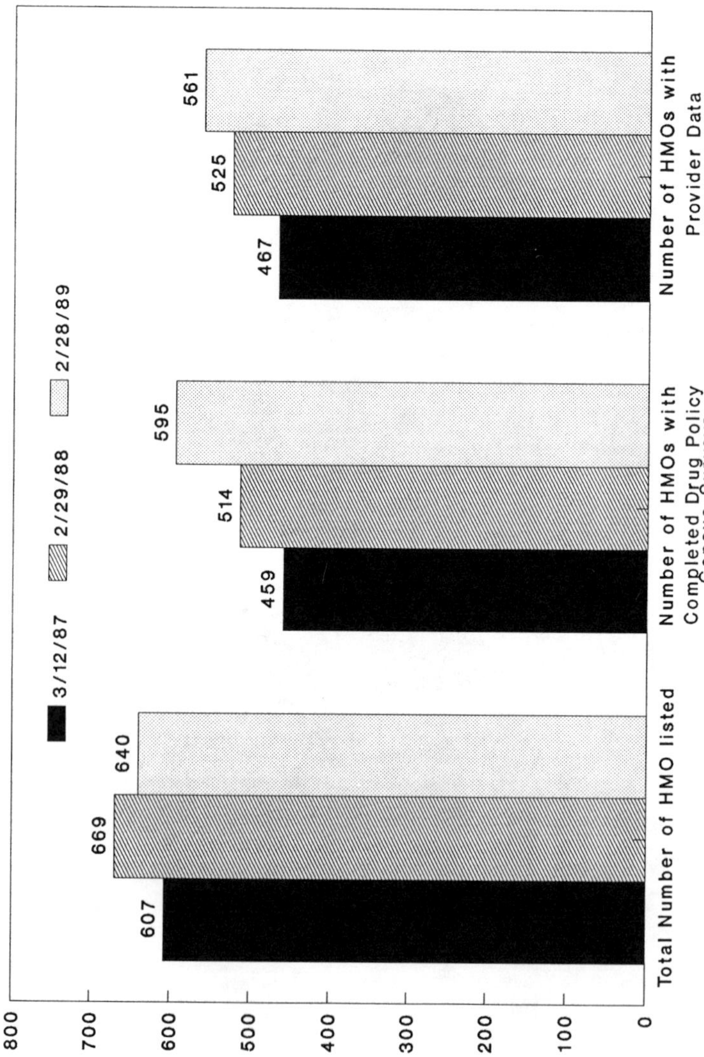

Source: HMO/PPO Census Database File, 1989.

Unduplicated Provider Counts on the HMO/PPO Census Database File

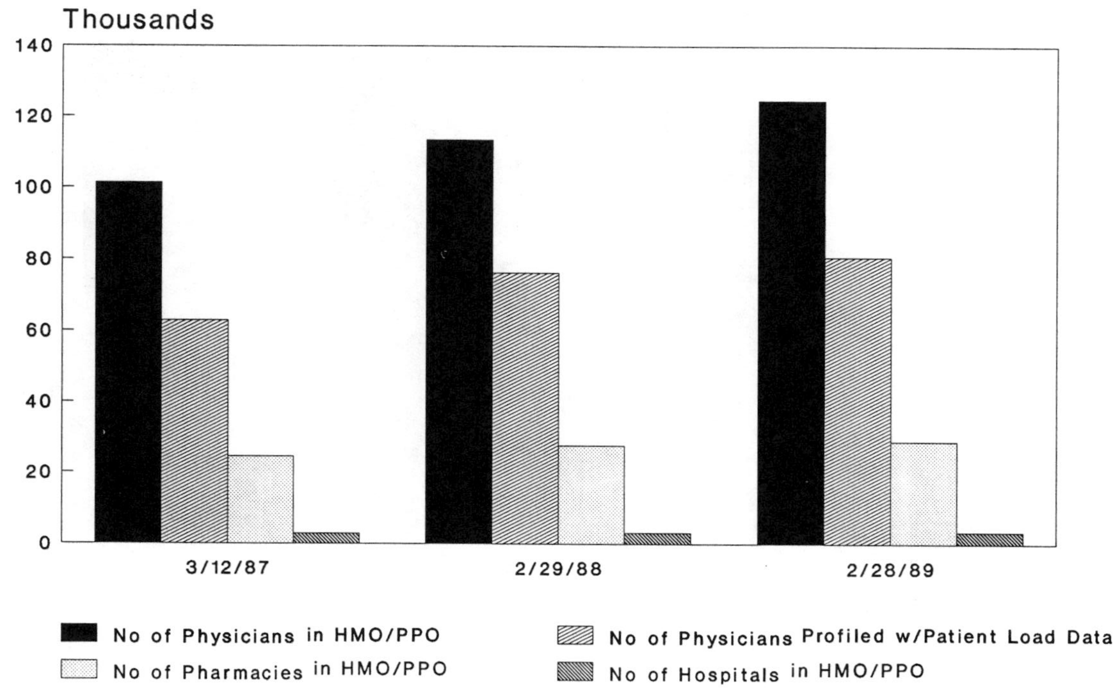

Source:HMO/PPO Census Database File, 1989.

Information on Preferred Provider Organization

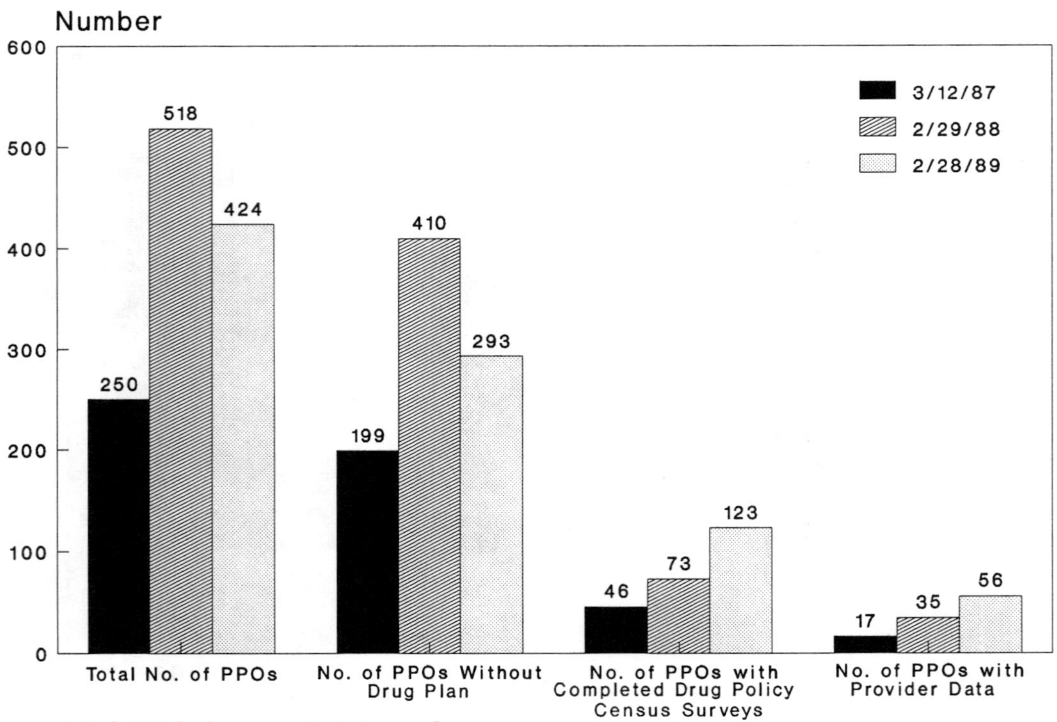

Source: HMO/PPO Census Database Survey, 1989.

HMO Enrollment
Top Ten States

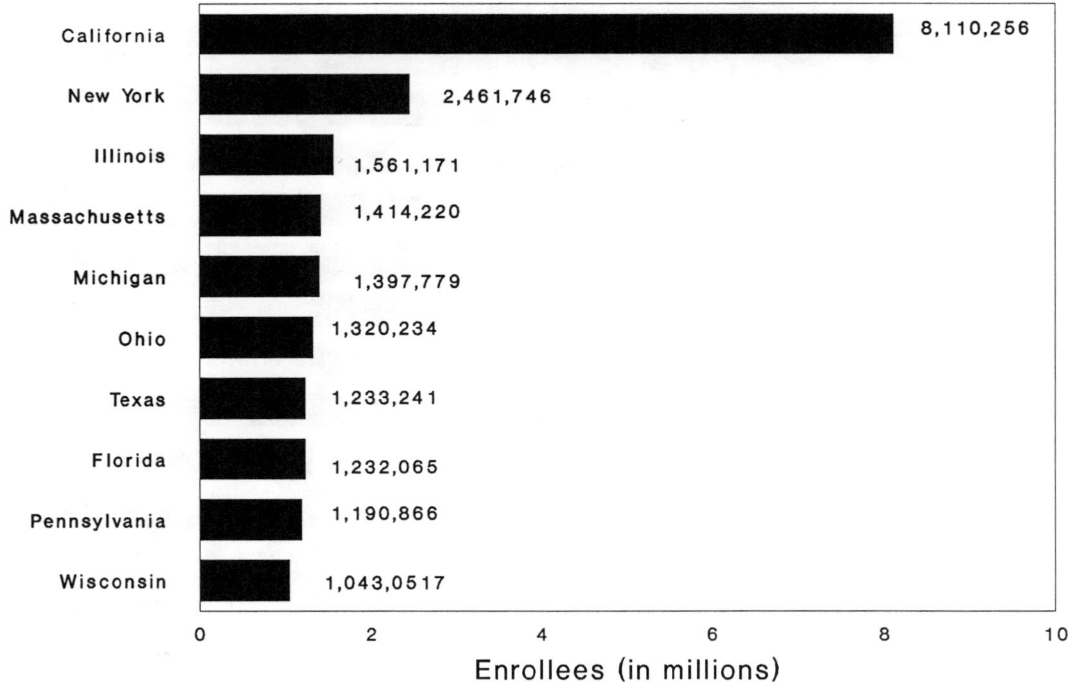

Source: InterStudy; Managed HealthCare, July 17, 1989.

States with Lowest HMO Enrollment

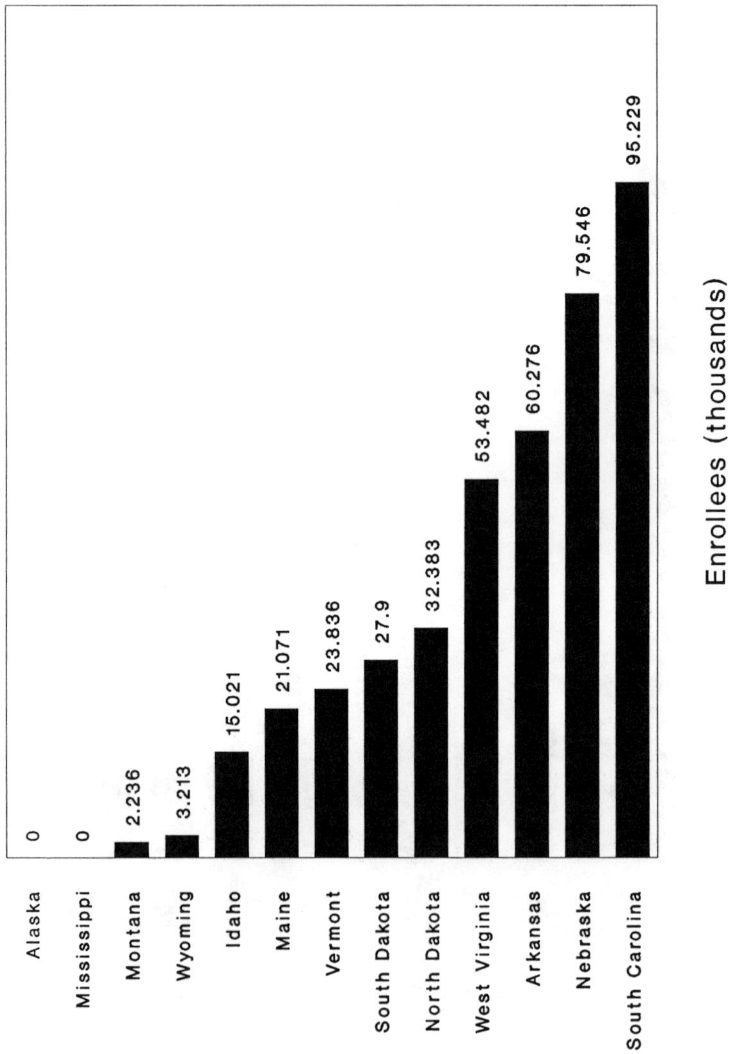

Source: Interstudy;Managed HealthCare, August 14, 1989.

HMO Enrollment as a Percentage of State Population
(Top 10 States)

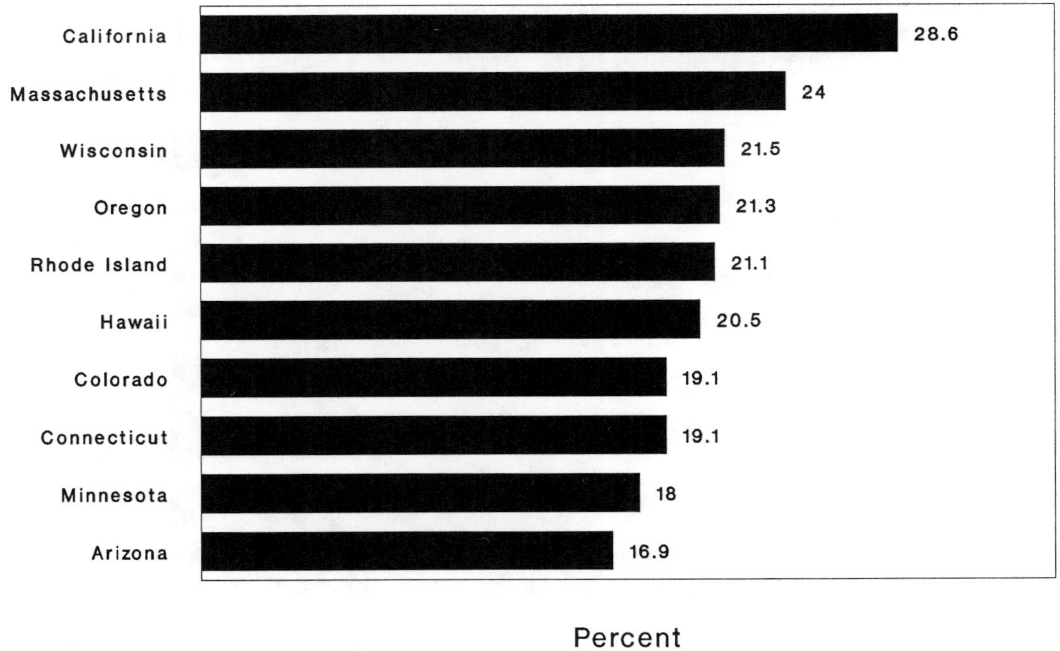

Source: InterStudy; Managed HealthCare, July 17, 1989.

HMO Enrollments
(by type of practice)

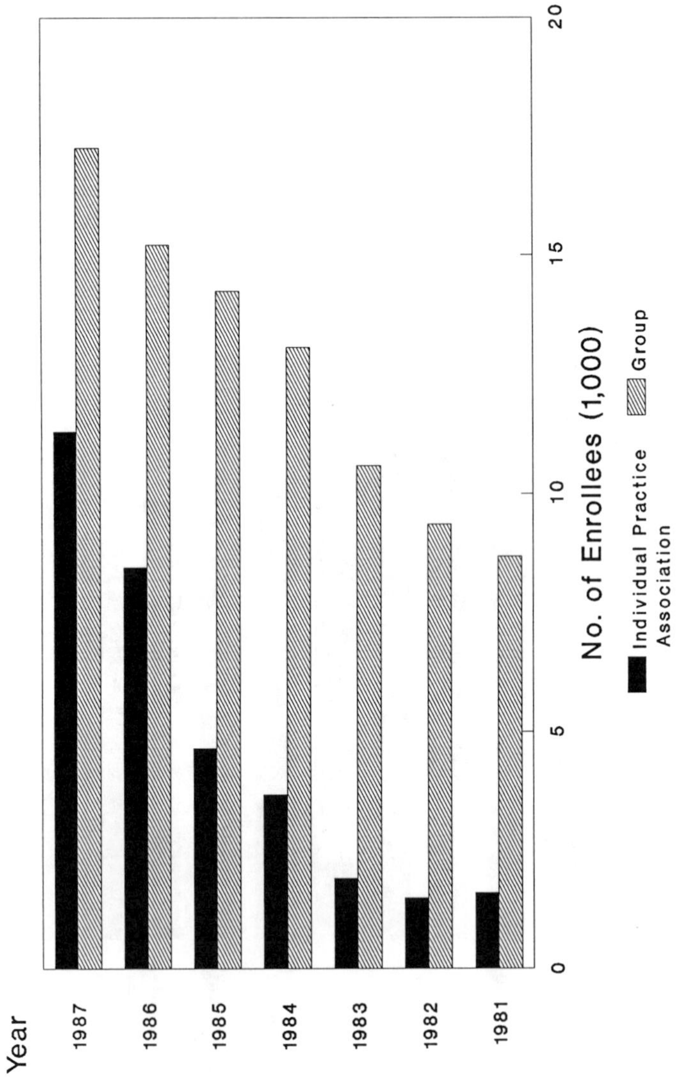

Source: Group Health Association of America, Inc., The Interstudy Edge, Fall 1987 and earlier publications.

Distribution of HMO Membership: 1988
(Plans Over Three Years Old)

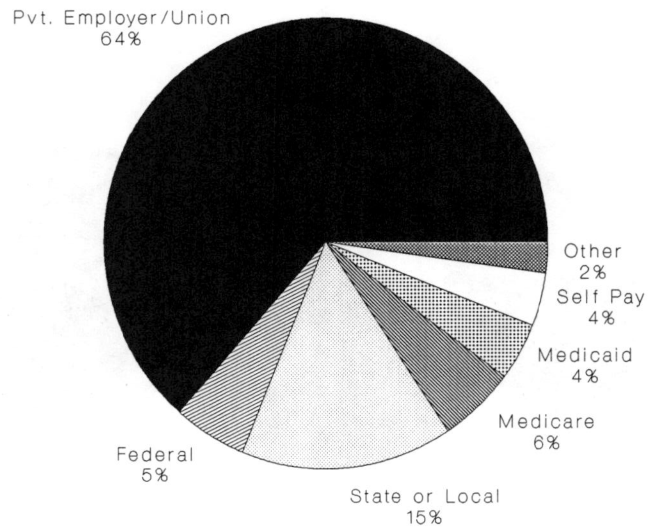

Source: GHAA's Annual HMO Industry Survey, June 1989.

Rating Method of HMO Plan Enrollees 1988

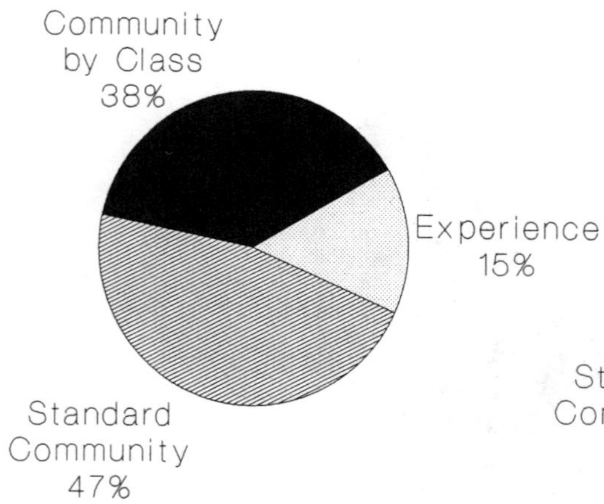

Plans Over Three Years Old

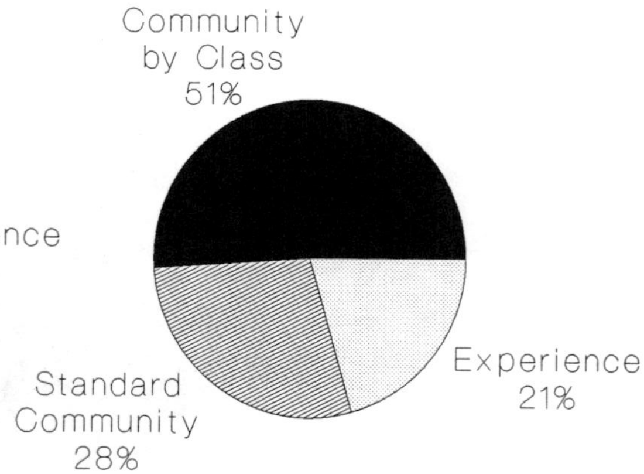

Plans Three Years or Younger

Source: GHAA's Annual HMO Industry Survey, June 1989.

HMO Ownership, 1988

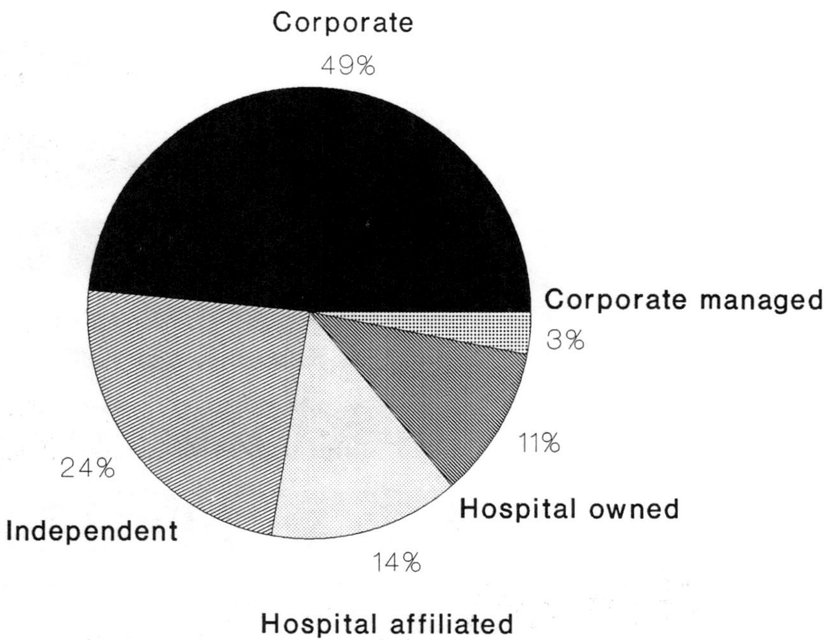

Source: Marion Managed Care Digest/SMG Marketing Group Inc.

Corporate Owned and Managed HMOs by Region, 1988

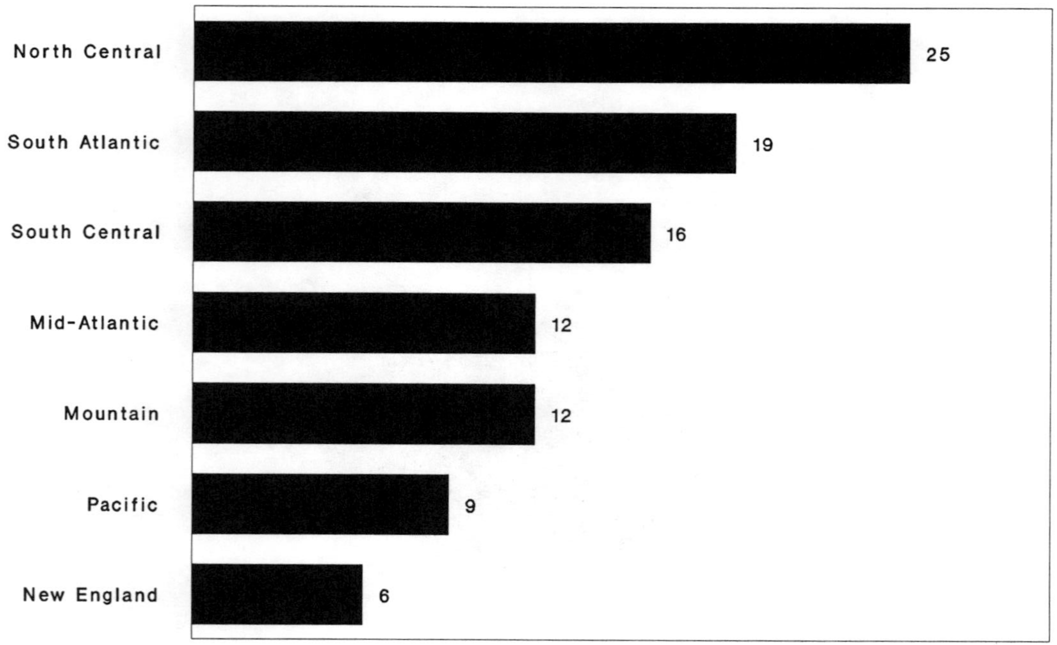

Source: Marion Managed Care Digest/SMG Marketing Group Inc., 1989.

Ten Largest Medicare HMOs

Plan name, city	Medicare enrollment
1. Humana Medicare Plan Inc., Miami	143,532
2. FHP of California, Long Beach	106,685
3. PacifiCare of California, Los Angeles	83,411
4. Kaiser Foundation-Southern California, Pasadena	76,913
5. Share Health Plan of Minnesota, Minneapolis	41,335
6. Physicians Health Plan of Minnesota, Minnetonka	40,588
7. Group Health Cooperative of Puget Sound, Seattle	39,451
8. Kaiser Foundation-Northwest, Portland, Ore.	30,819
9. Share of Illinois, Itasca	26,611
10. Health Insurance Plan of Greater New York	25,359

Source: HCFA; Managed HealthCare, Oct. 10, 1989.

HMO Diversification Activities: 1988
(Plans Over Three Years Old)

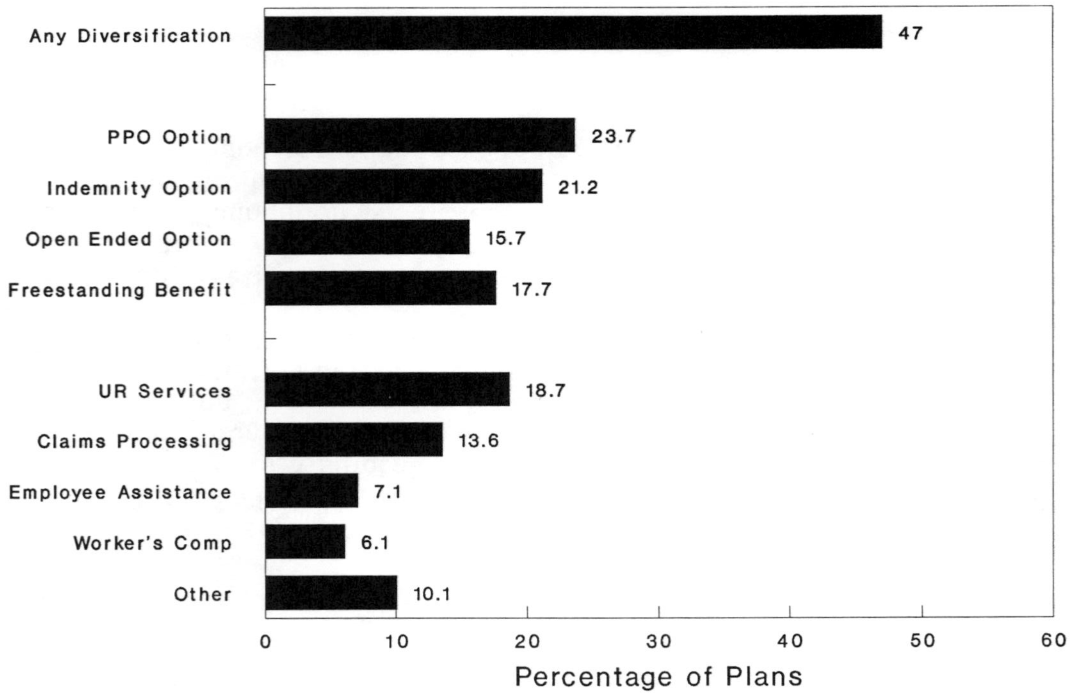

Source: GHAA's Annual Industry Survey, June 1989.

Selected Characteristics of HMO Accounts
(Plans Over Three Years Old)

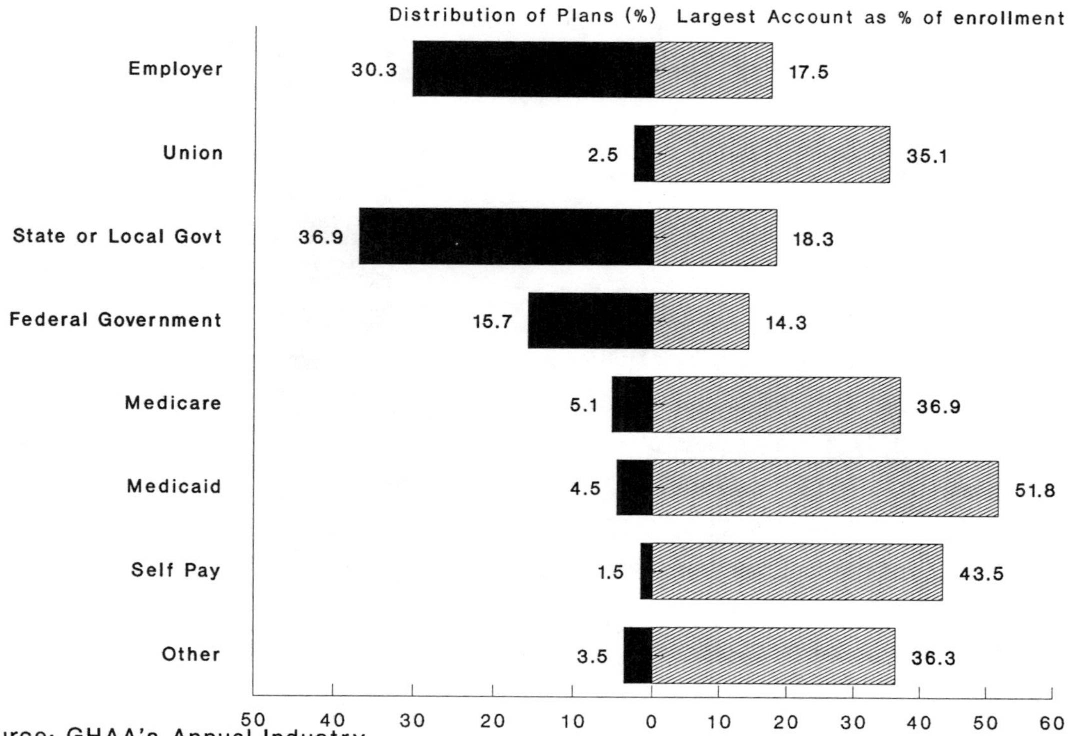

Source: GHAA's Annual Industry Survey, June 1989.

Coverage of Various Preventive Services in Best Selling Benefit Package: 1988
(Plans Over Three Years Old)

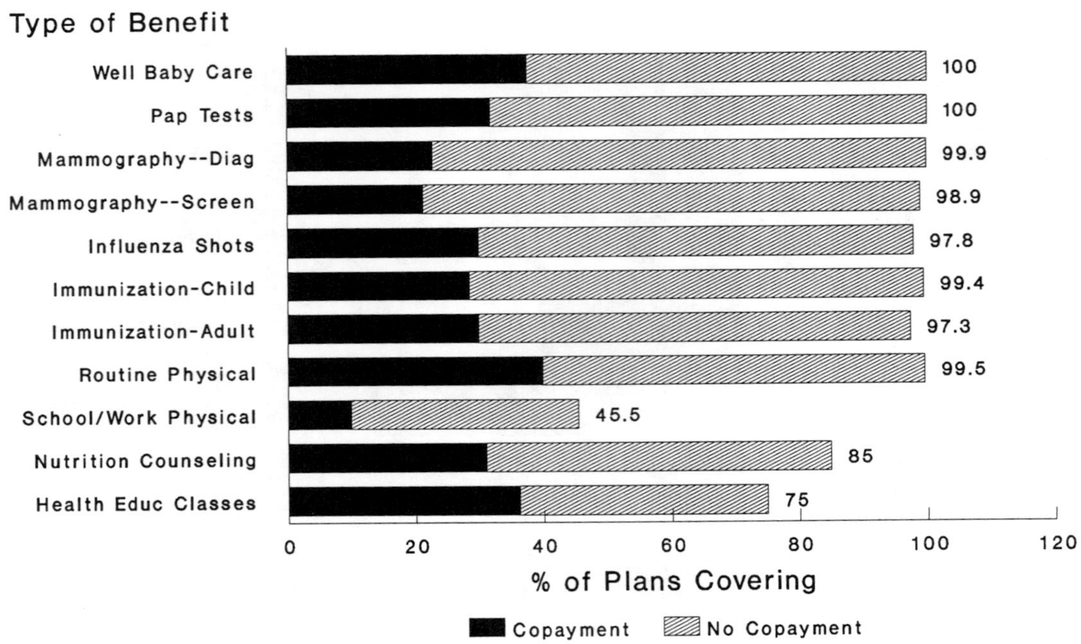

Source: GHAA's Annual HMO Industry Survey, June 1989.

*Best selling: Benefit package to which the largest proportion of the plan's enrollees subscribe.

Percent of Plans Using Copayments for Selected Basic Benefits, by Plan Age

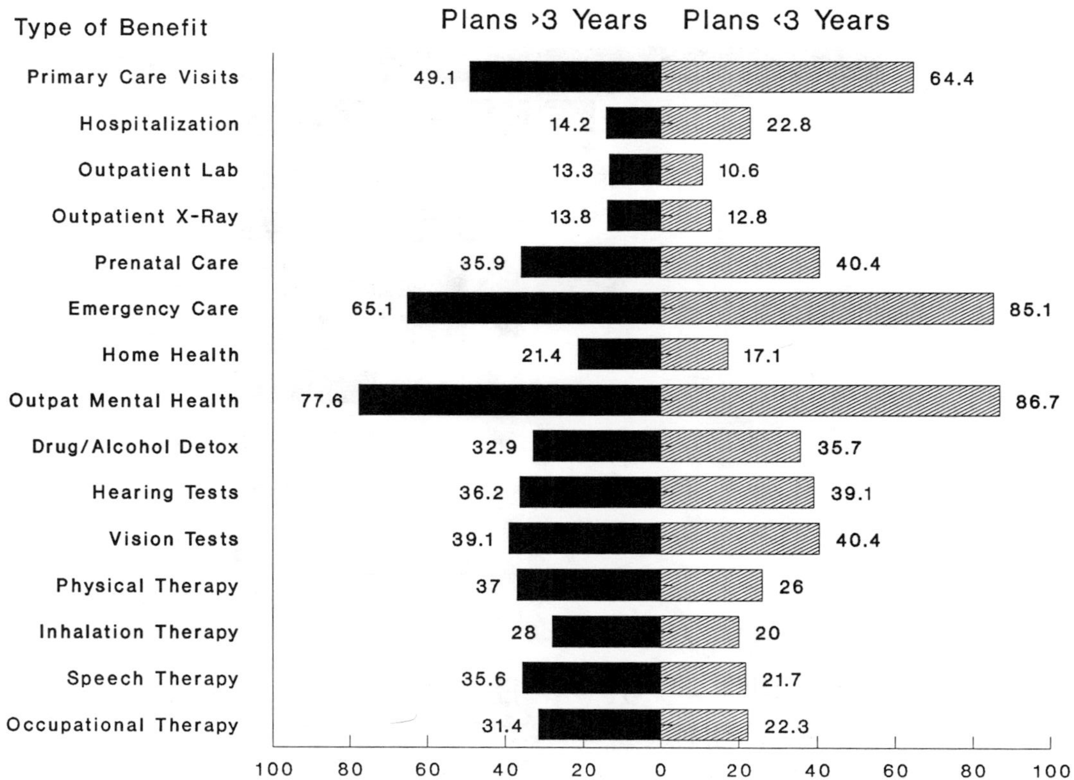

Percentage of HMO Enrollment in Best Selling Benefit Package, Distribution of Plans, Plans Over Three Years Old, 1988

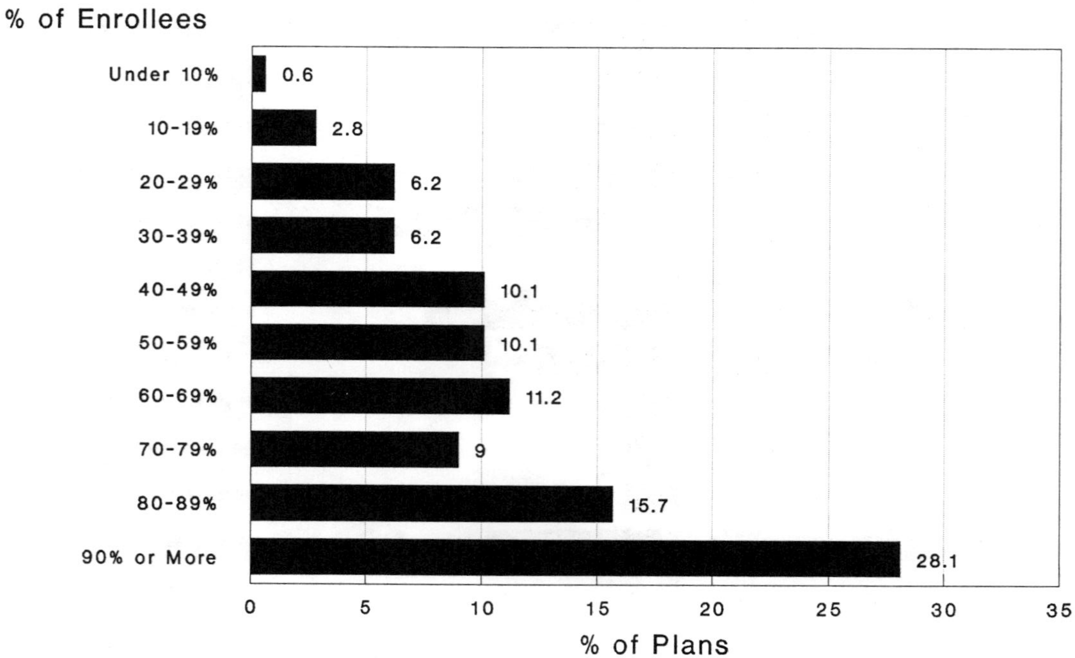

Source: GHAA's Annual HMO Industry Survey, June 1989.

*Best selling: Benefit package to which the largest proportion of the plan's enrollees subscribe.

Extent of Agreements with Other HMOs to Address Employer Needs, Plans Over Three Years Old, 1988

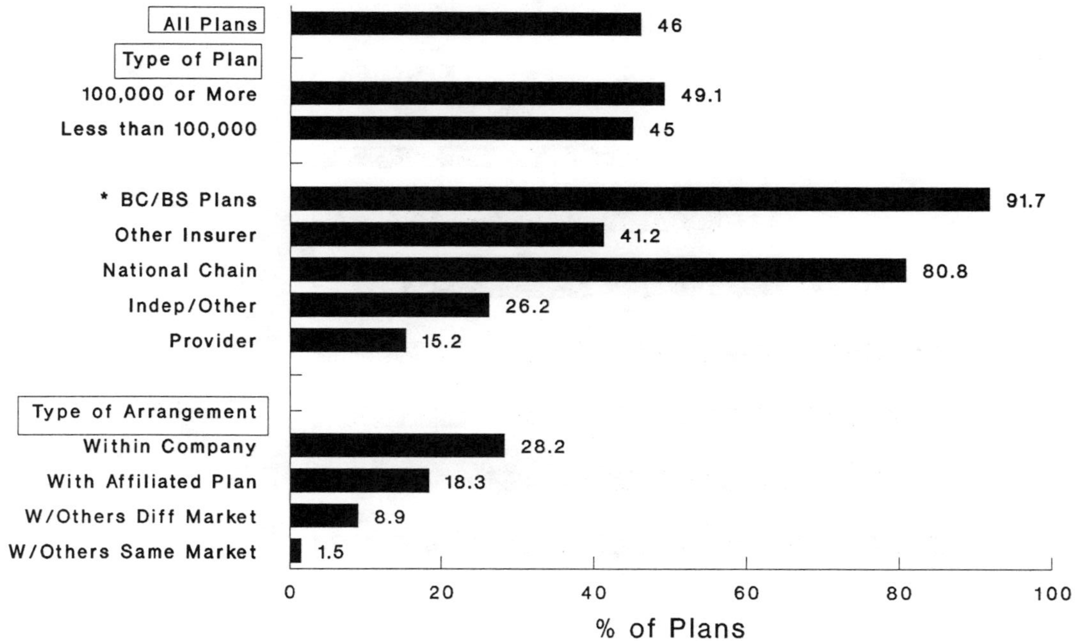

Source: GHAA's Annual Industry Survey, June 1989.

*BC/BS= Blue Cross-Blue Shield

Transplant Coverage by Type: 1988

(Plans Over Three Years Old)

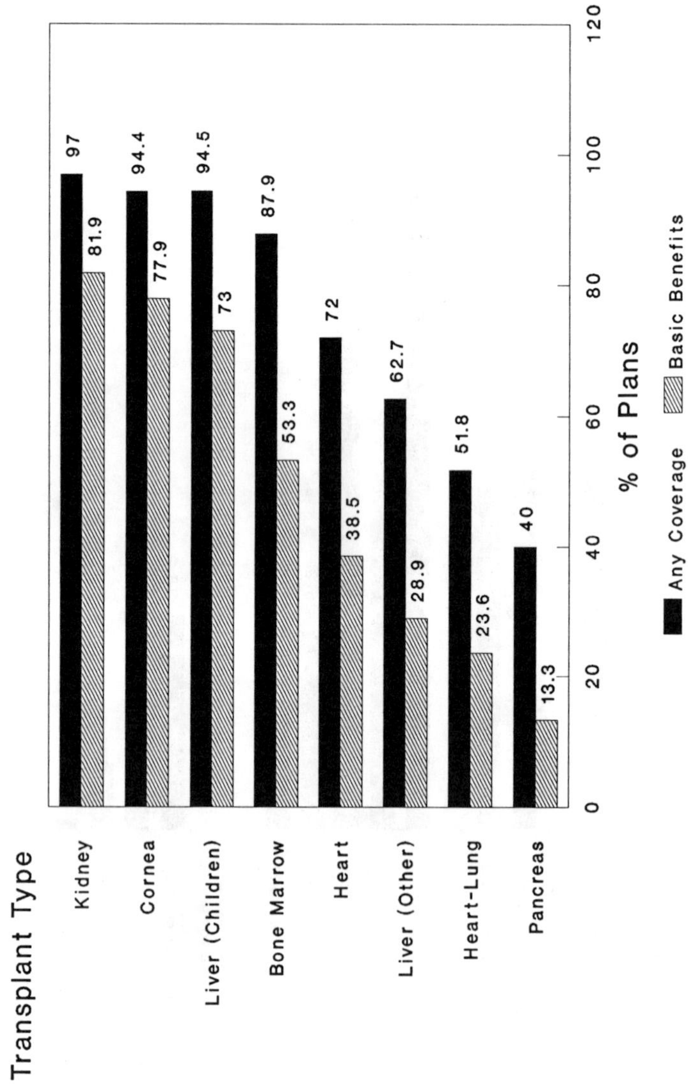

Source: GHAA's Annual HMO Industry Survey, June 1989.

Factors Cited as Contributions to Rising HMO Premiums: 1988-1989

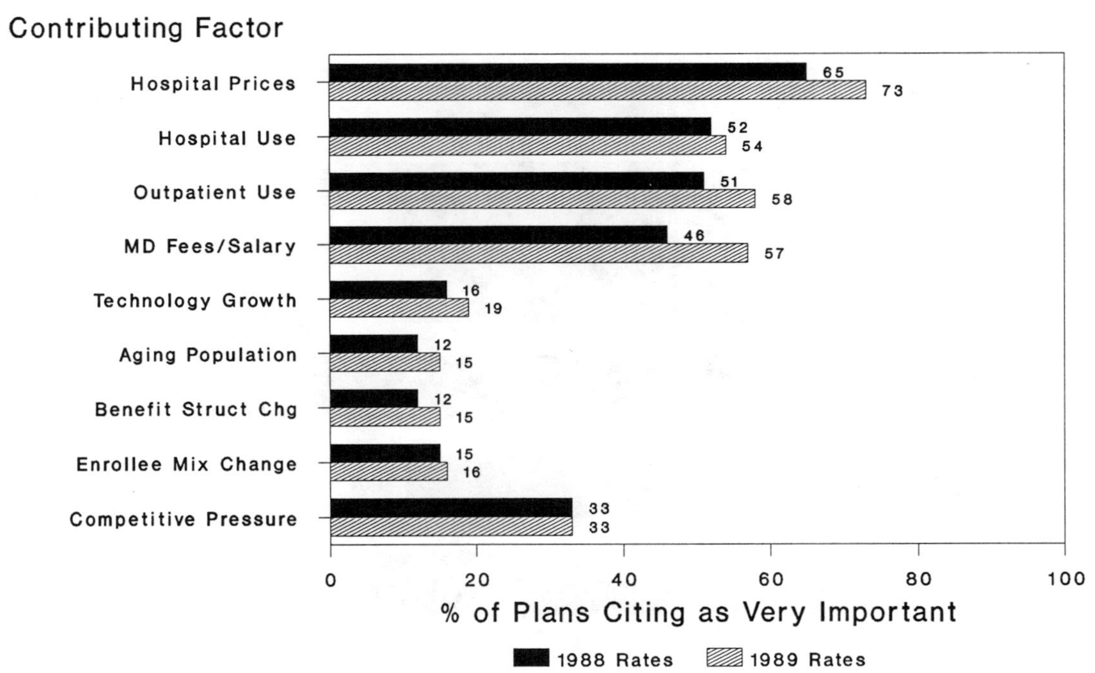

Source: GHAA's Annual HMO Industry Survey, June 1989.

Monthly HMO Premium Increases 1988-1989

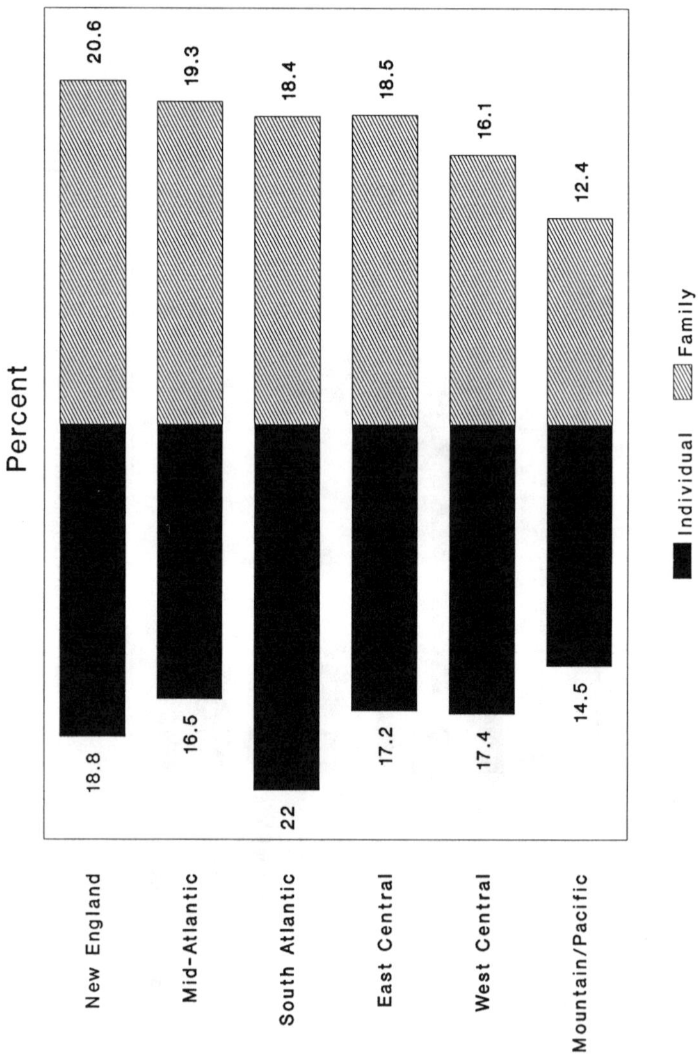

Source: GHAA; Managed HealthCare, October 10, 1989.

Average HMO Premium Increase

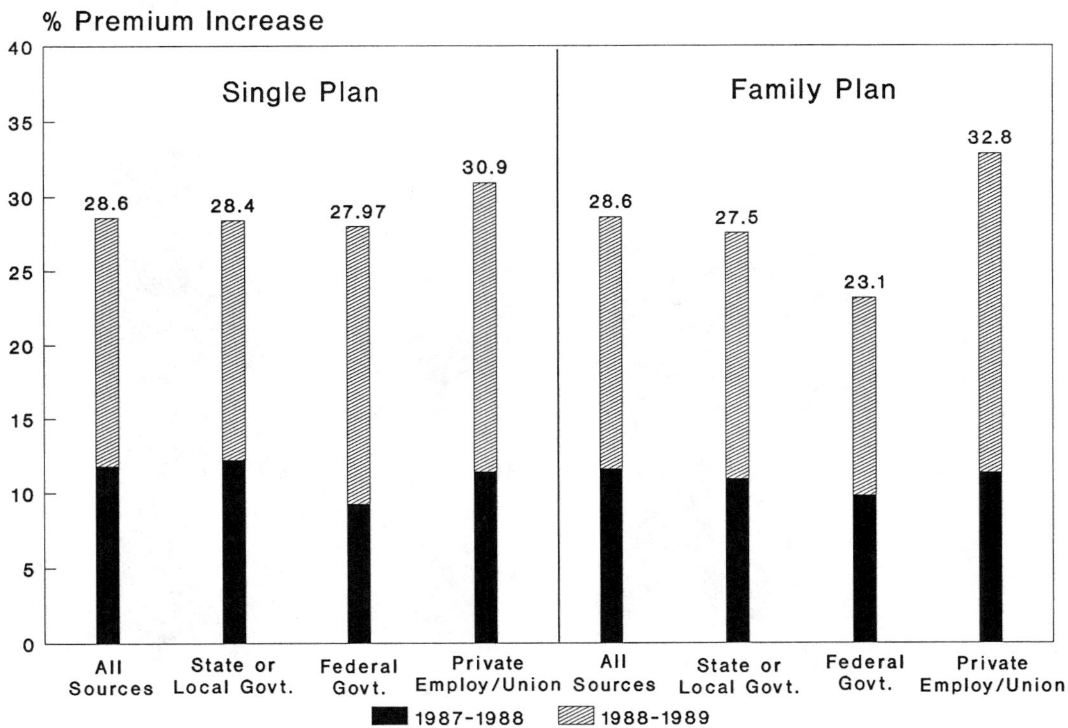

Source: GHAA's Annual HMO Industry Survey, June 1989.

Average HMO Premium Increase 1987-1988

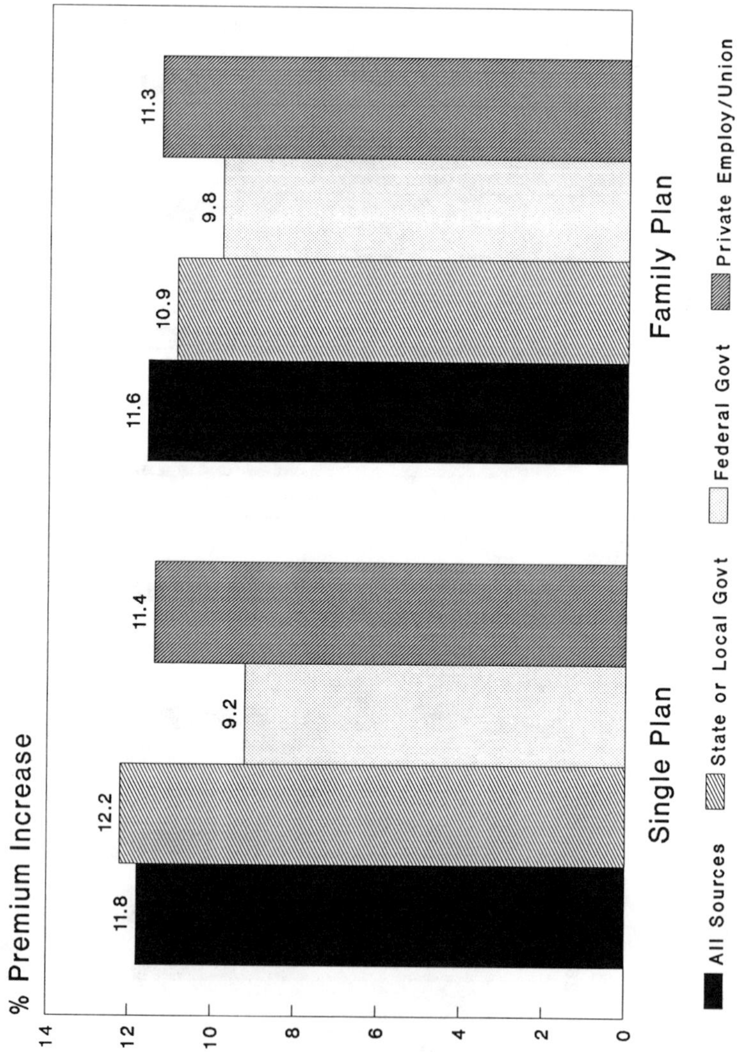

Source: CHAA's Annual HMO Industry Survey

Generic vs. Branded Drugs by Model Type

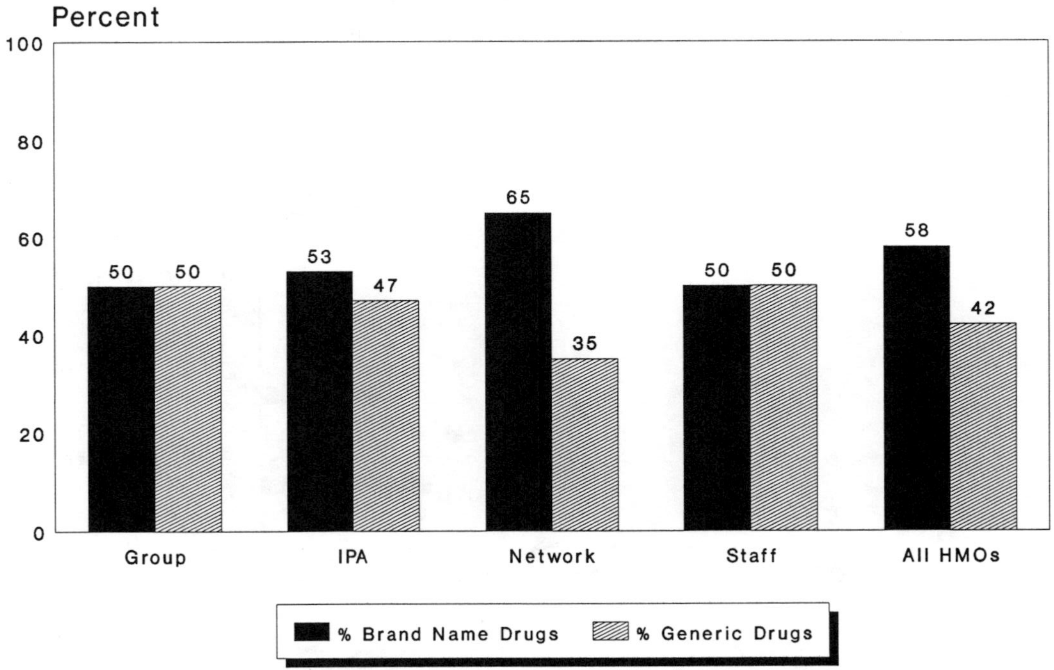

Source: Marion Laboratories/SMG Marketing Group Inc.; Managed HealthCare October 10, 1989.

Major Health Care Service Provider Companies

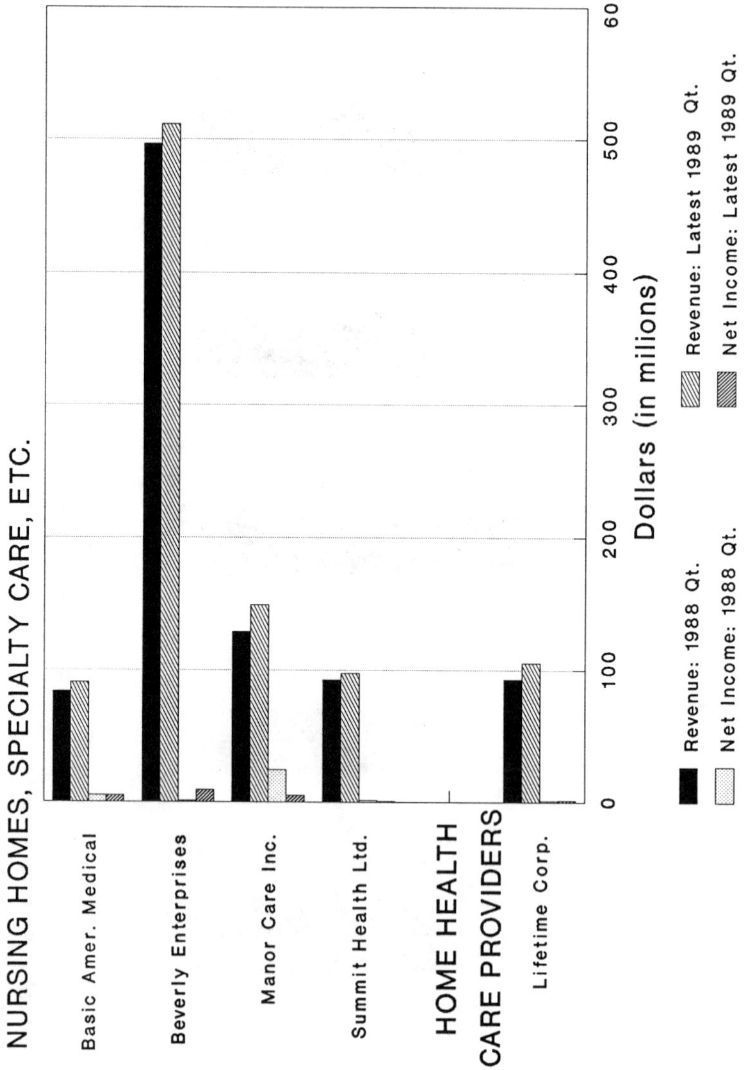

Source: Health Commerce Line, Issue 5, 1989.

Anticipated Growth of Freestanding Ambulatory Centers

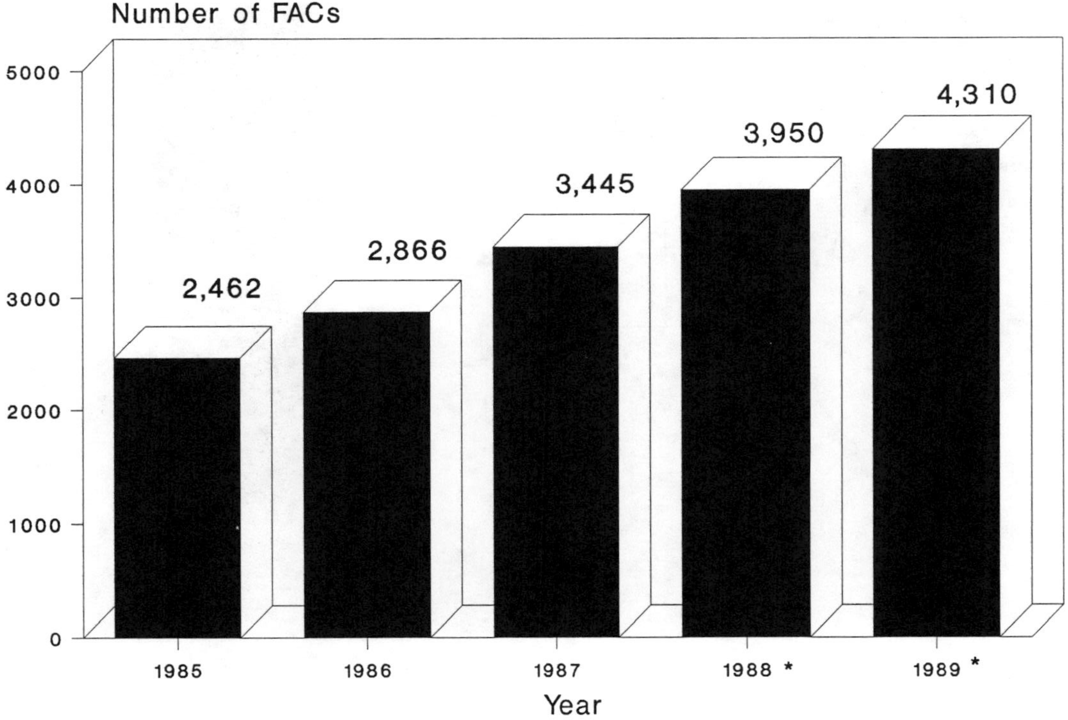

Source: SMG Marketing Group, 1989

*estimated

Percent Ambulatory Encounters by Provider

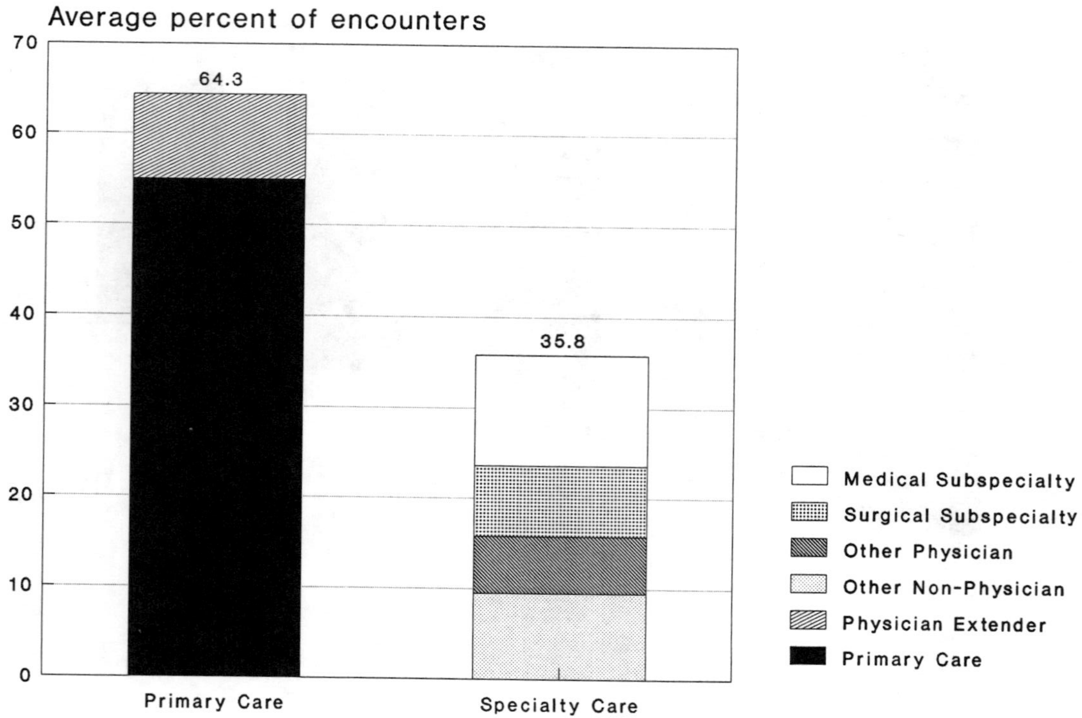

Source: GHAA, 1988

Chapter 5

DRUG DEVELOPMENT AND PRODUCTION

Graphs are presented of new drug entities in the market, drug lag, drug production and drug exports.

The Steps Toward Drug Approval

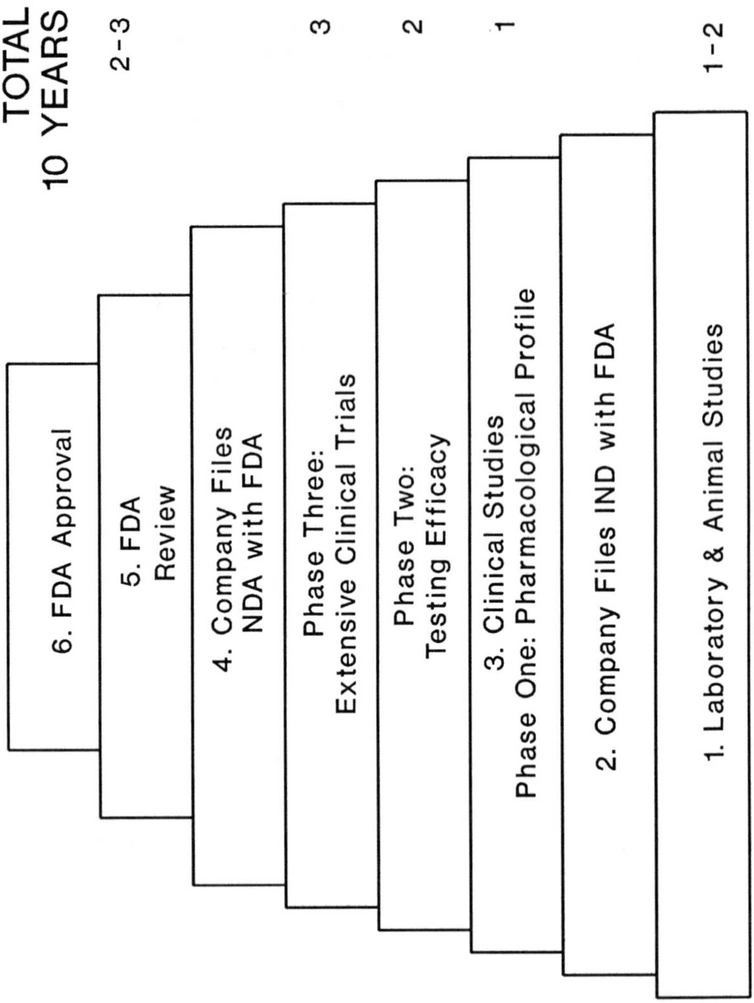

Source: PMA Annual Survey Report, 1988.

National Support for Health
R&D by Source: 1977-1987

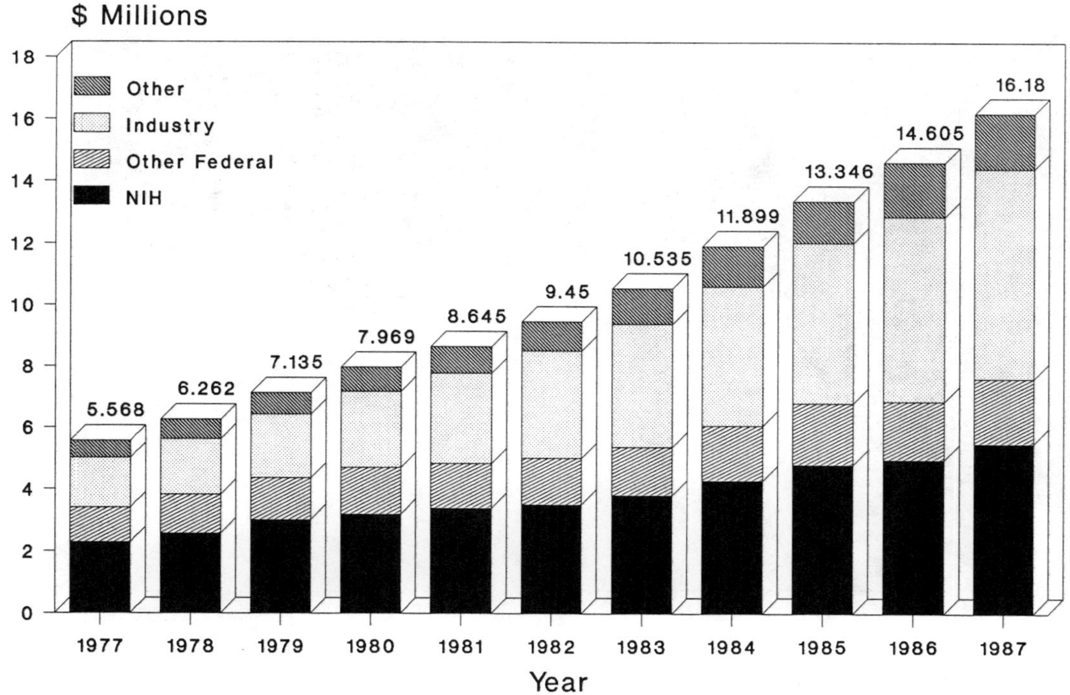

Source: National Institutes of Health
1987.

U.S. Pharmaceutical R&D Expenditures as a Percentage of U.S. Pharmaceutical Sales

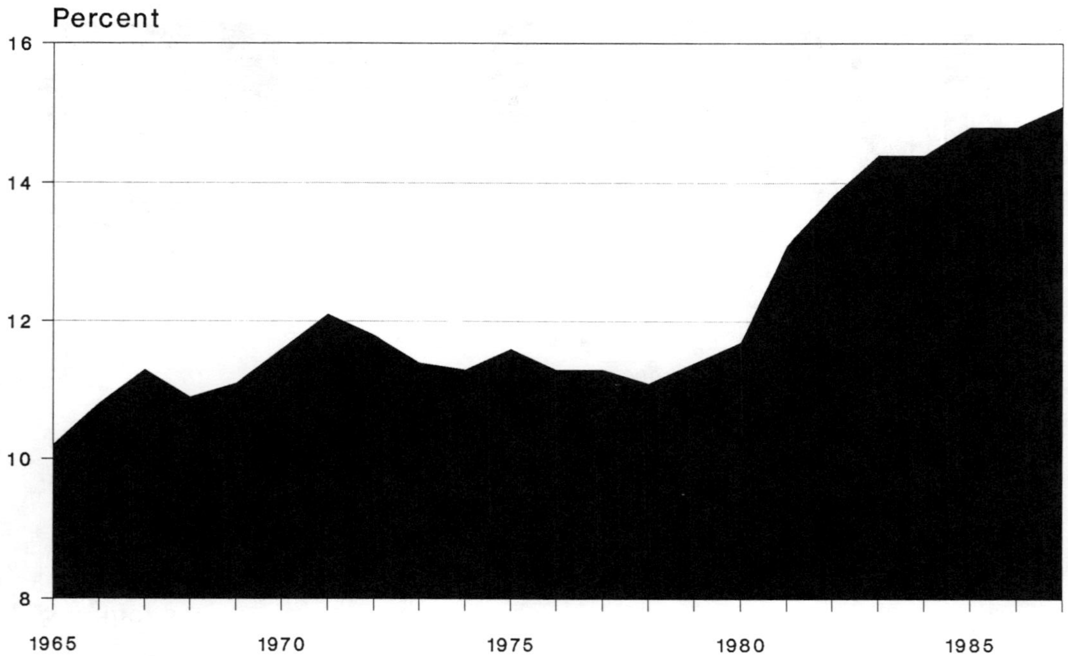

Source: PMA Annual Survey Report, August 1988.

R&D Expenditures for Human Use Ethical Pharmaceuticals 1974-1987

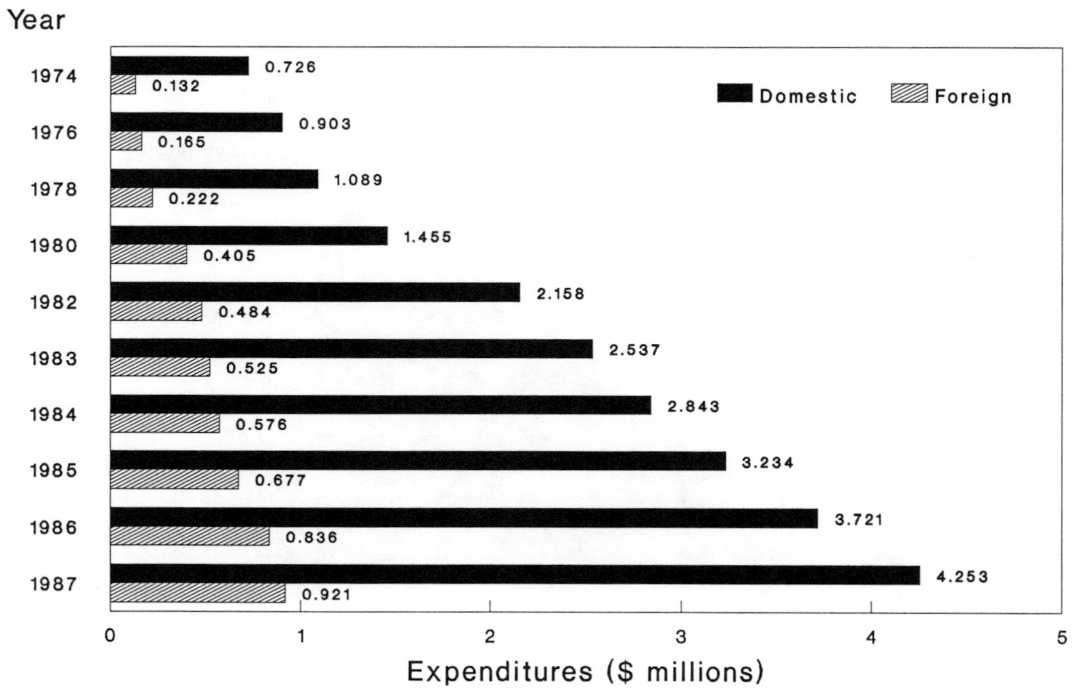

Source: PMA Annual Survey, August 1988.

U.S. Pharmaceutical R&D Expenditures by Product Class: 1986

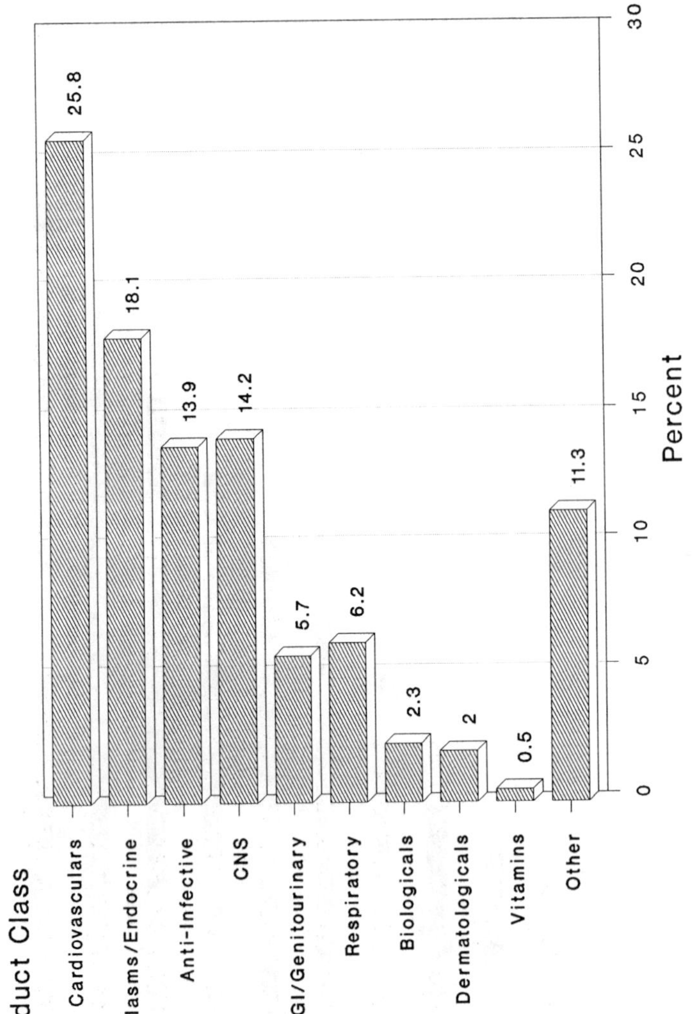

Source: PMA Annual Survey Report, August 1988.

U.S. Patents for Drugs and Medicines

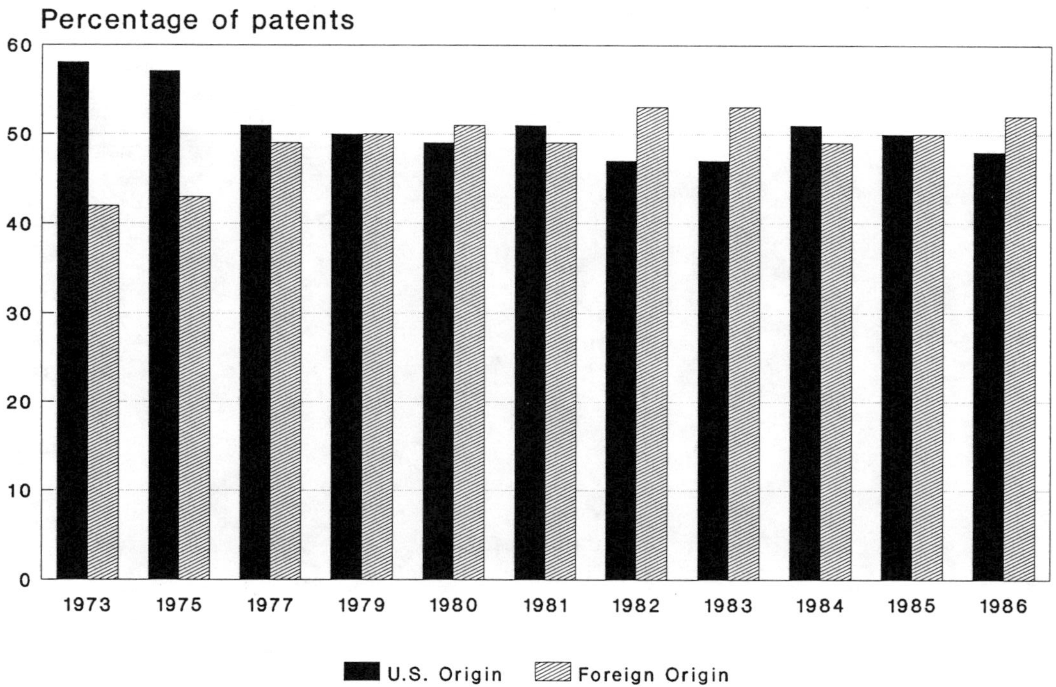

Source: U.S. Patent and Trademark Office, 1986.

Number of New U.S. Patents for Drugs and Medicines by Origin 1973-1986

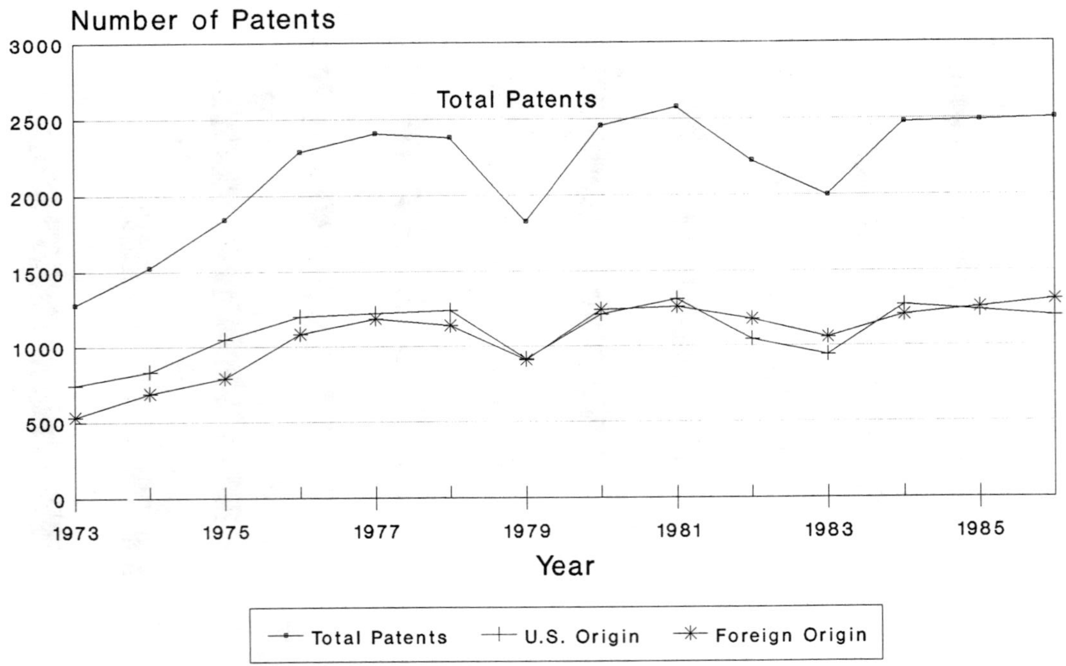

Source: U.S. Patent and Trademark Office 1986.

New Single Chemical Entity Drugs Introduced to U.S. Market 1940-1987 by Country of Origin

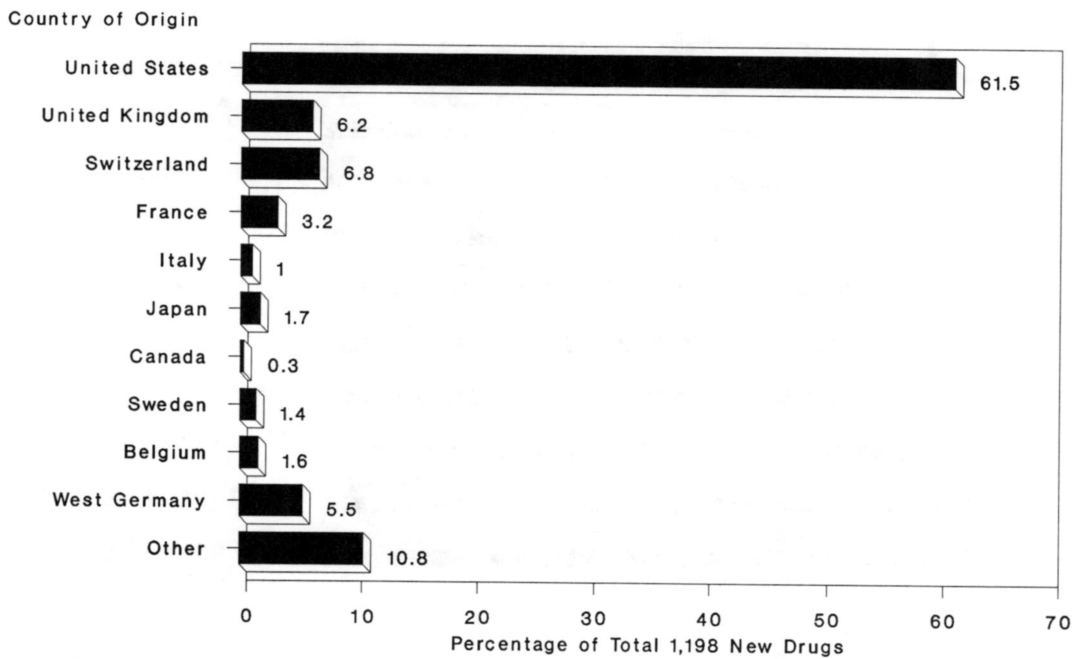

Source: PMA Analysis of Paul De Haen Data, 1987.

Top 10 Companies Worldwide in R&D Compounds: 1987

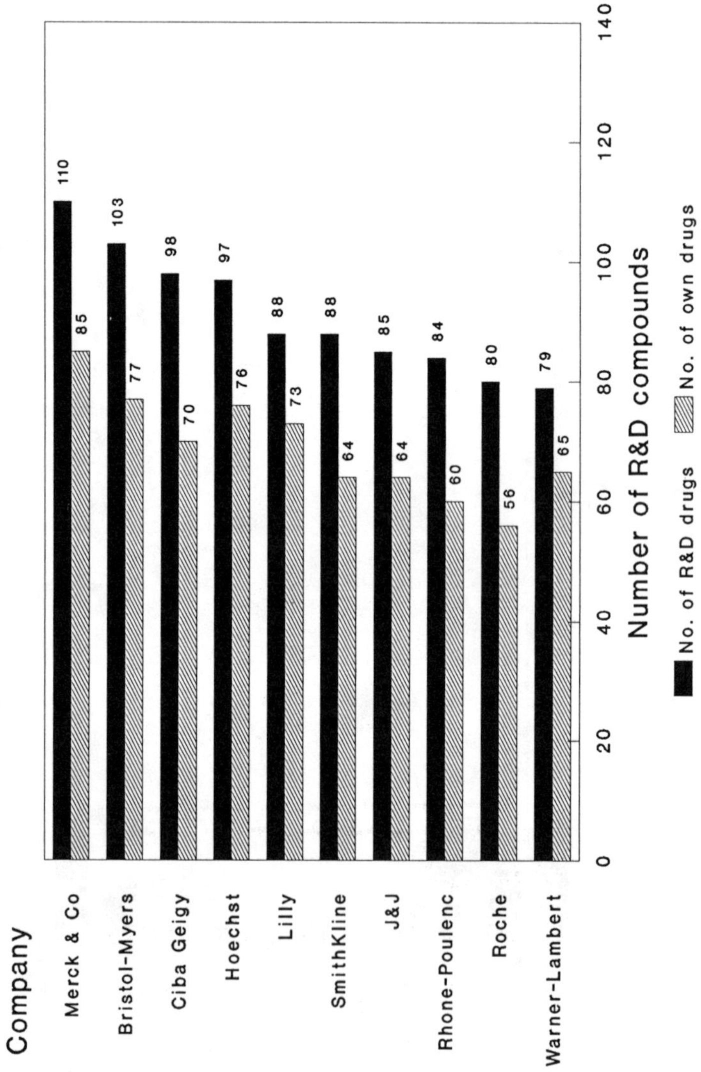

Source: Health U.S., 1988

Listing of Important ("A"-Rated) New Drugs Introduced by the Top 25 U.S. Drug Manufacturers

1981-1988

	BRAND NAME	GENERIC NAME	INDICATION (USE)
1.	Accutane	(Isotretinoin)	Severe acne
2.	Alprostadil	(Prostin VR)	Heart problems in premature babies
3.	Blocadren	(Timolol)	Chest pain, High blood pressure
4.	Carioplegic Solution		Heart surgery
5.	Cytotec gastric ulcers	(Misoprostol)	For Drug-induced
6.	Ifex	(Ifosfamide)	Cancer
7.	I.V. Indocin	(Indomethacin)	Heart problems in premature babies
8.	Lamprene	(Clofazimine)	Leprosy
9.	Mevacor	(Lovastatin)	High cholesterol
10.	Rogaine	(Minoxidil)	Hair growth stimulant
11.	VePesid (Intravenous solution)	(Etoposide)	Cancer
12.	VePesid (Oral capsule)	(Etoposide)	Cancer

U.S. Senate Special Committee on Aging, July 1989.

Top 25 Manufacturers' Annual Production of New Drugs by FDA Therapeutic Classification

(Number and Percentage of Total)

Year	Drug Classication			Year	Drug Classification		
	A	B	C		A	B	C
1981	2 4%	11 23%	35 73%	1985	1 2%	6 13%	39 85%
1982	2 5%	2 5%	35 90%	1986	2 3%	11 18%	48 79%
1983	1 4%	- -	25 96%	1987	1 3%	4 11%	31 86%
1984	- -	8 13%	54 87%	1988	3 10%	2 7%	25 83%
				Total 1981-88	12 3%	44 13%	292 84%
				Grand Total 1981-88			348 New Drugs

U.S. Senate Special Committee on Aging, July 1989.

New Drugs from Top 25 Drug Companies as Proportion of New Drugs from All Companies, 1981-88

		FDA Therapeutic Categories			
Year	*Companies*	*A*	B	C	*Total*
1981 #	All	3	17	76	96
#(%)	Top	2 (67)	11 (65)	35 (46)	48 (50)
1982 #	All	7	7	97	111
#(%)	Top	2 (29)	2 (29)	35 (36)	39 (35)
1983 #	All	5	3	86	94
#(%)	Top	1 (20)	--	25 (36)	26 (26)
1984 #	All	2	15	125	142
#(%)	Top	--	8 (53)	54 (43)	62 (44)
1985 #	All	5	17	78	98
#(%)	Top	1 (20)	6 (35)	39 (50)	46 (46)
1986 #	All	2	18	78	98
#(%)	Top	2 (100)	11 (61)	48 (63)	62 (62)
1987 #	All	2	10	57	69
#(%)	Top	1 (50)	4 (30)	31 (54)	36 (62)
1988 #	All	5	7	54	66
#(%)	Top	3 (60)	2 (29)	25 (46)	30 (45)
Total: #	All	31	94	651	776
Total: #(%)	TOP	12(39)	44(45)	292(45)	348(45)

U.S. Senate Special Committee on Aging, July 1989.

Individual Drug Manufacturer Track Record: Number of Therapeutic Breakthroughs Between 1981-1988

Company	A (%)	B (%)	C (%)	Total
1. Abbott.....	1 (1)	4 (4)	103 (95)	108
2. Bristol....	3 (60)	2 (20)	5 (50)	10
3. Ciba-Geigy.	1 (8)	2 (15)	10 (77)	13
4. Glaxo......	-	3 (14)	18 (86)	21
5. Lederle....	-	1 (14)	6 (86)	7
6. Lilly......	-	4 (20)	6 (80)	10
7. Mead.......	-	-	1 (100)	1
8. Merck......	3 (11)	6 (21)	19 (68)	28
9. Merrell....	-	2 (50)	2 (50)	4
10. Pfizer.....	-	1 (13)	7 (88)	8
11. Roche......	1 (7)	5 (33)	9 (60)	15
12. Robins.....	-	1 (17)	5 (83)	6
13. Roering....	-	-	2 (100)	2
14. Rorer......	-	1 (100)	-	1
15. Ross.......	-	-	-	-
16. Schering...	1 (3)	3 (10)	25 (86)	29
17. Searle.....	-	-	8 (100)	8
18. Smithkline.	-	2 (40)	3 (60)	5
19. Squibb.....	-	3 (15)	17 (85)	20
20. Syntex.....	-	2 (20)	8 (80)	10
Total......	10 (3)	42 (13)	264 (84)	316

U.S. Senate Special Committee on Aging, July 1989.

Average Development Time: New Molecular Entities First Approved Abroad 1987

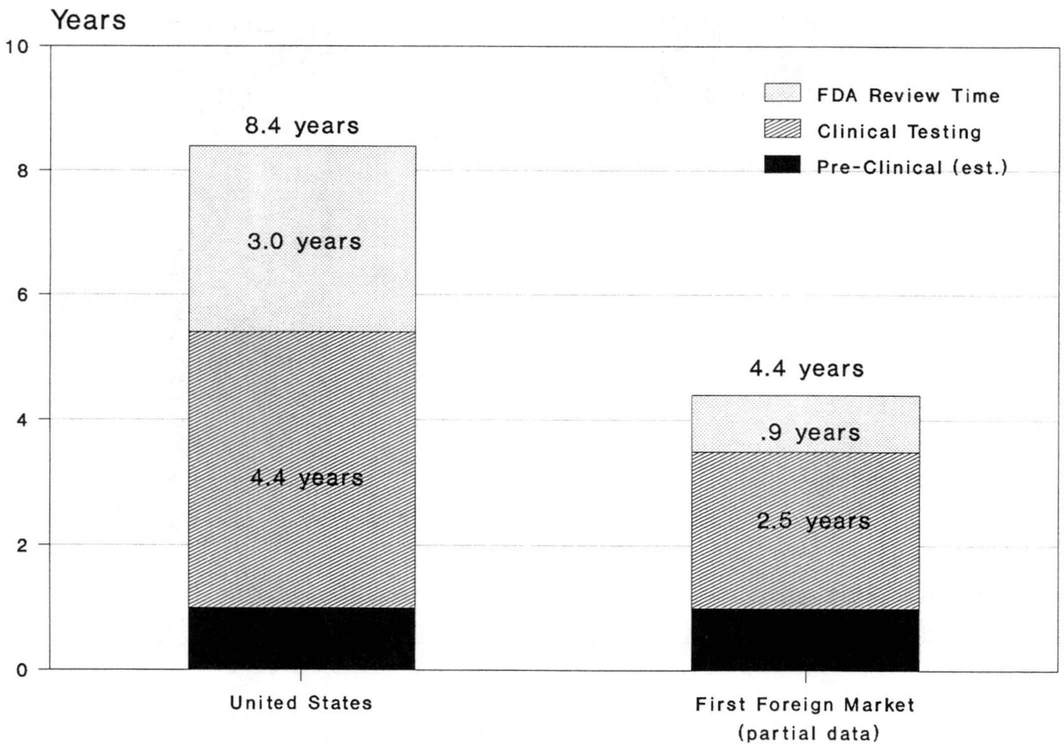

Source: PMA Survey , 1987.

New Molecular Entities Marketed Abroad Prior to U.S. Approval

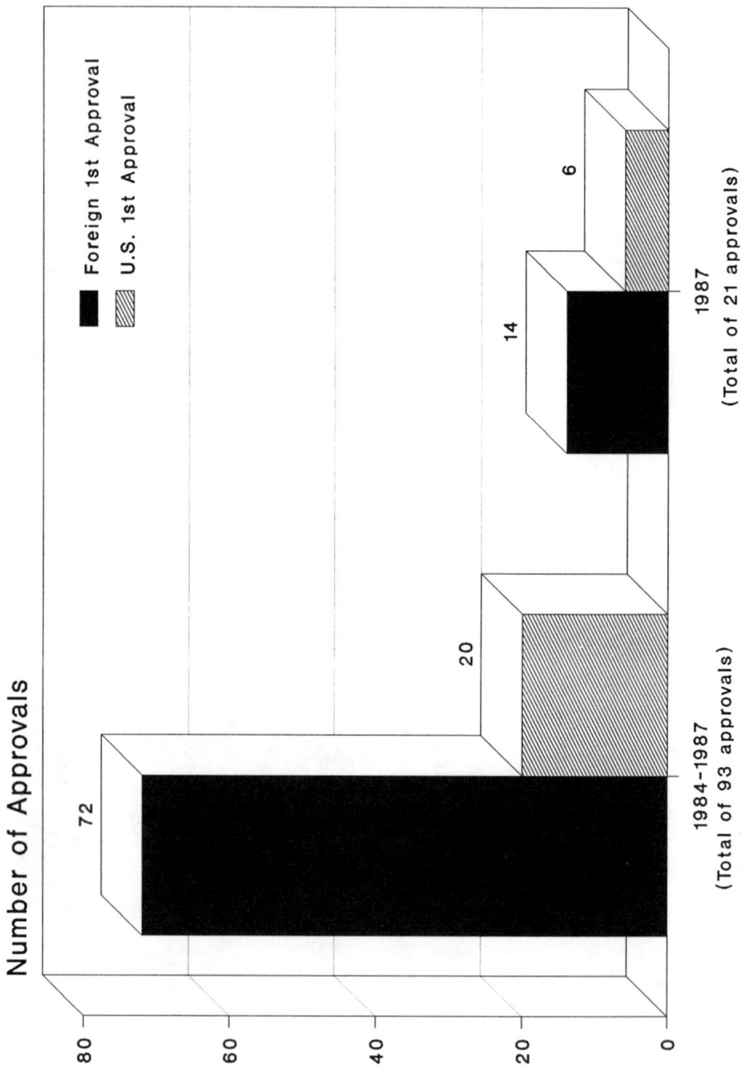

Source: PMA Survey, 1987.

Number of New Drug Applications (NDA) an
New Molecular Entities (NME) Approved
1975-1987

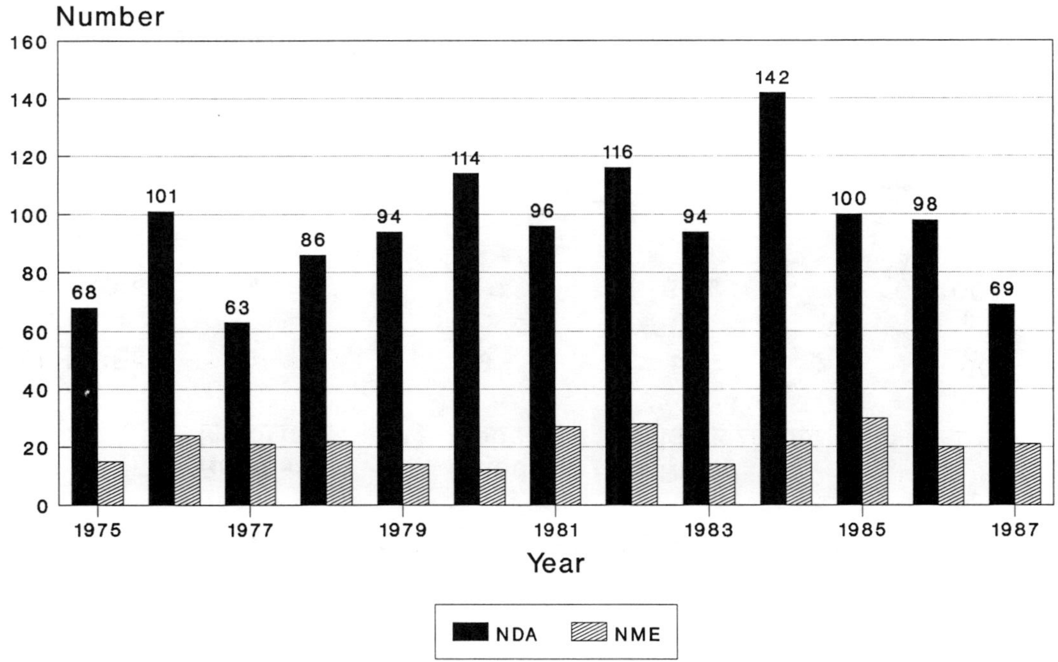

Source: Pharmacoepidemiology
(An Introduction), 1987.

New Molecular Entities (NMEs) Introduced by 25 Largest U.S. Rx Drug Manufacturers, 1981-1988

	Potential Contribution to Existing Therapies			
	Rated-Important	Rated-Modest	Rated-Little/None	Total
Number of NMEs	7	29	54	90
Percent of NMEs	8%	32%	60%	100%

(Source: FDA New Drug Evaluations Statistical Reports, Ratings of New Drugs by Therapeutic Potential.)

U.S. New Molecular Entity Approvals Per Year

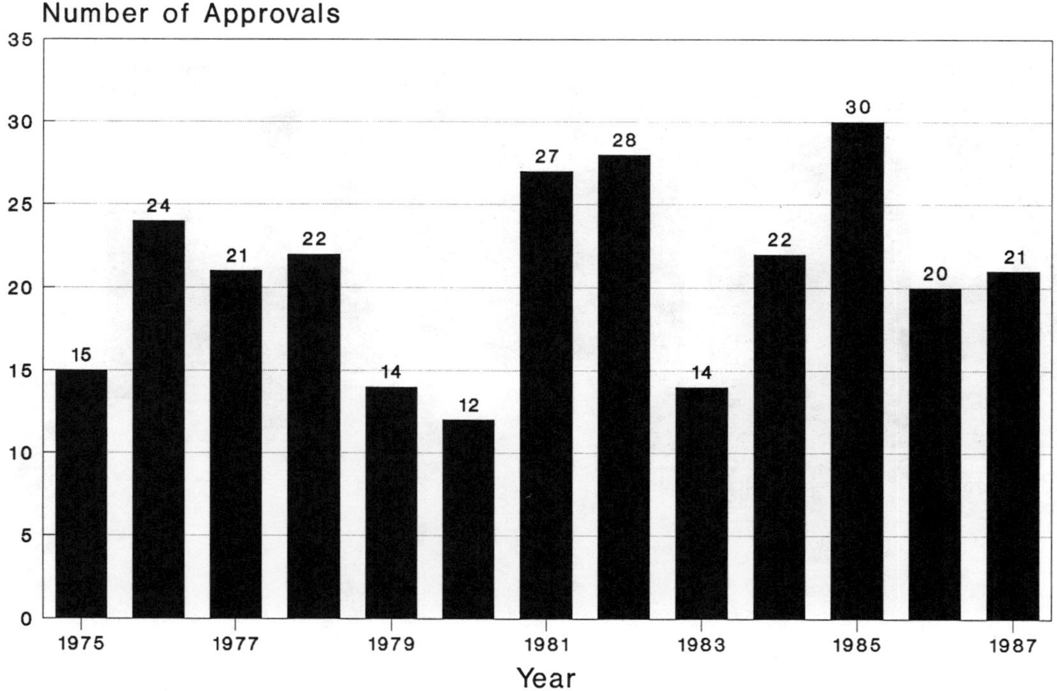

Source: U.S. Food and Drug Administration, 1987.

New Molecular Entity Backlog

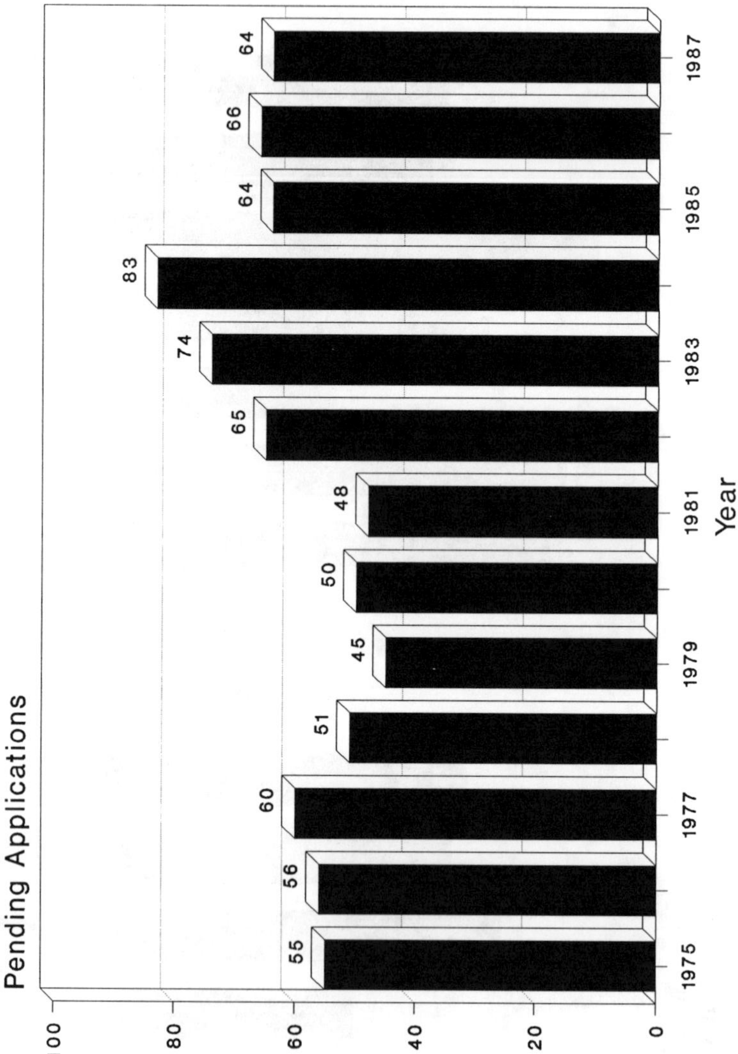

Source: U.S. Food and Drug Administration, 1987

New Single Entity Drug Introductions to U.S. Markets

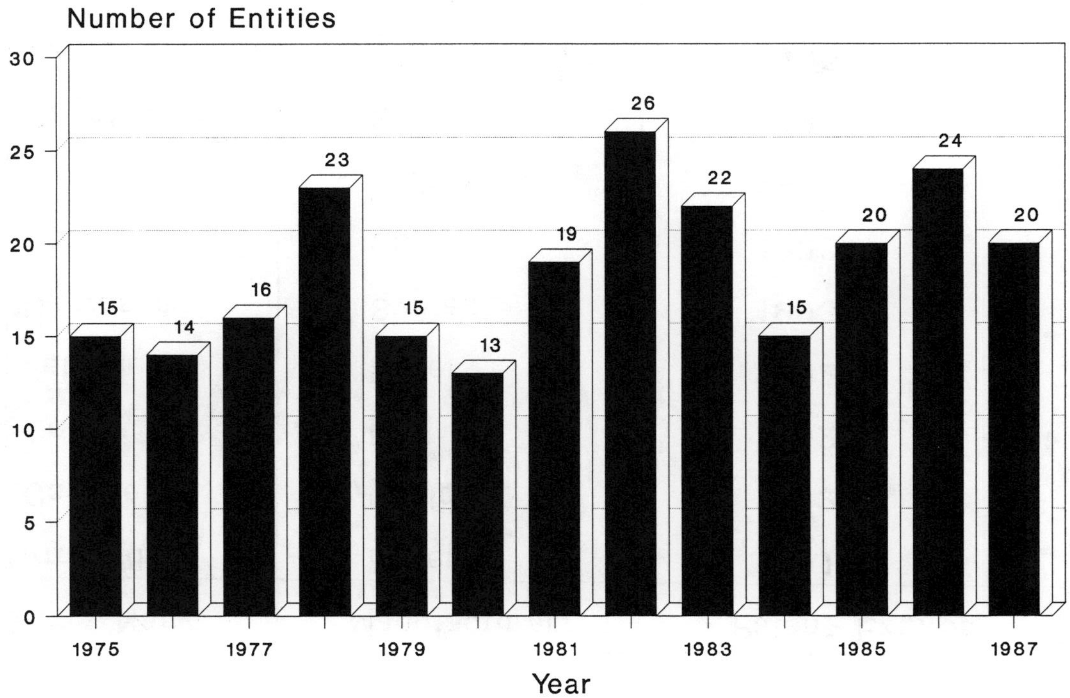

Source: PMA Analysis of Paul De Haen Data, 1987.

Patent Expirations on Prescription Drugs

Brand Name	Manufacturer	Patent Expires
Procardia	Pfizer	1991
Cardizem	Marion	1992
Ceclor	Lilly	1992
Feldene	Pfizer	1992
Naprosyn	Syntex	1993
Xanax	Upjohn	1993
Tagamet	SmithKline	1994
Capoten	Squibb	1995
Zantac	Glaxo	1995
Vasotec	Merck	2000

Source: David Saks, Wedbush Morgan Securities, 1989.

Total Value of Drug Imports and Exports 1980-1989

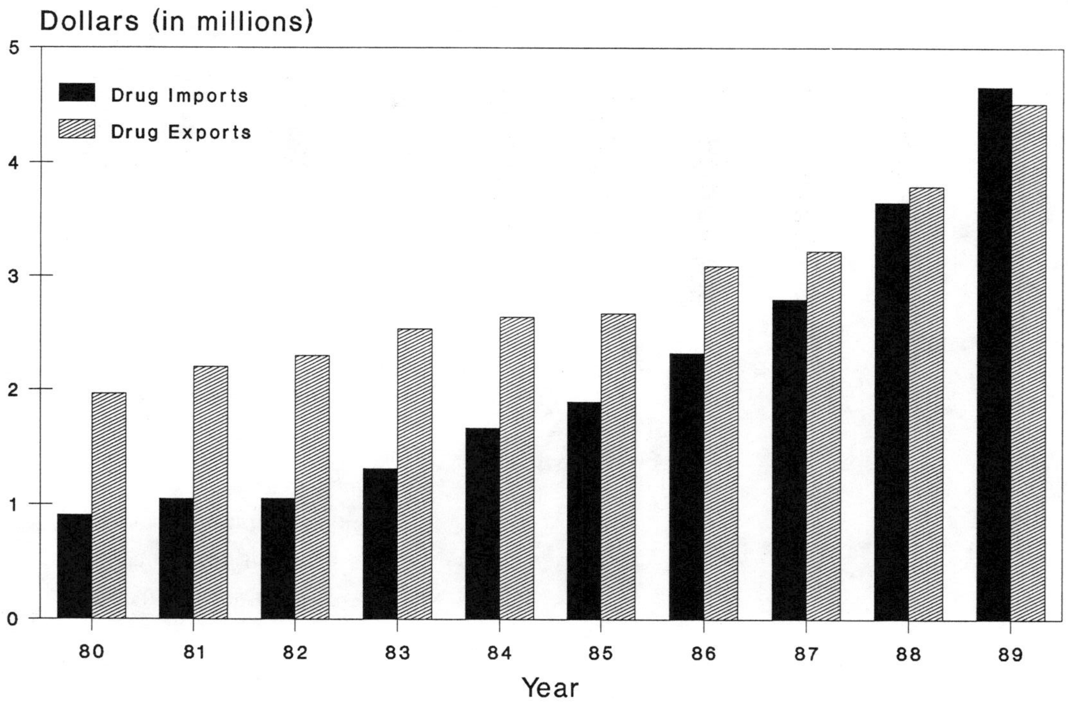

Source: U.S. Department of Commerce
1989 Industrial Outlook

Value of Drug Imports by Category 1980-1989

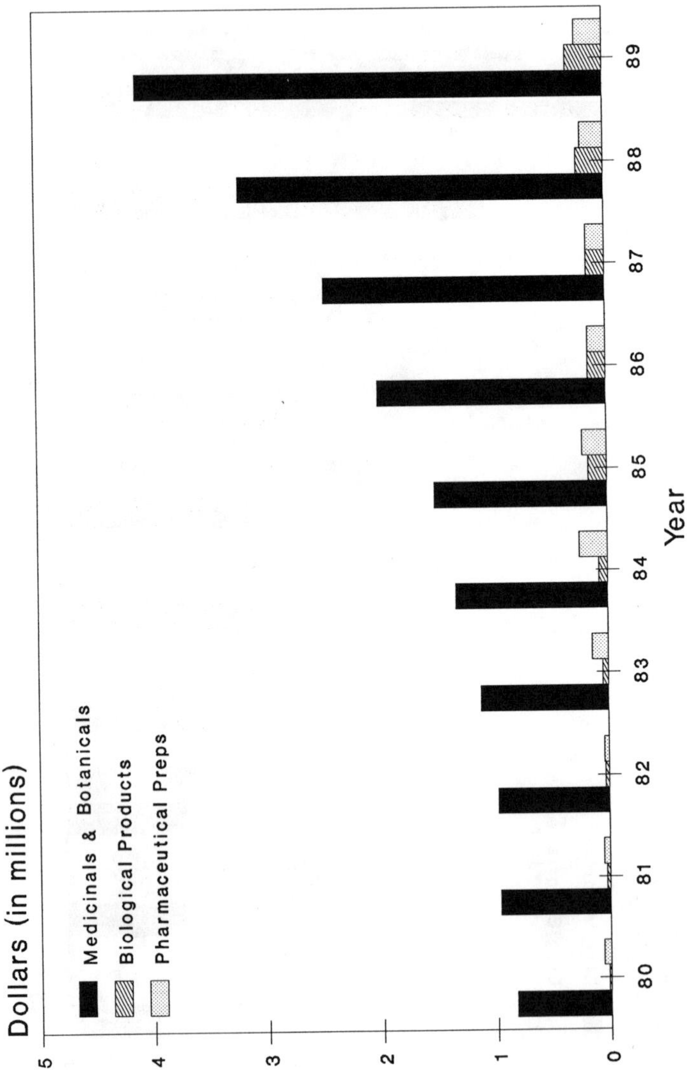

Source: U.S. Department of Commerce
1989 Industrial Outlook

Value of Drug Exports by Category 1980-1989

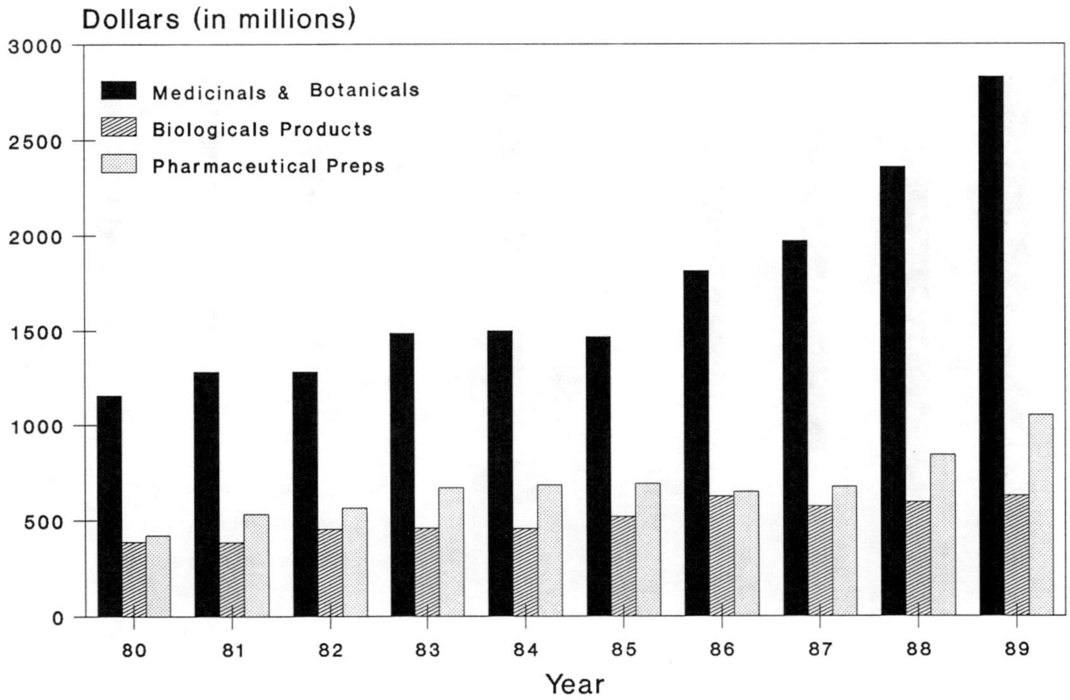

Source: U.S. Department of Commerce,
1989 Industrial Outlook

Pharmaceutical Imports as Percentage of Total Supply: 1977-1986
(by category)

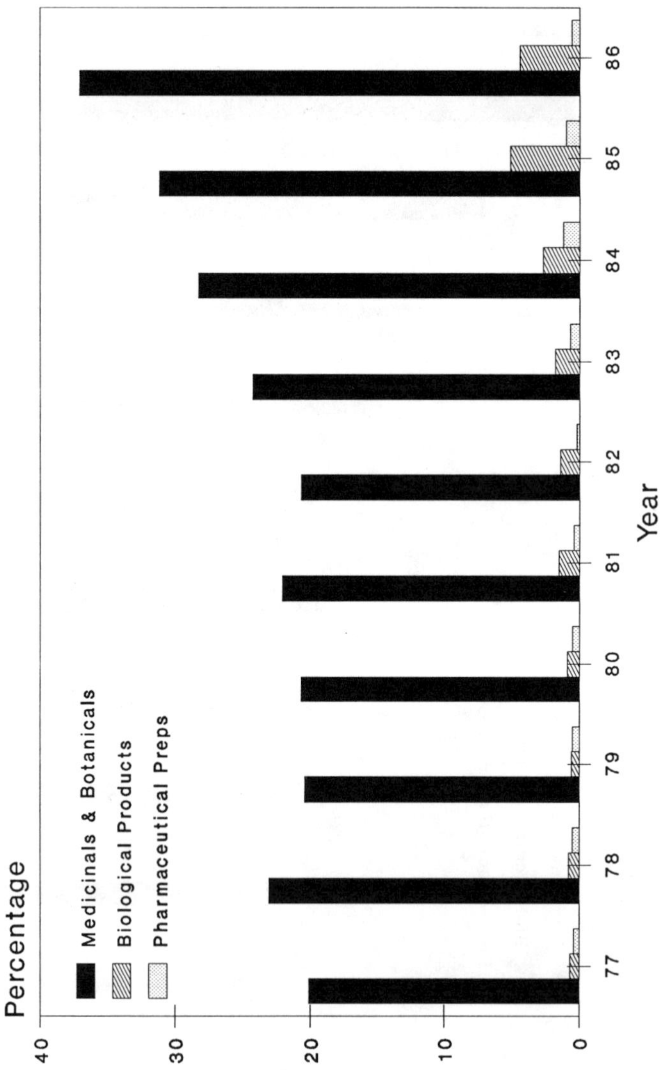

Source: U.S. Department of Commerce, 1989 Industrial Outlook

Exports as a Percent of Total Shipments (by category)

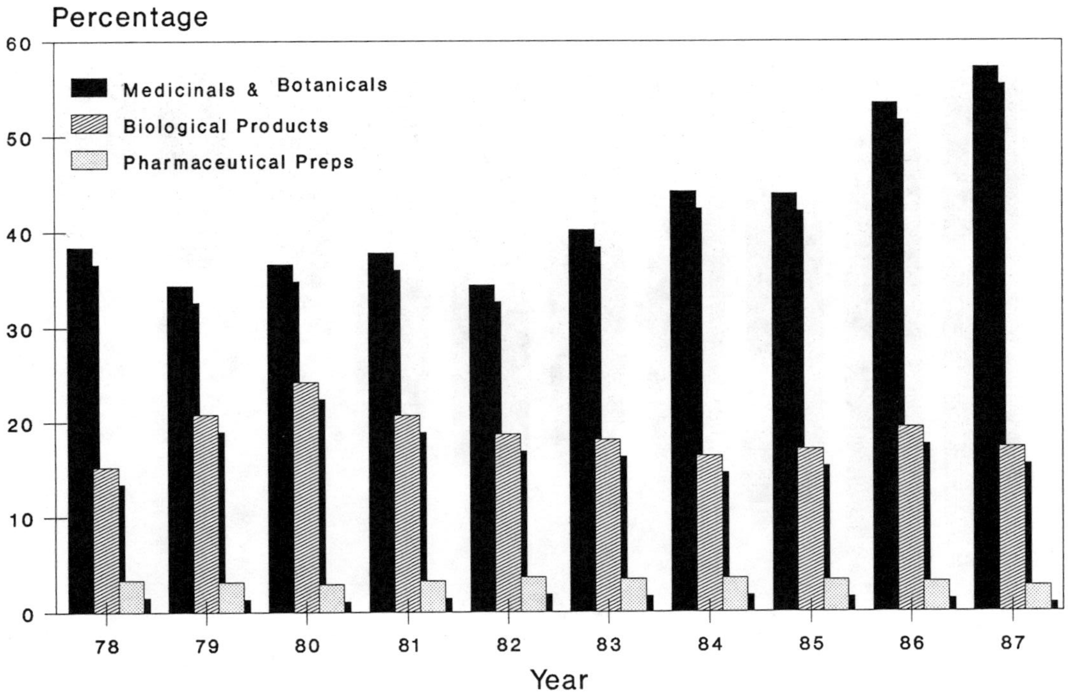

Source: U.S. Department of Commerce
1989 Industrial Outlook

Value of Biological Products Produced
1979-1988

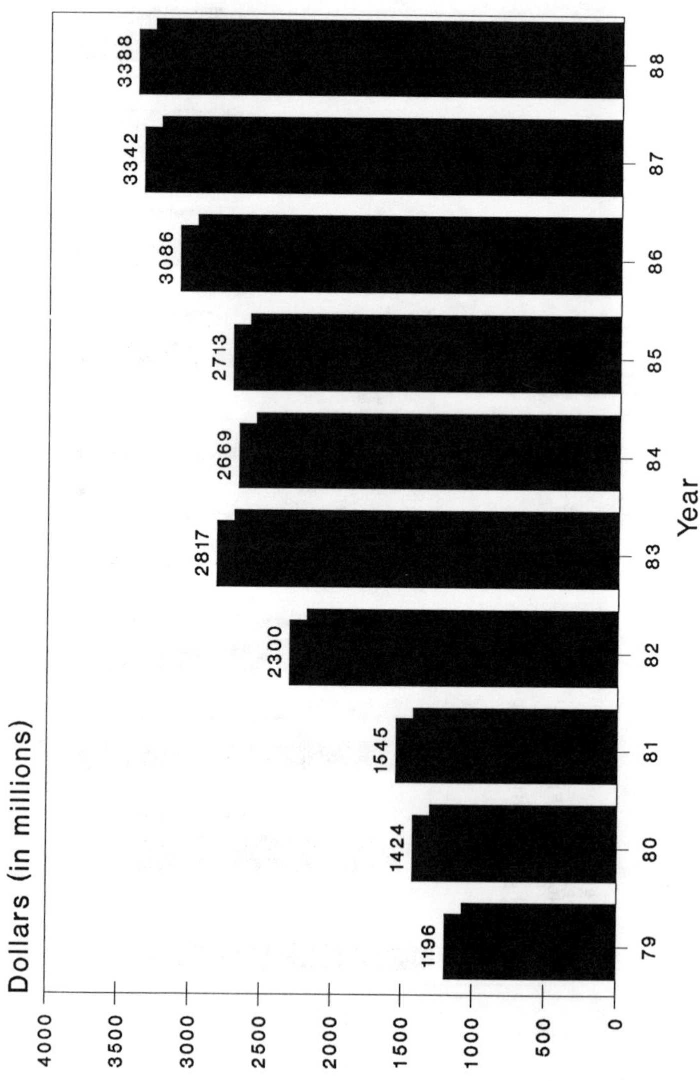

Source: U.S. Department of Commerce
1989 Industrial Outlook

Value of Medicinals and Botanicals Produced from 1979-1988

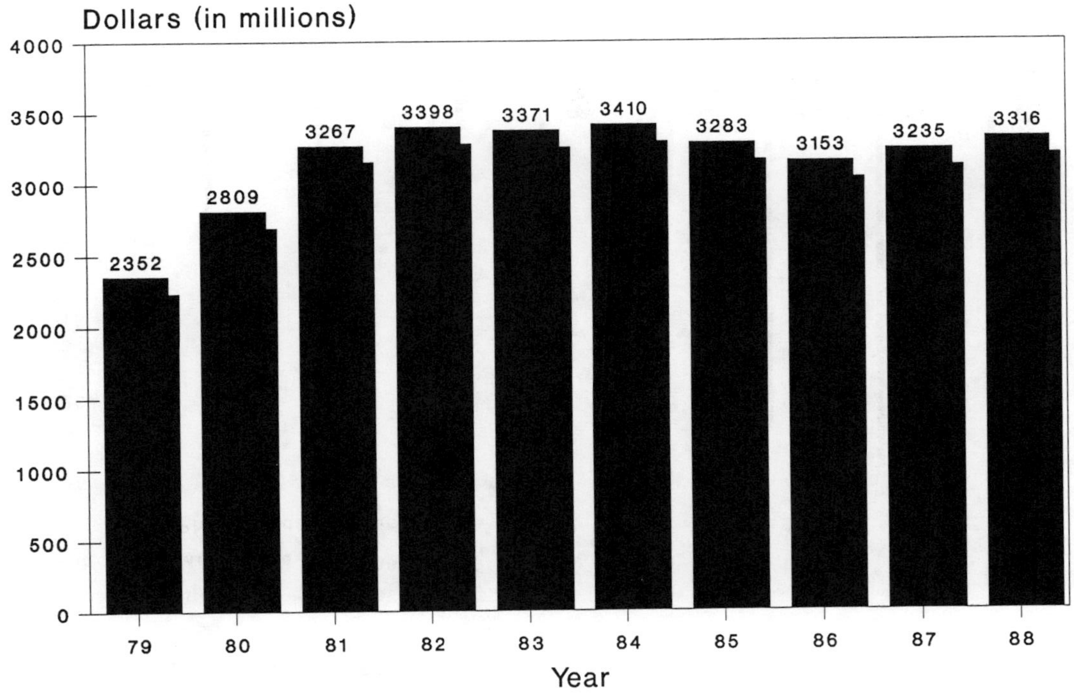

Source: U.S. Department of Commerce
1989 Industrial Outlook

Value of Shipments Sold by the Drugs Industry

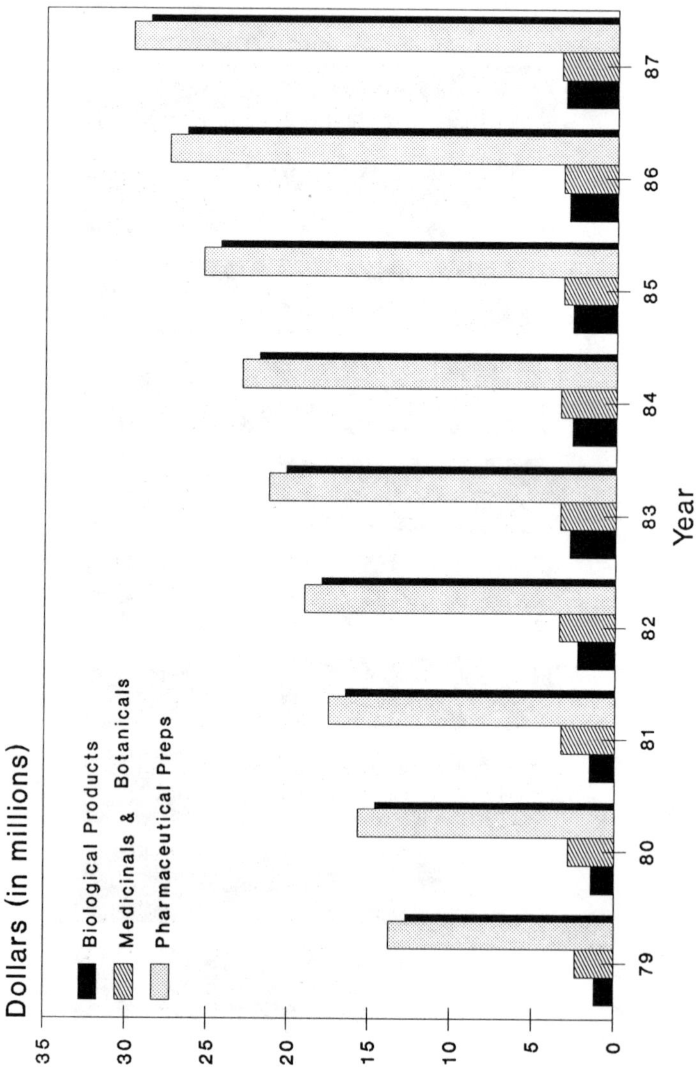

Source: U.S. Department of Commerce 1989 Industrial Outlook

Chapter 6

PHARMACEUTICAL

Provides information on the structure of the pharmaceutical distribution system, including pharmaceutical manufacturers, wholesalers and retail outlets.

U.S. and Foreign Pharmaceutical Sales: PMA Member Firms

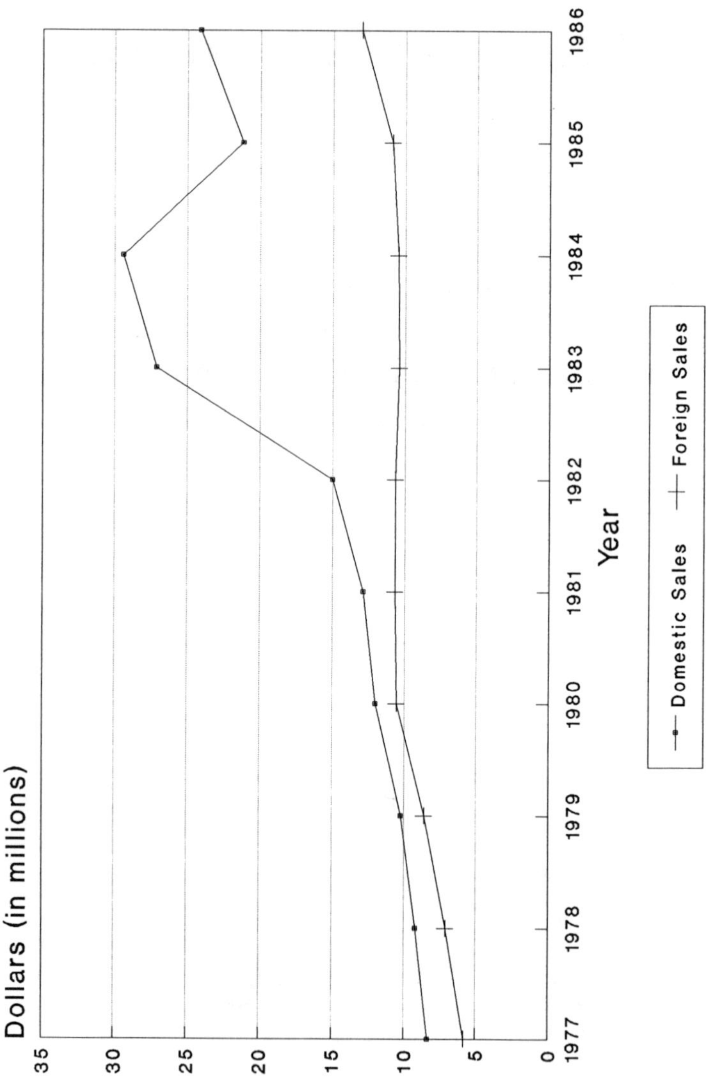

Source: PMA Annual Survey, August 1988.

Manufacturers' Domestic Sales of Ethical Drugs for Human Use by Product Class

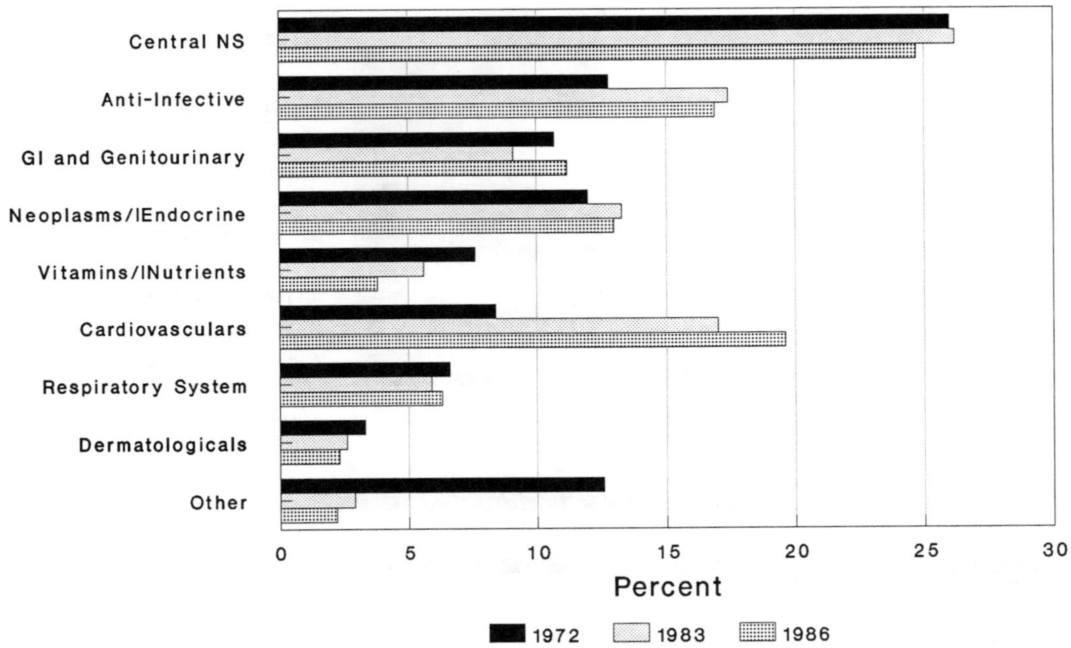

Source: PMA Annual Survey Report, 1988.

Foreign Sales of Ethical Drugs for Human Use by Product Class

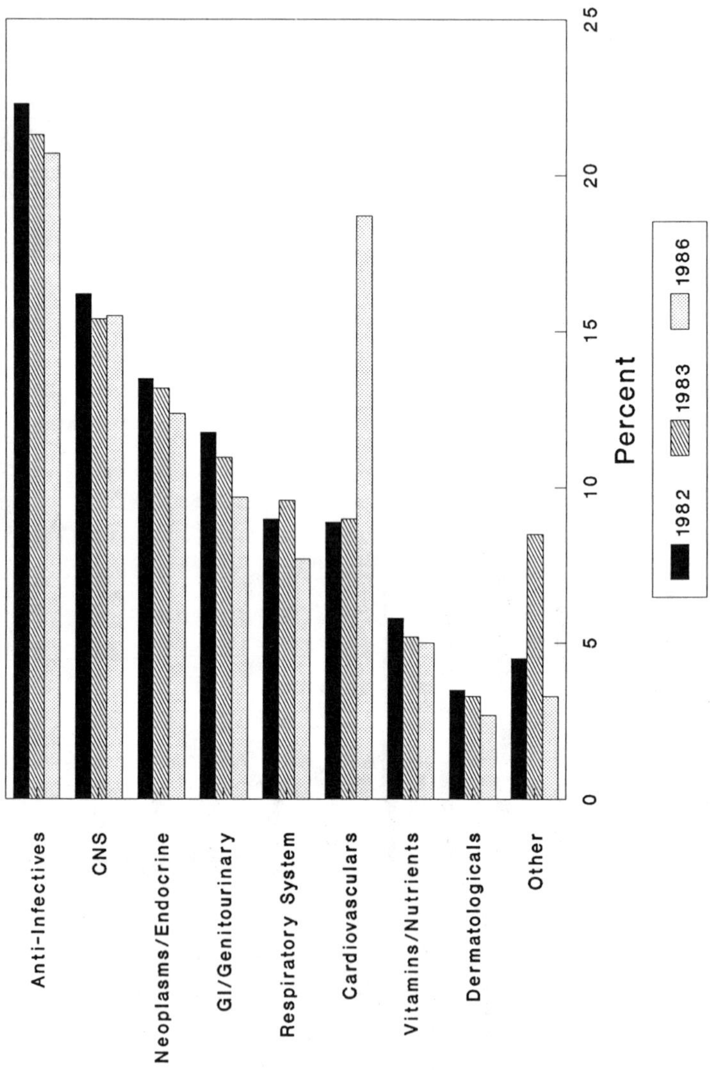

Source: PMA Annual Survey, 1988.

Foreign Sales of Ethical Pharmaceuticals by U.S.- Owned PMA Member Firms

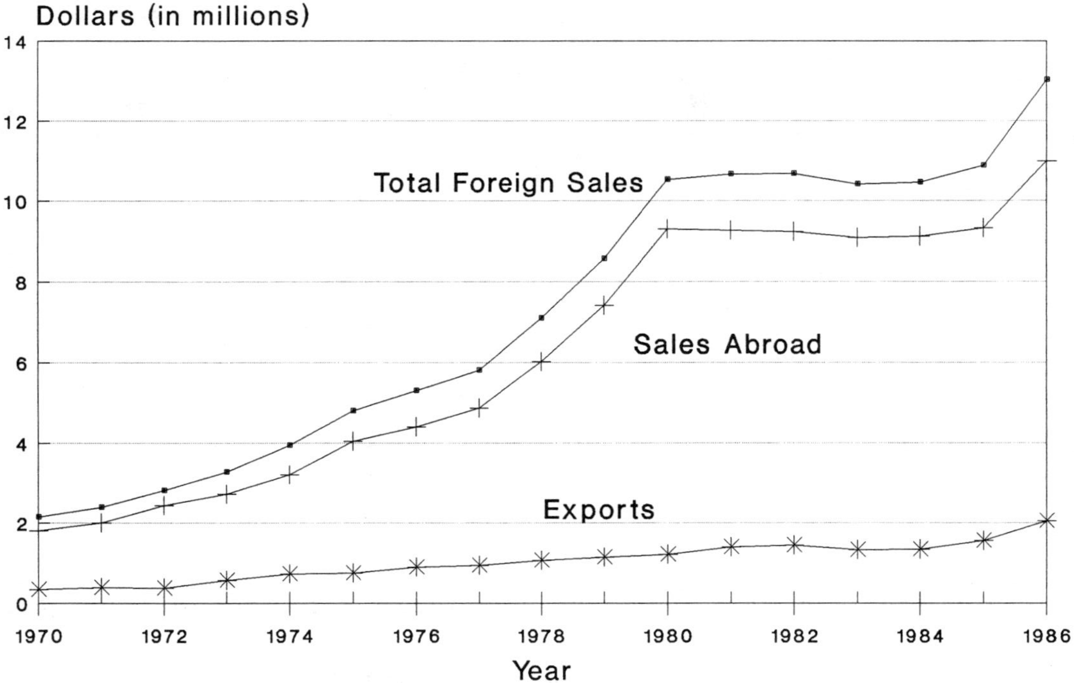

Source: PMA Annual Survey, various years.

Relative Profitability Trends as Measured by After-Tax Return on Net Worth, 1980-1988

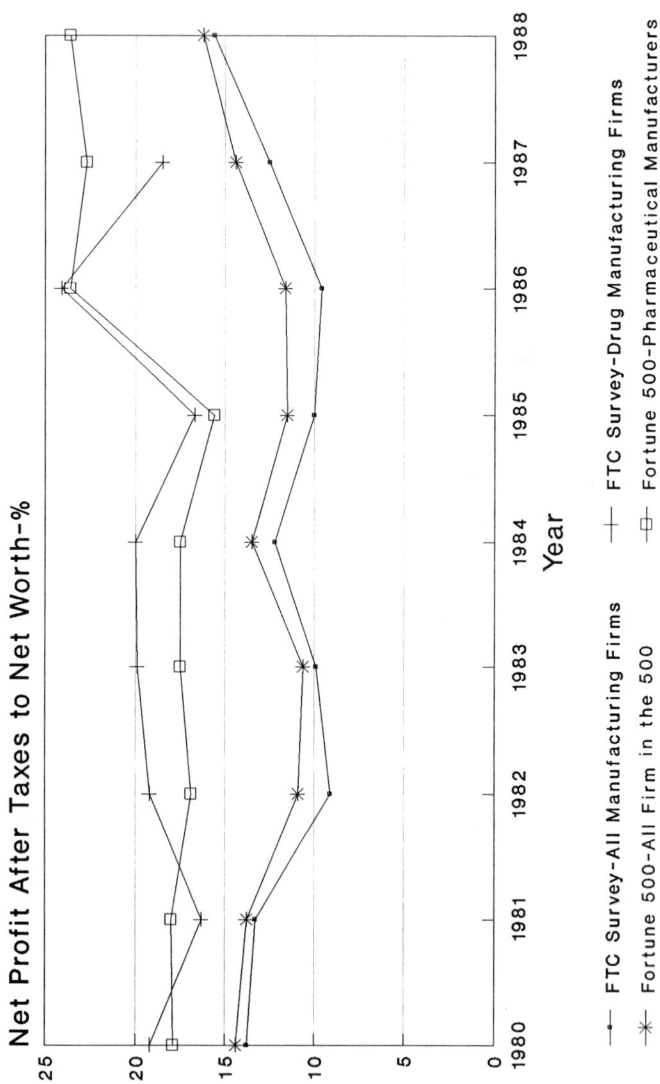

Source: FTC Survey and Fortune 500

Biotech Firms: Product Plans

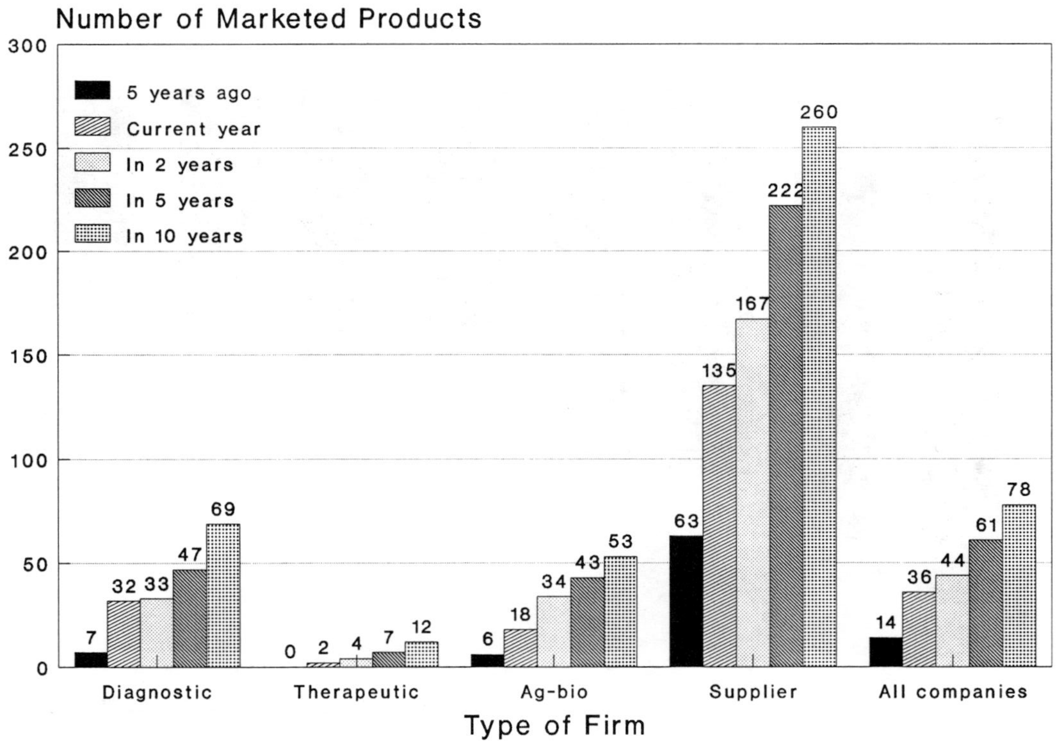

Source: Technology Statistics,
The Wall Street Journal, November 1989.

Estimated Total Wholesale Industry Sales Growth, 1981-1988

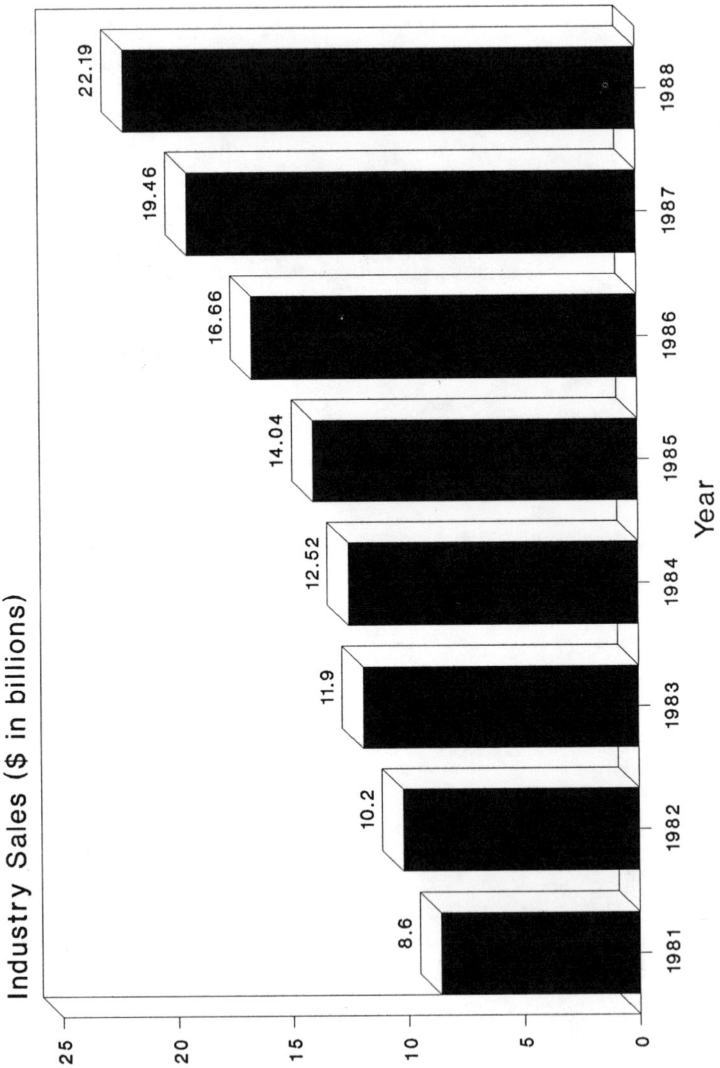

Source: NWDA Operating Survey, 1988

Expense Trends for Wholesalers 1981-1988

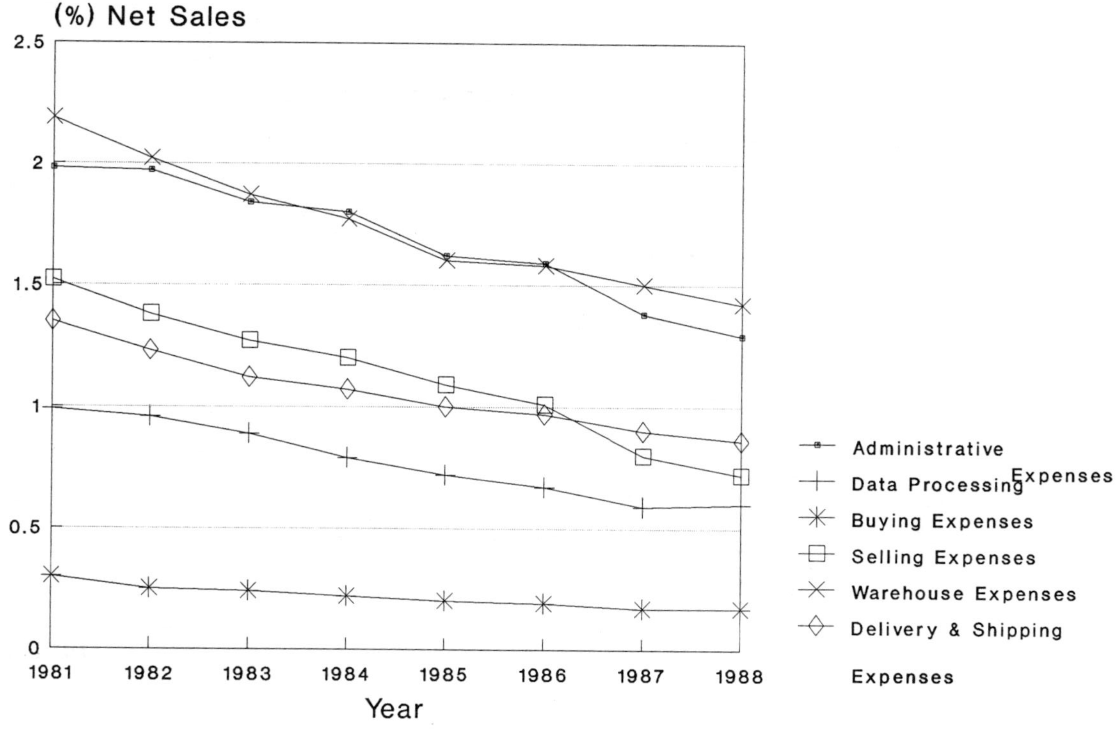

Source: NWDA Operating Survey, 1988

Wholesalers Gross Margin and Operating Expense Trends, 1982-1988

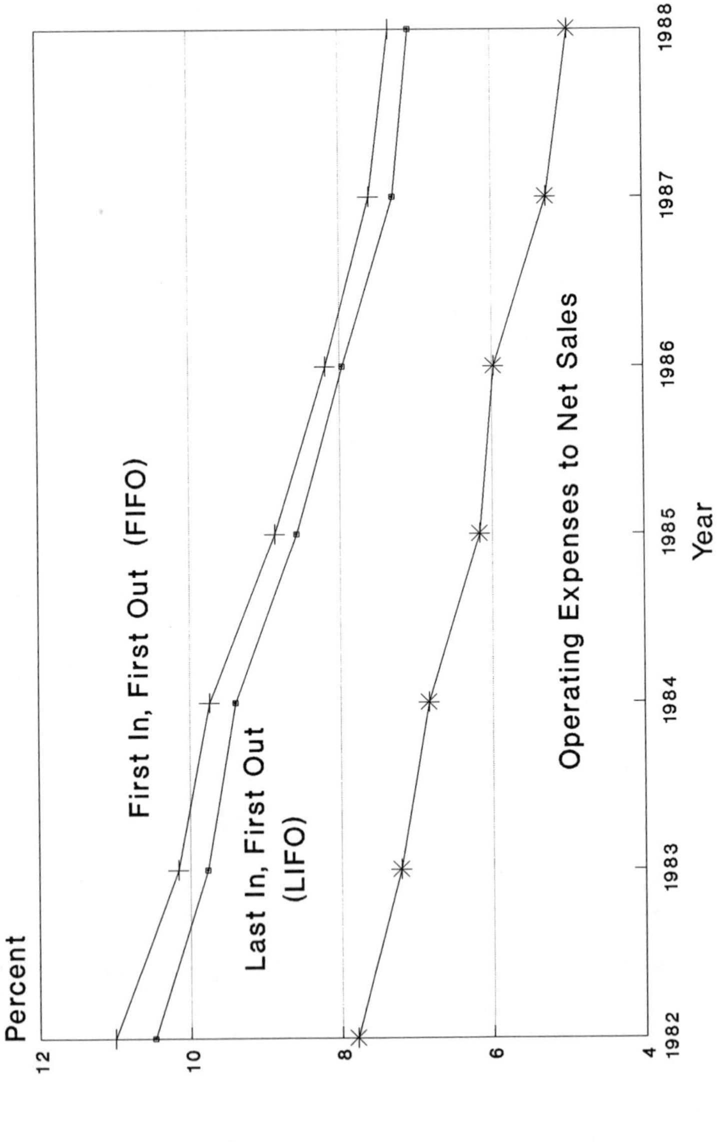

Source: NWDA Operating Survey, 1988

Percentage Net Profit Margin Trend for Pharmaceutical Wholesalers

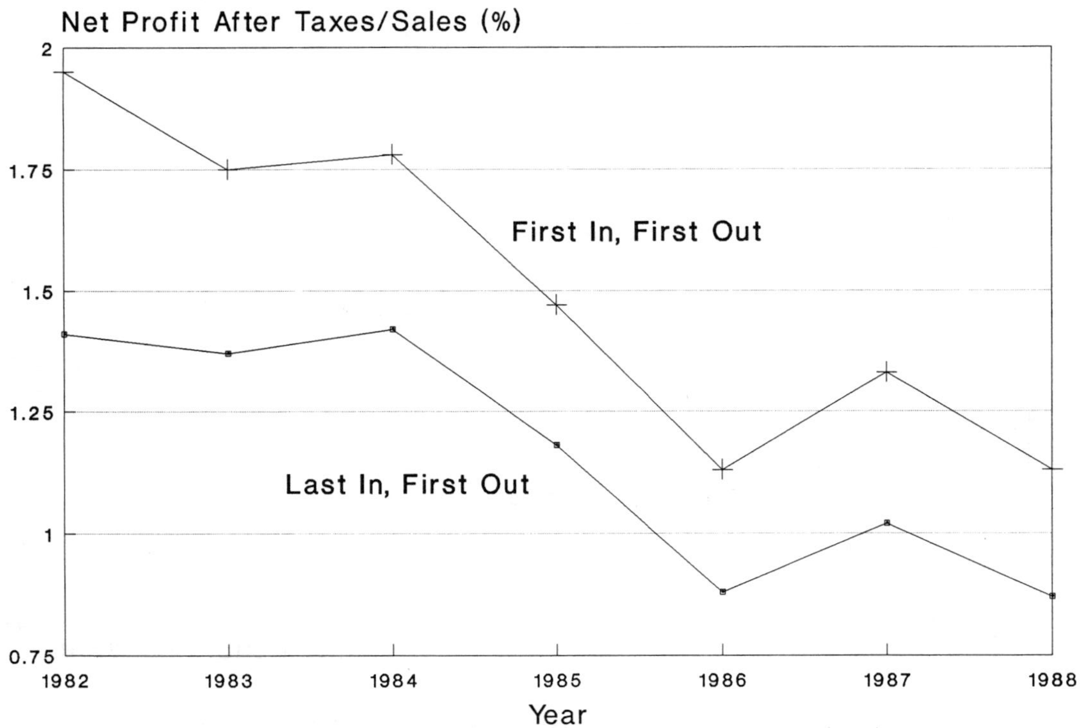

Source: NWDA Operating Survey, 1988

Operating Profit Margin Trend for Pharmaceutical Wholesalers, 1982-1988

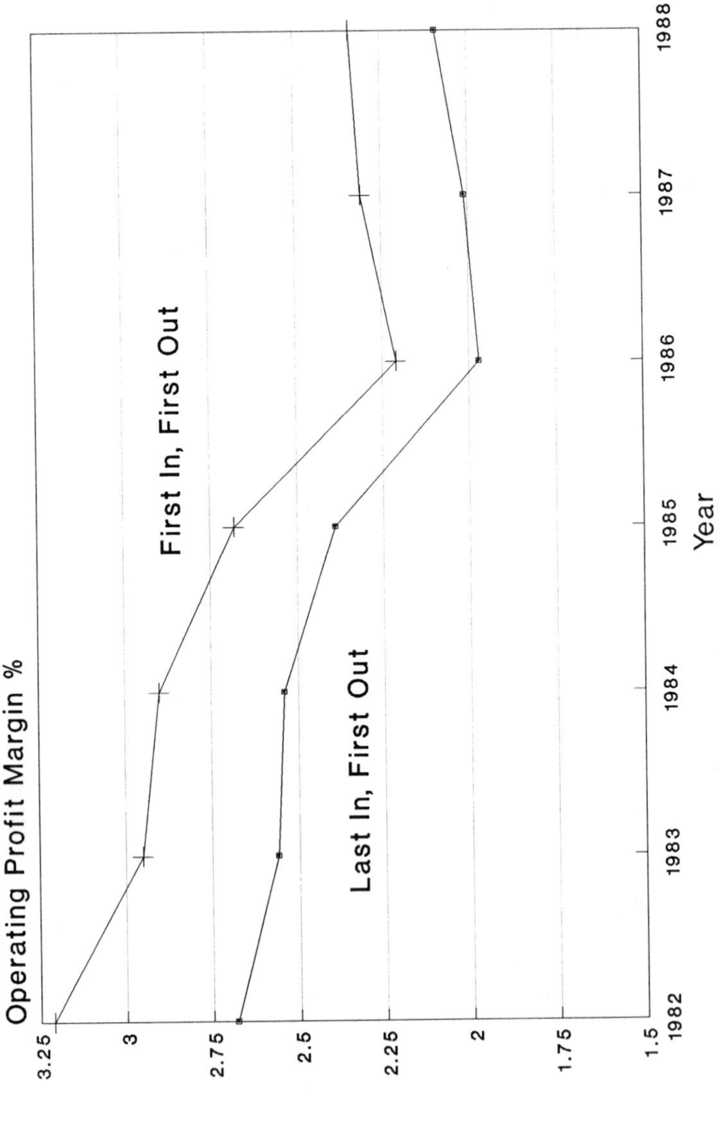

Source: NWDA Operating Survey, 1988

Return on Net Worth Trend for National Wholesale Druggists' Association Firms: 1981-1988

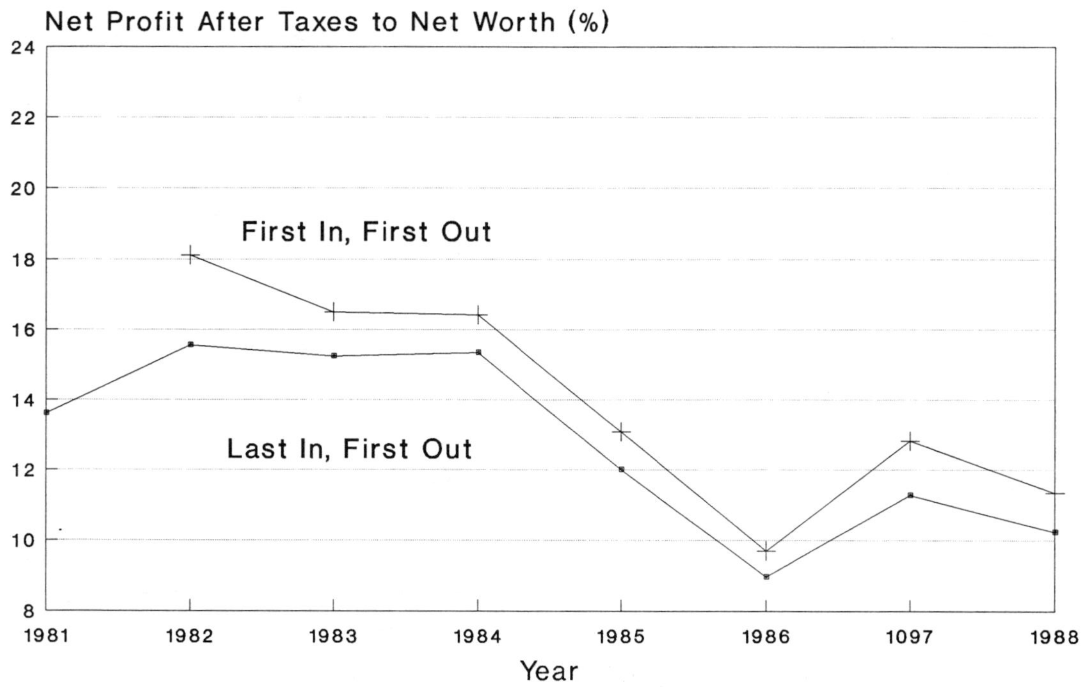

Source: NWDA Operating Survey, 1988

Financial Leverage Trend for Wholesalers
Total Assets to Net Worth, 1981-1988

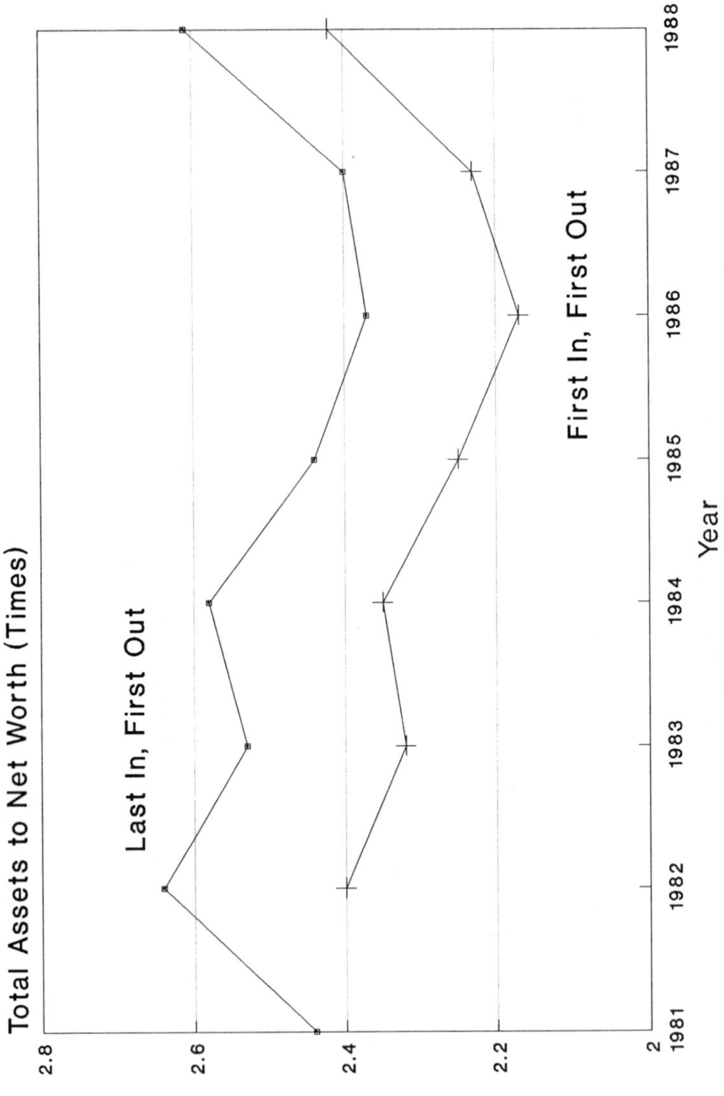

Source: NWDA Operating Survey, 1988

Total Operating Expenses as a Percent of Gross Profit for Pharmaceutical Wholesalers, 1981-1988

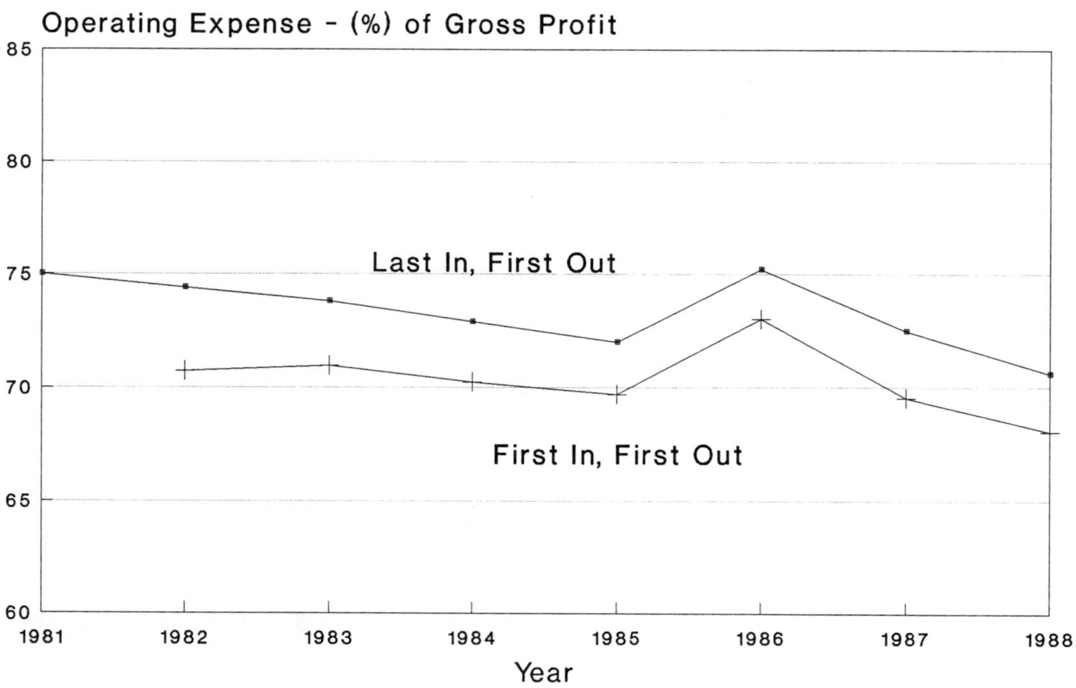

Source: NWDA Operating Survey, 1988

Total Asset Turnover Trend for Wholesalers, 1981-1988

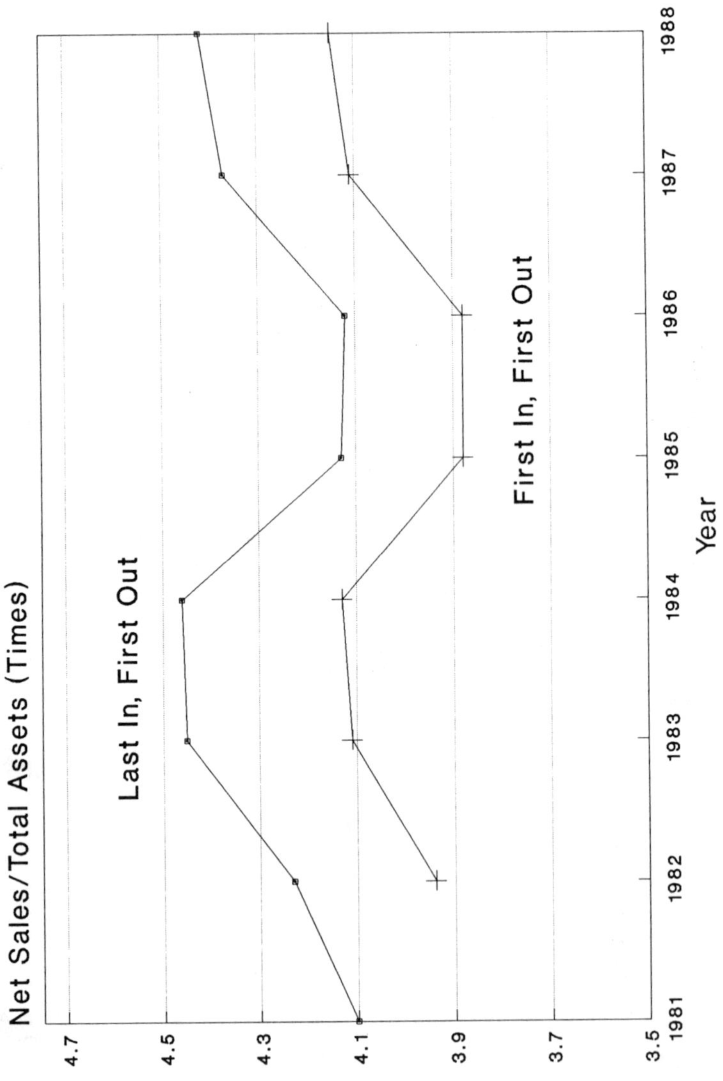

Source: NWDA Operating Survey, 1988

Return on Total Assets for All National Wholesale Druggists' Association Firms, 1981-1988

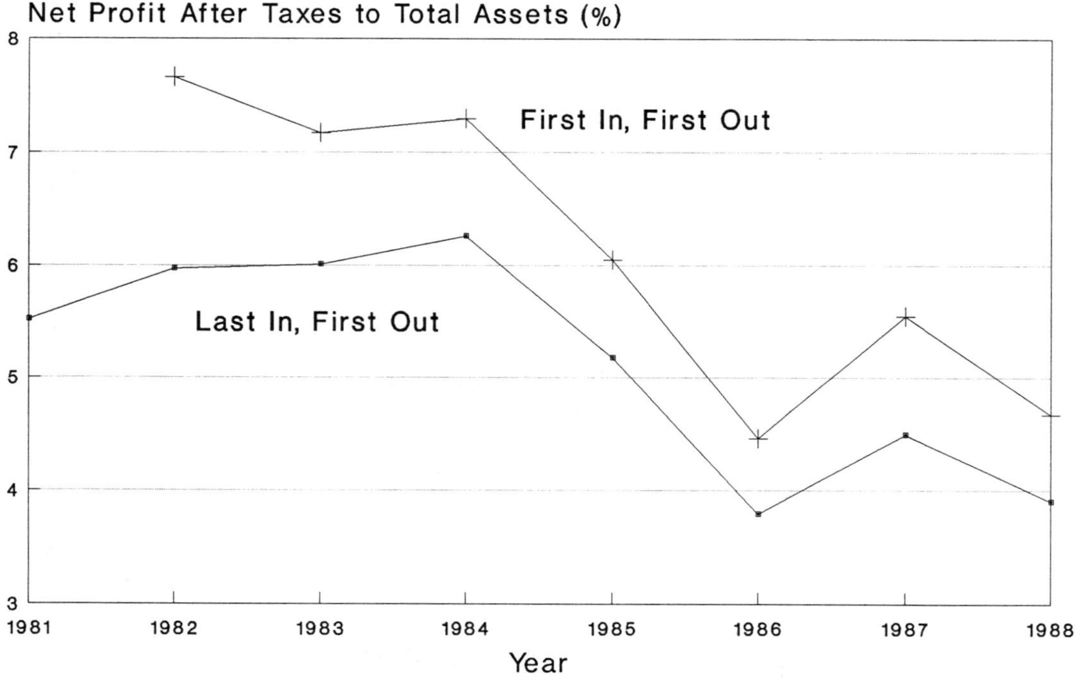

Source: NWDA Operating Survey, 1988

Average Collection Period and Average Days' Sales in Inventory Trends for Wholesalers, 1980-1988

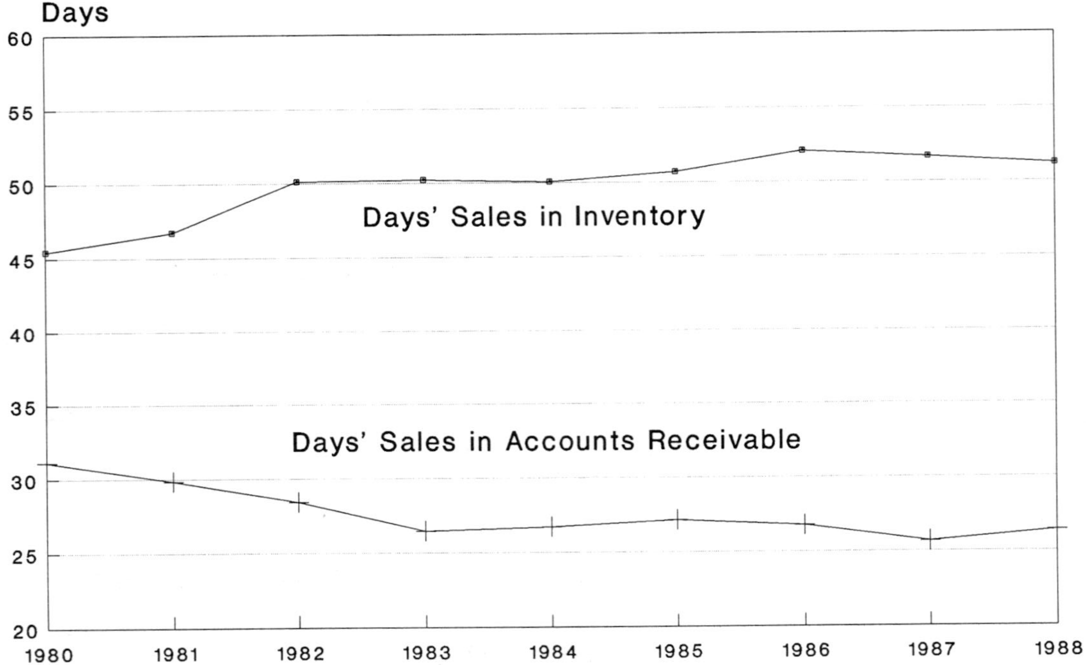

Source: NWDA Operating Survey, 1988

Pharmaceutical Wholesalers: Customer Sales Mix

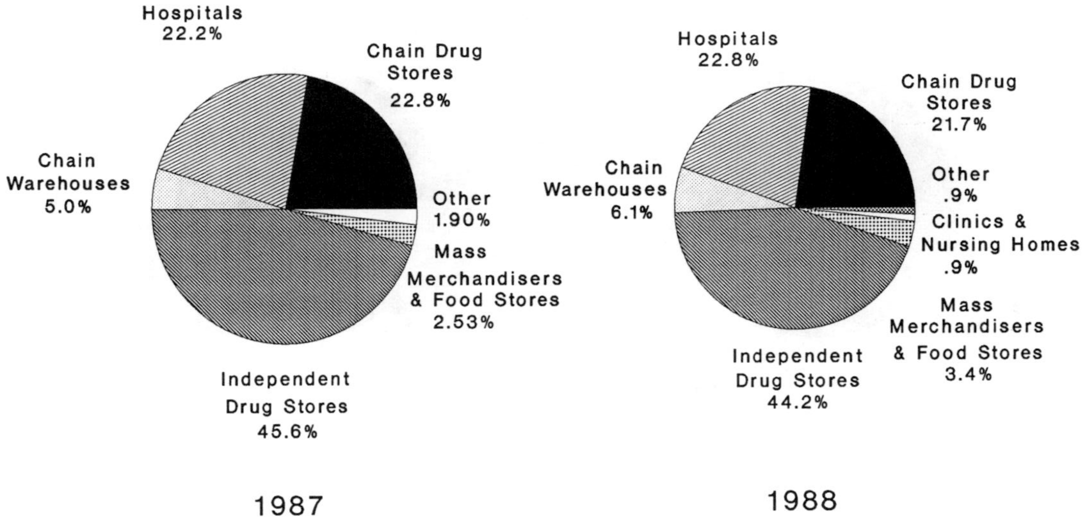

Source: NWDA Operating Survey, 1988

Pharmaceutical Wholesalers: Product Sales Mix

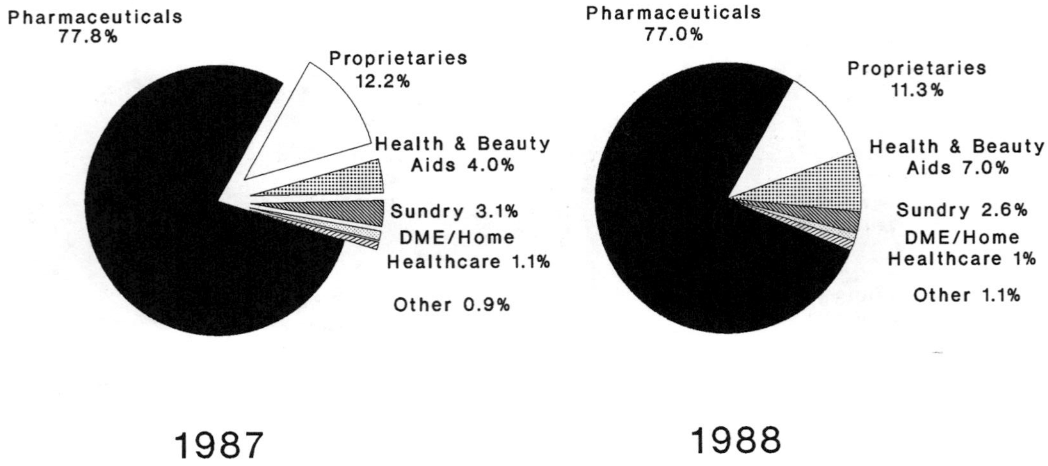

Source: NWDA Operating Survey, 1988

U.S. Retail Prescription Drug Sales 1976-1987

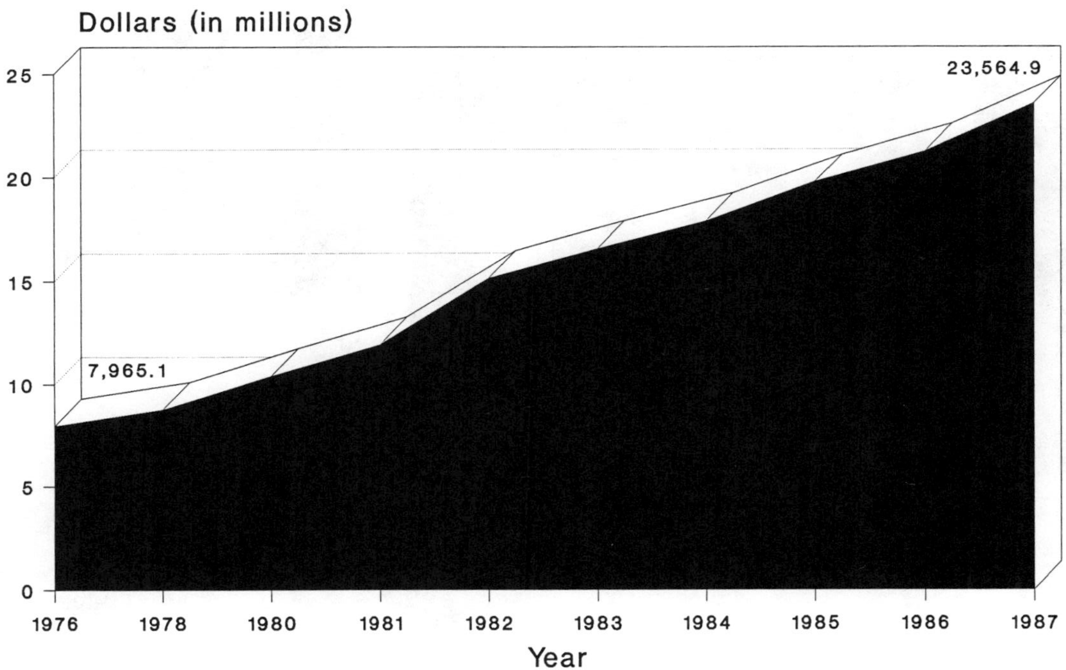

Source: American Druggist, 1979, 1982, 1983, 1984, 1985, 1986, 1987 and 1988.

Retail Sales Figures for Chain Drug Stores

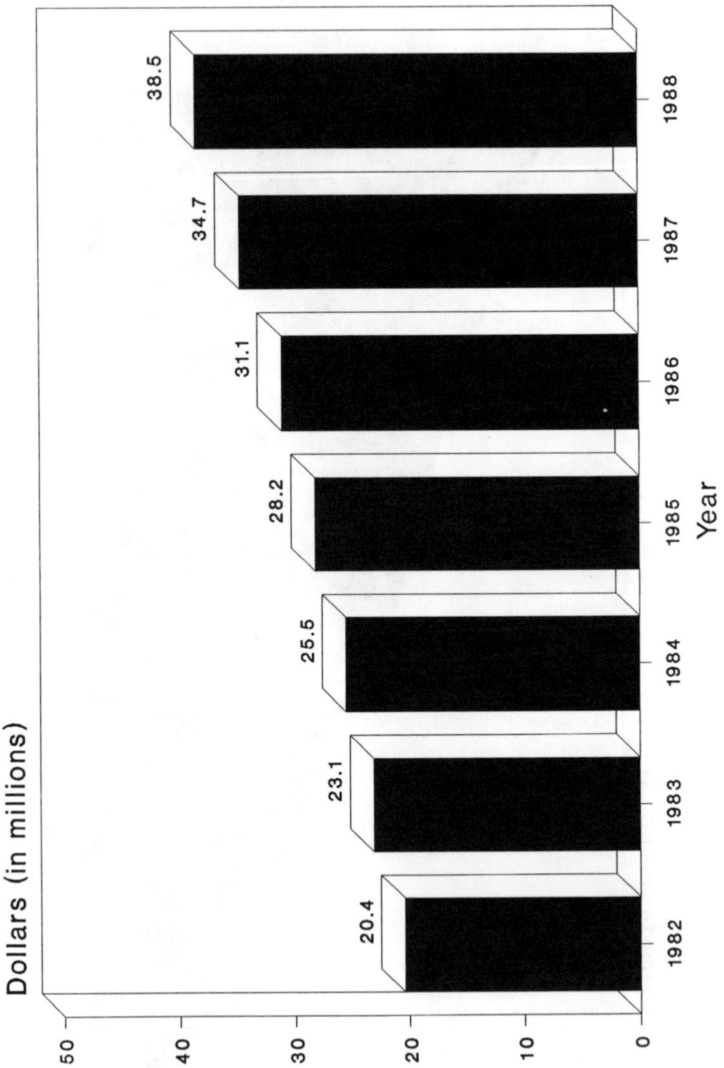

Source: NACDS Annual Report 1988

Top 10 American Drug Chains:
1988 Store Totals

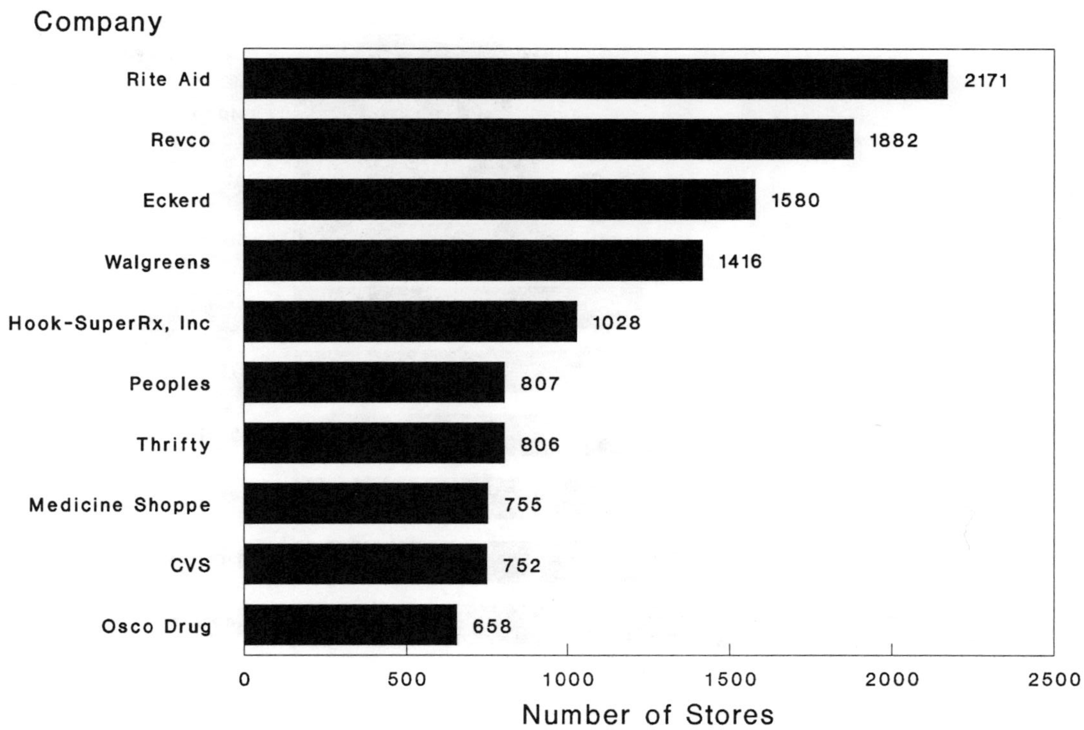

Source: Drug Store News, May 1, 1989

Top 10 American Drug Chains: 1988 Dollar Volume

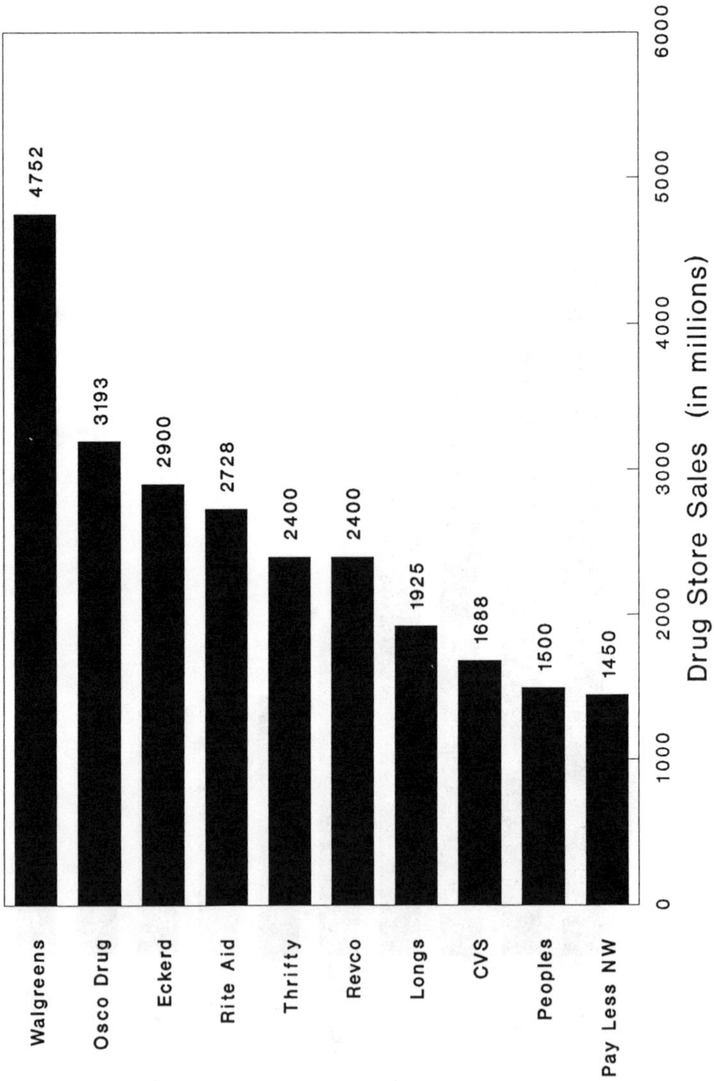

Source: Drug Store News, May 1, 1989

1988 Drug Chains:
Sales per Average Store

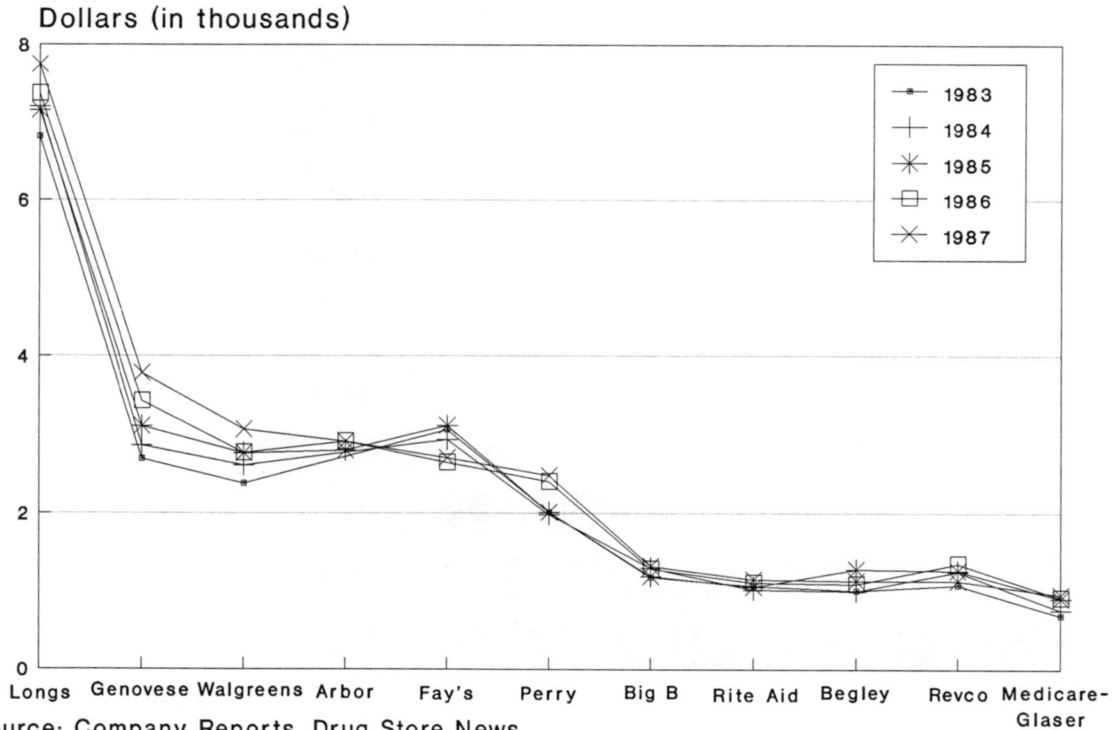

Source: Company Reports, Drug Store News
April 11, 1988.

Top Deep Discounters

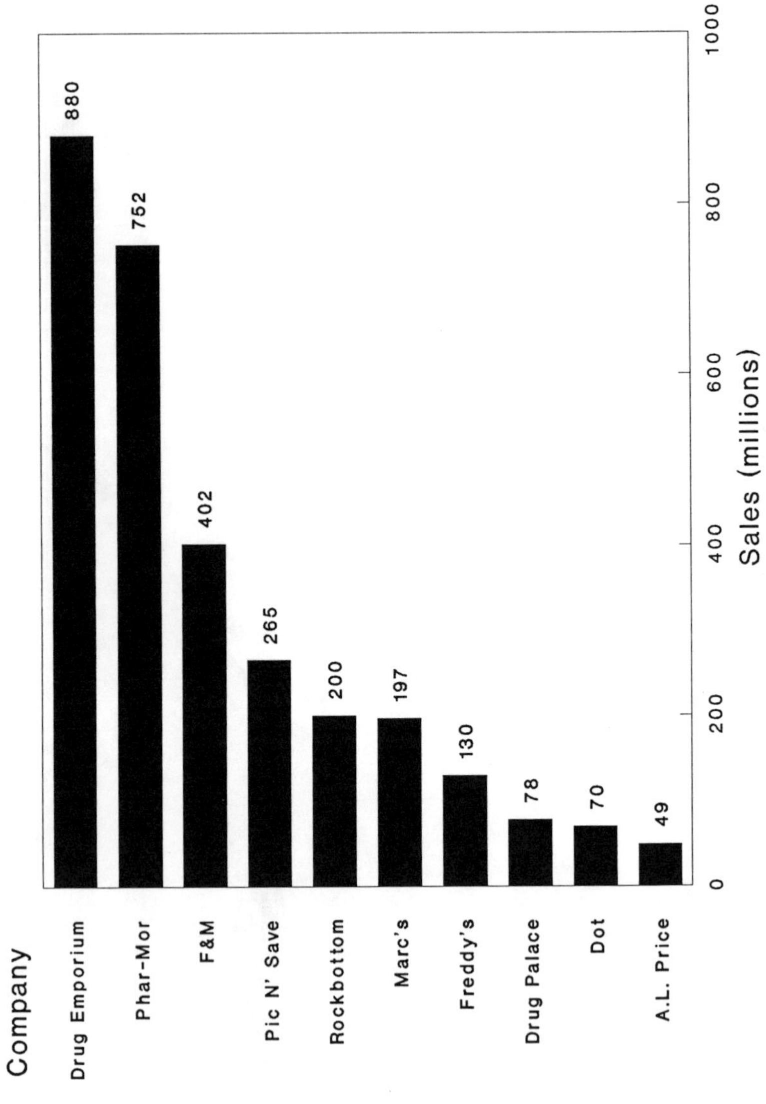

Source: Drug Store News, May 1, 1989

1988 Drug Chains: Growth in Units

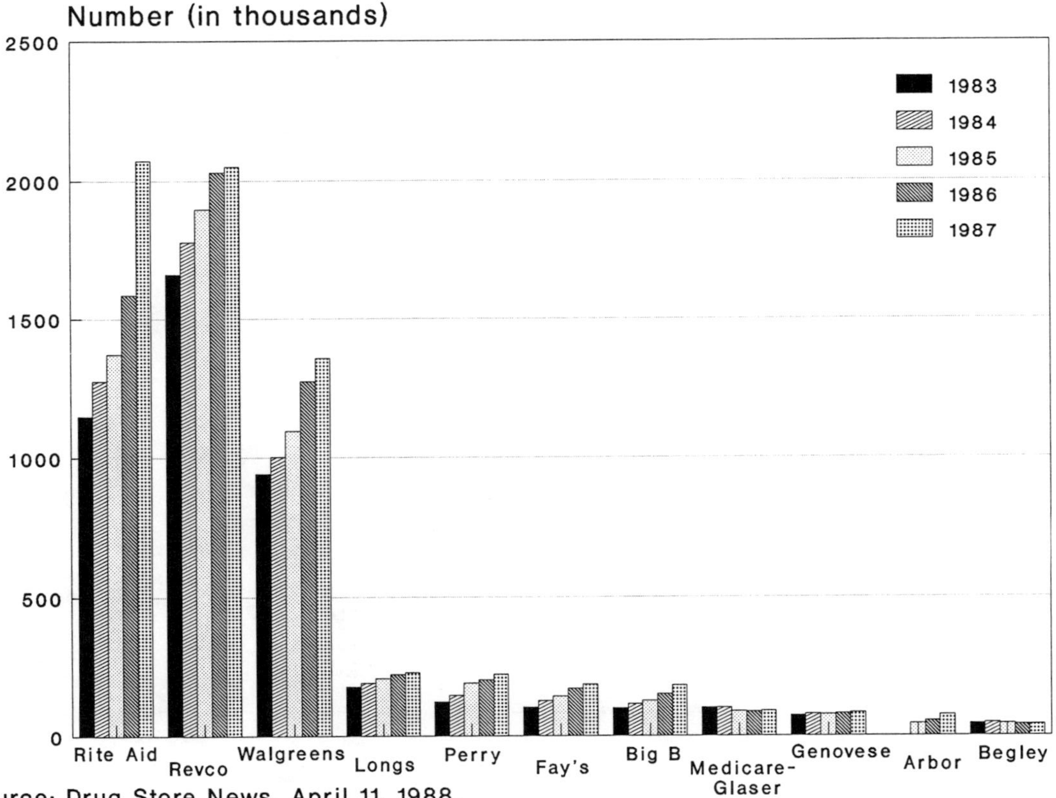

Source: Drug Store News, April 11, 1988.

Average Sales Gain for Chain Drug Stores

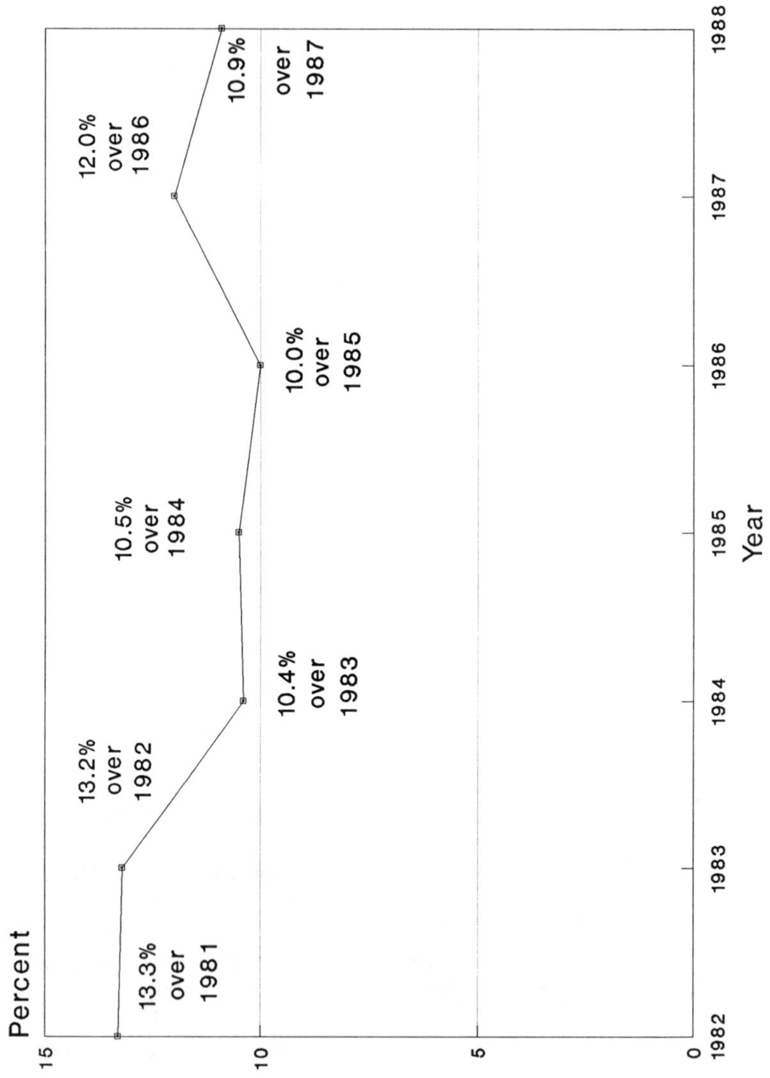

Source: NACDS Annual Report 1988

Ethical Pharmaceutical Sales: Leading Companies for Drug Stores

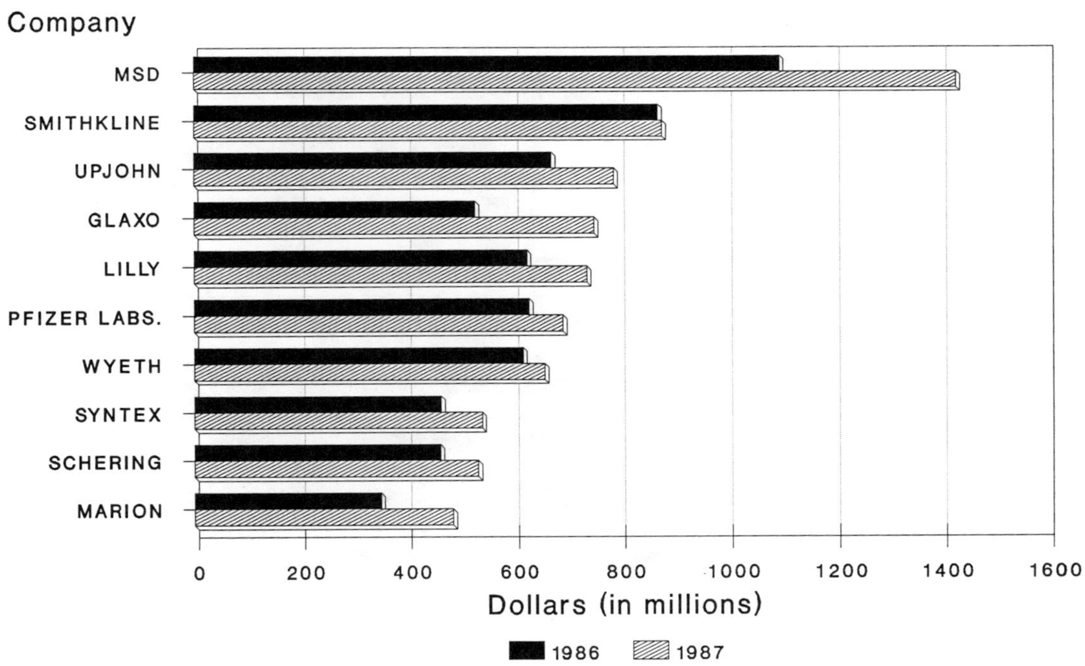

Source: Year In Review, 1987
IMS America, LTD., 1988.

Top Ten Companies: U.S. Retail Sales to Drug Stores

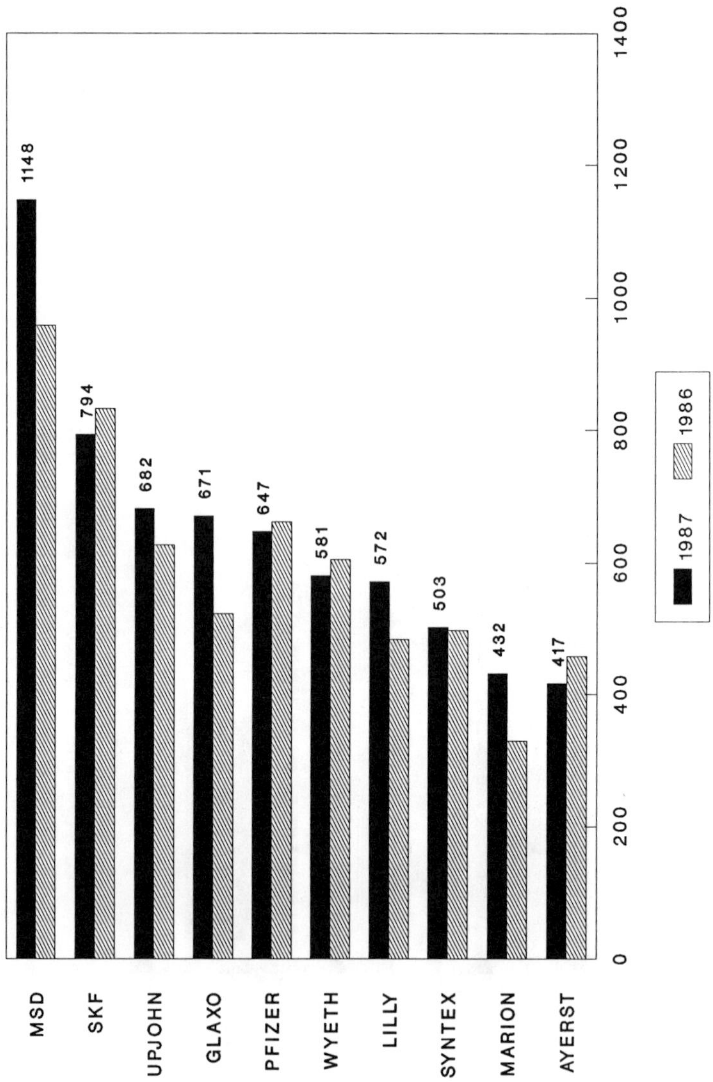

Source: PSD, 1987 Industry Review

Ethical Pharmaceuticals: Leading Product for Drug Stores

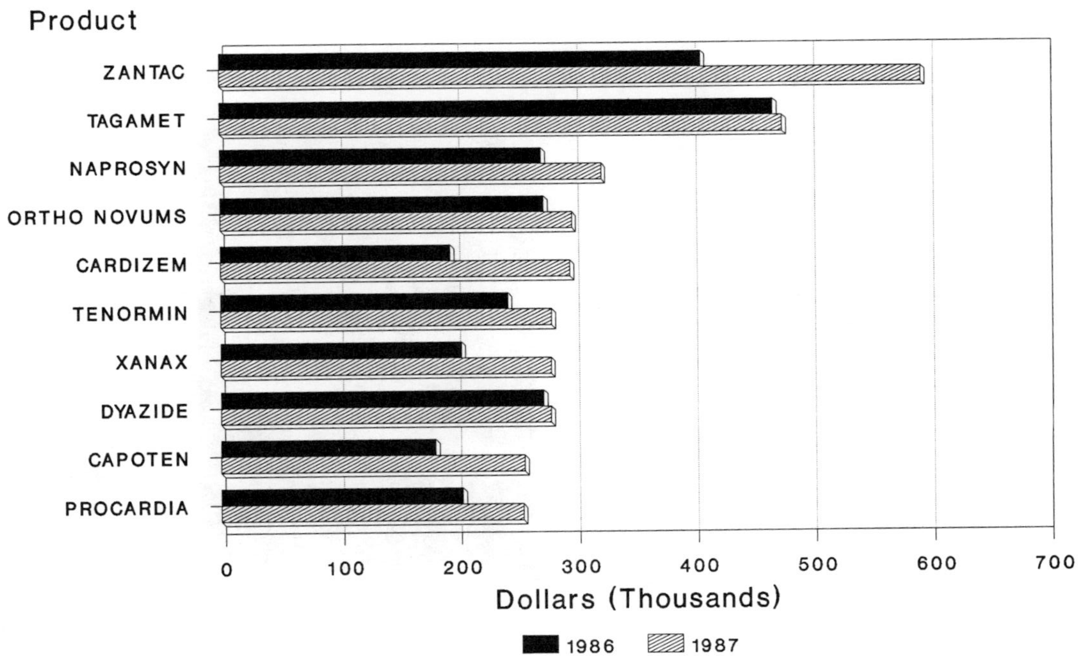

Source: Year In Review, 1987:
IMS America, Ltd., 1988.

Breakout of 1988 Chain Drug Sales: 1988 Total Chain Sales

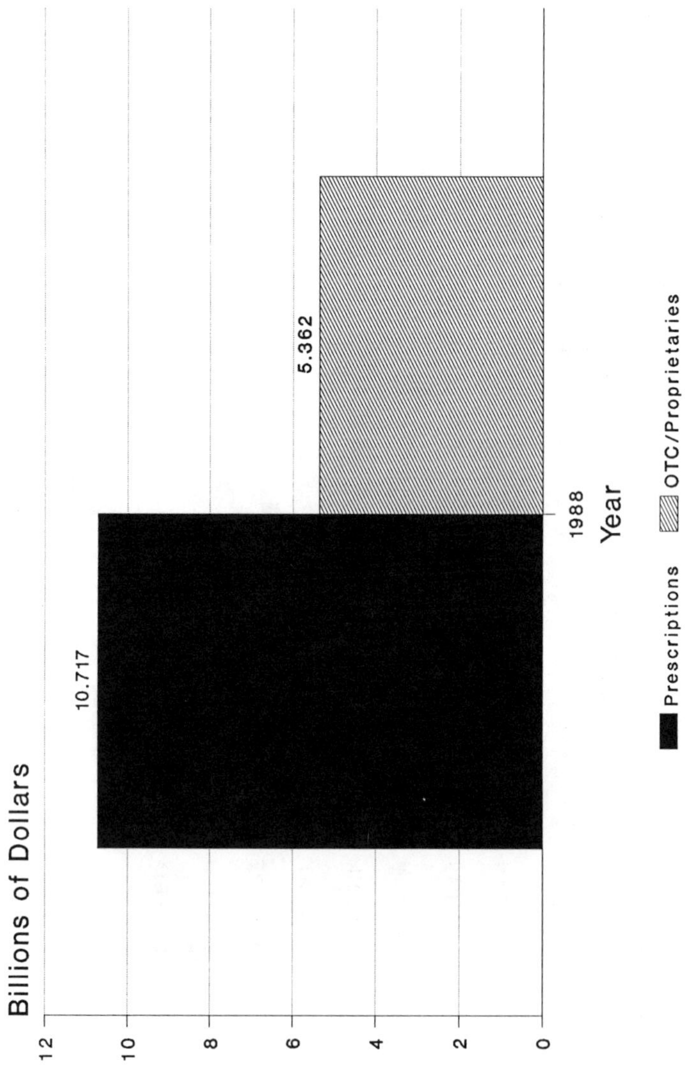

Source: Drug Store News 1989 survey of drug chains.

Chain Drug Store Average Sales Mix: 1987

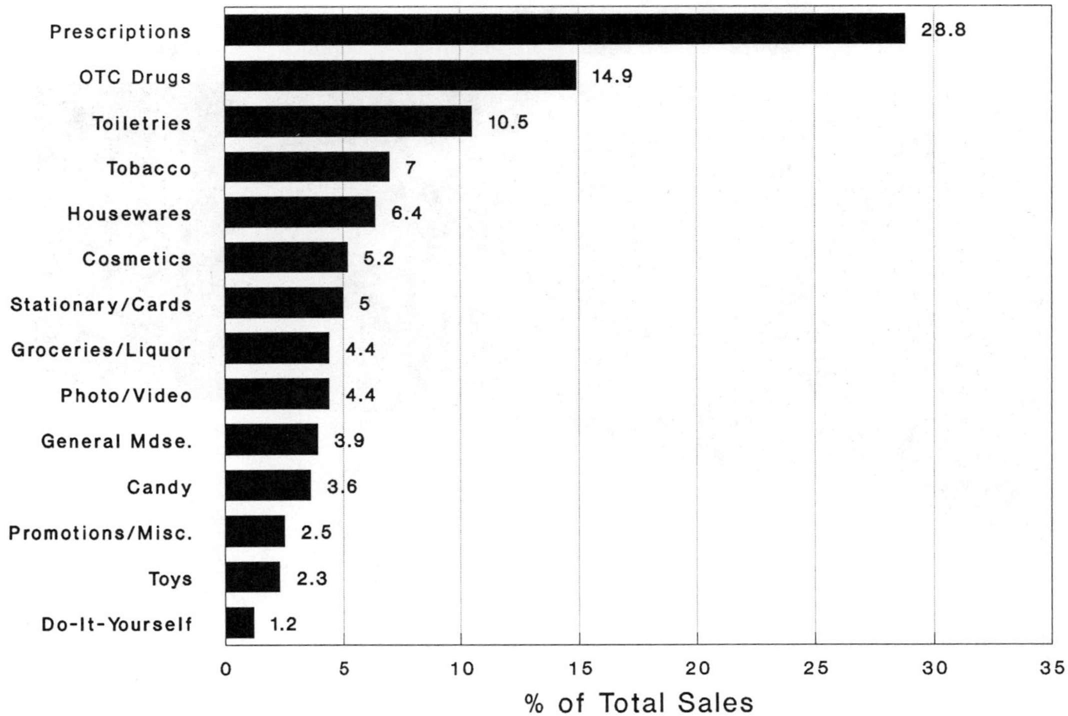

NACDS Resource Guide, The Chain Drug Store Industry and the Retail Prescription Market.

Percent of Prescriptions Filled by Chains

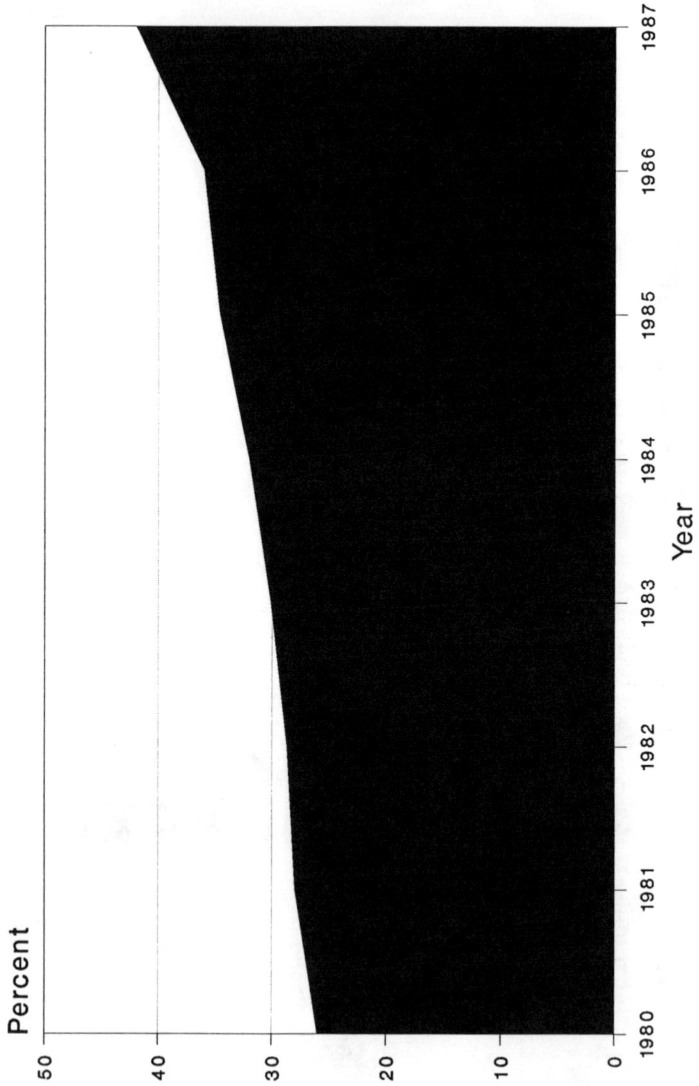

Source: National Association of Chain Drug Stores, Inc. 1987

Total Dollar Sales: Independent vs. Chain

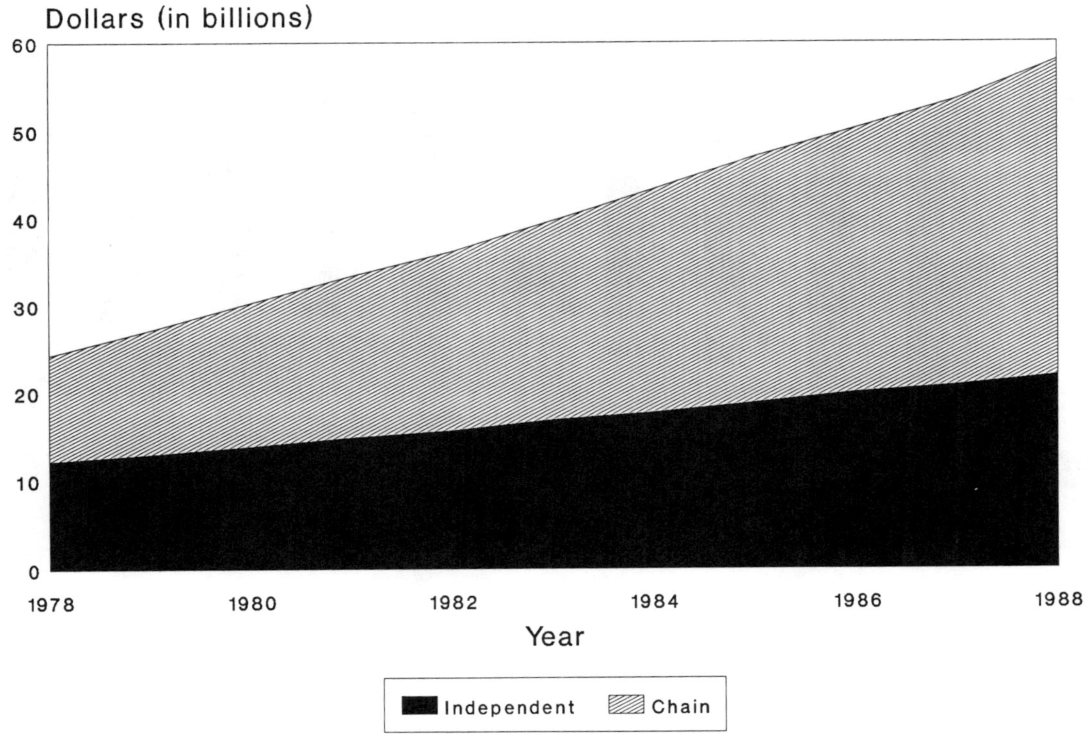

Source: A.C. Nielson Co.

Total Number of Independent and Chain Pharmacies, 1978-1987

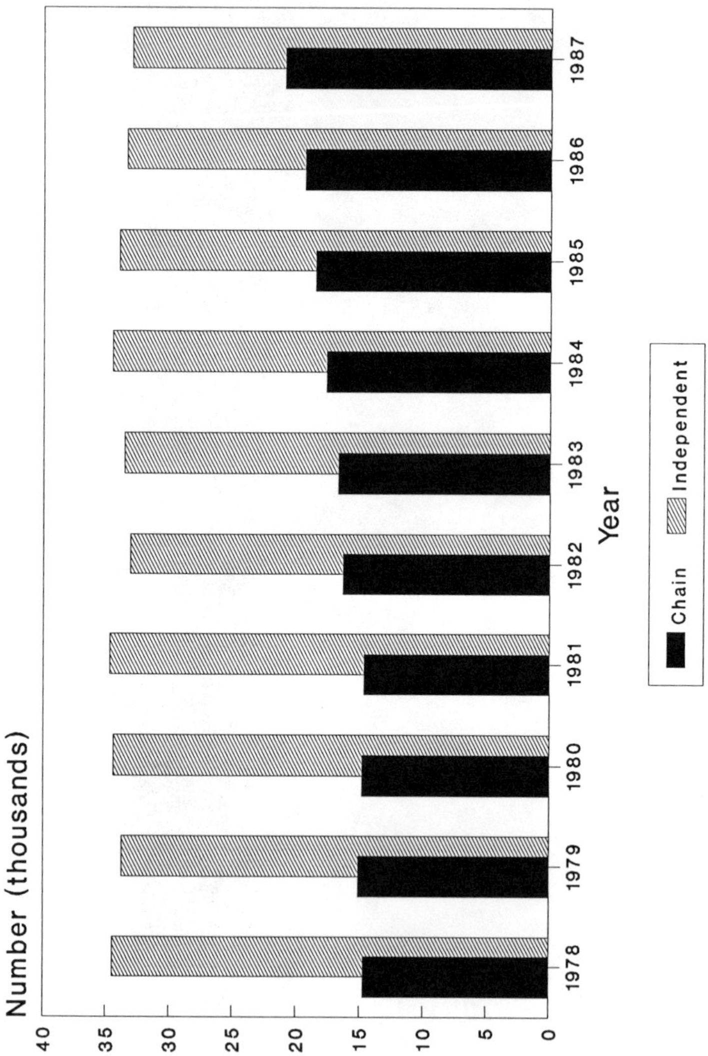

Source: Chain Store Guides and Census Bureau, 1988.

U.S. Retail Drug Store Sales
Chain vs. Independent

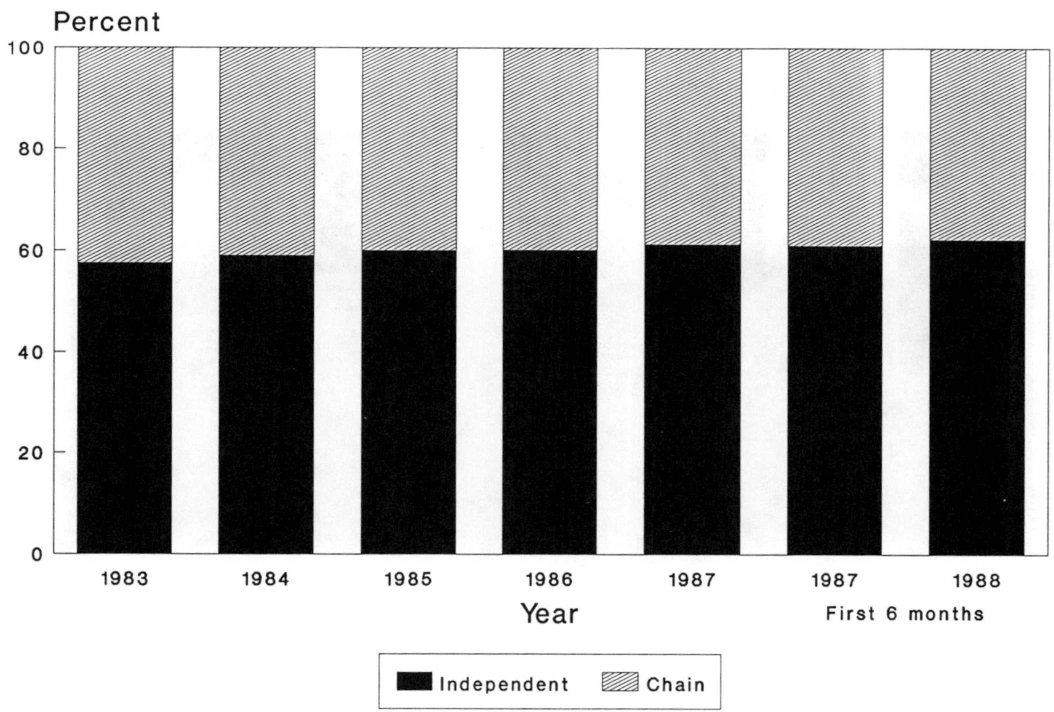

Source: Nielsen Marketing Research
Estimates, 1988.

U.S. Retail Drug Store Sales
Chain vs. Independent

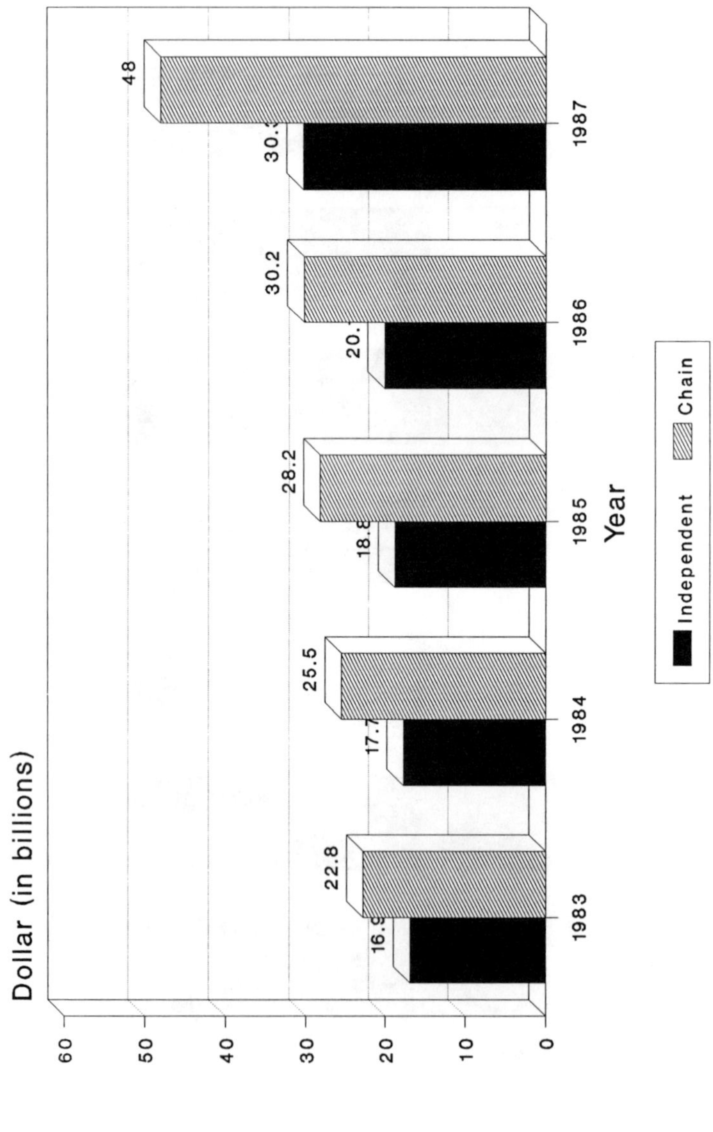

Source: Nielson Marketing Research Estimates, 1988

Daily Prescription Output: 1st Qtr. 1989

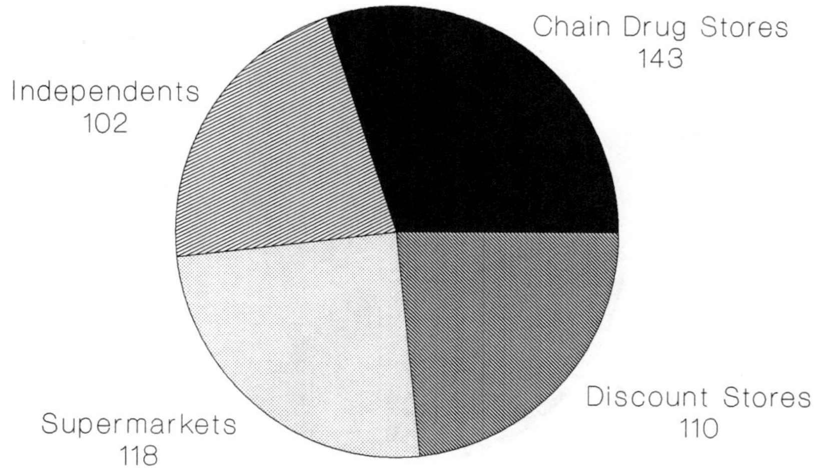

Source: Chain Drug Review, July 3, 1989.

Prescription Output (1st Qtr. 1989)
Total No. Scripts Filled: 420 million

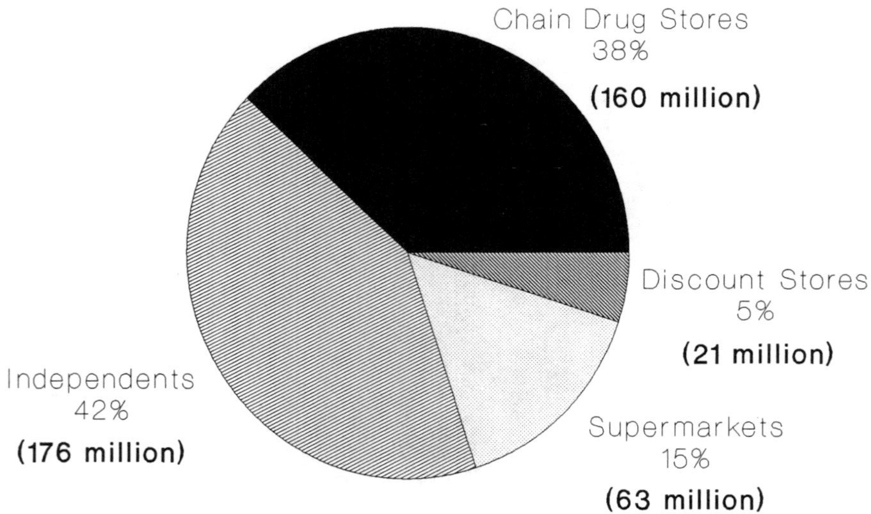

Source: Chain Drug Review, July 3, 1989

1988 Drug Chains: Net-to-Sales Ratio

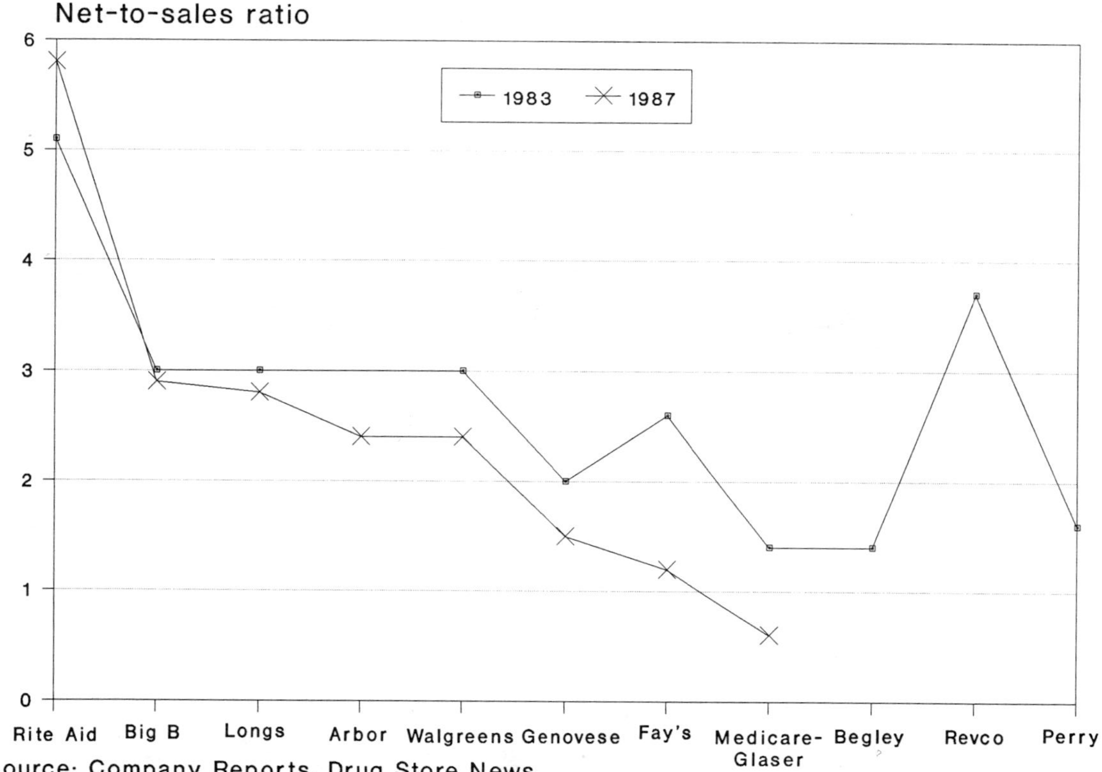

Source: Company Reports, Drug Store News April 11, 1988.

1988 Drug Chains: Expense Ratio*

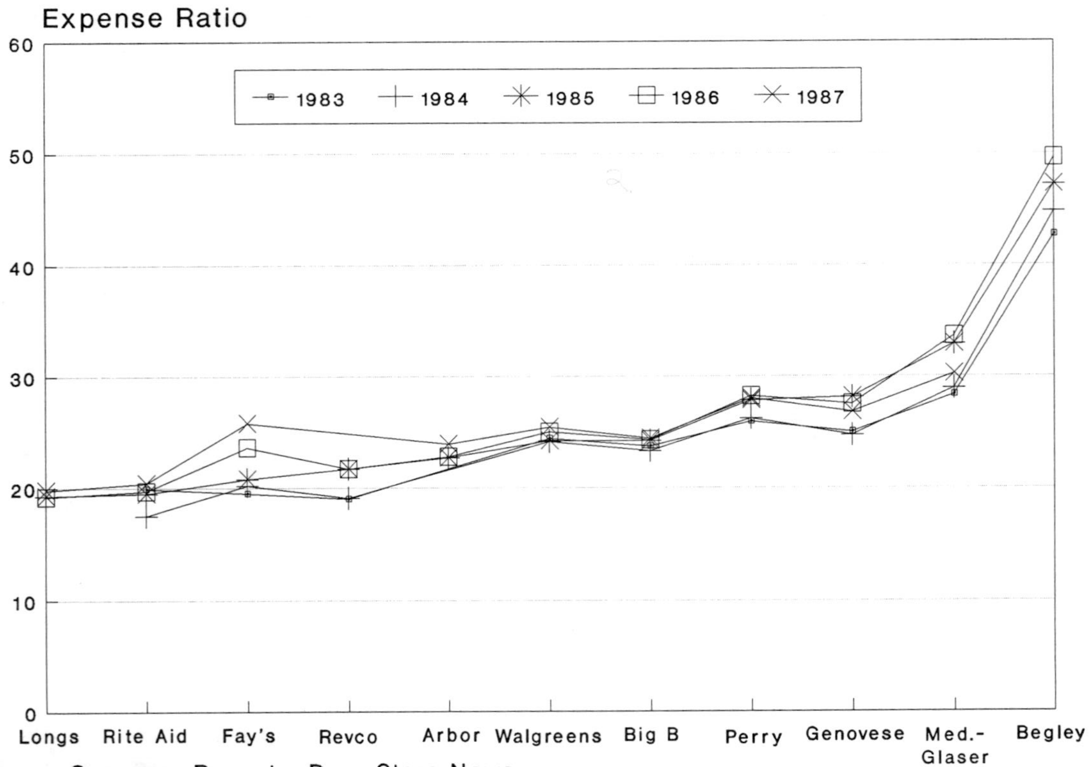

Source: Company Reports, Drug Store News April 11, 1988.

*Excludes depreciation and amortization costs

Pharmacy Sales by Number of Prescriptions Dispensed Daily in 1987

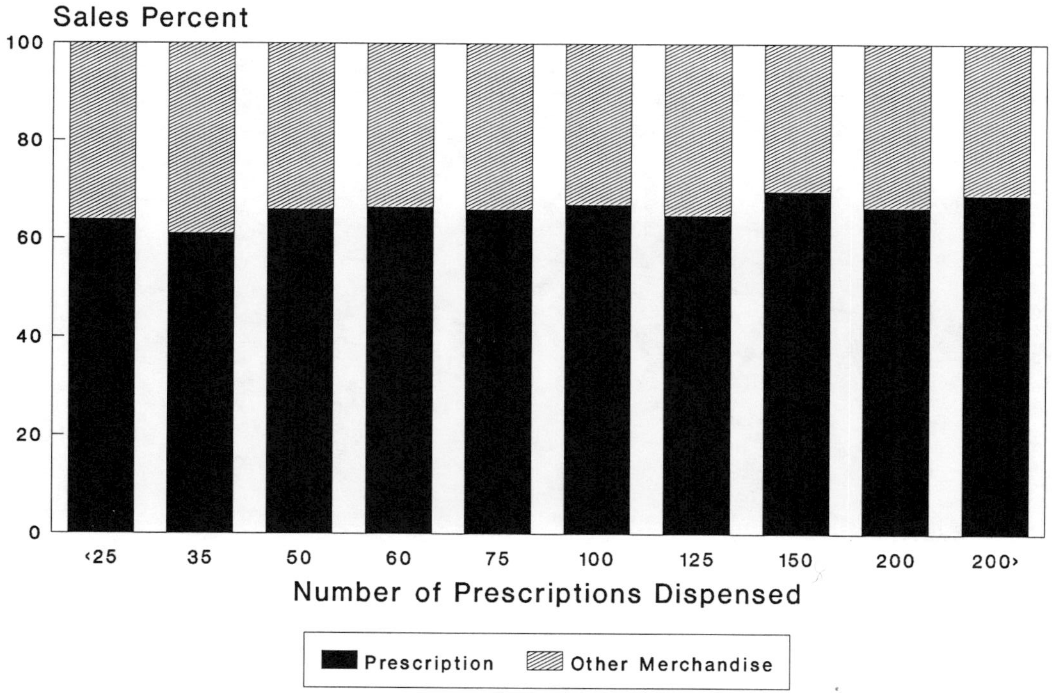

Source: Lilly Digest, 1988

10-Year Sales Trends
(1985 base equals 100)

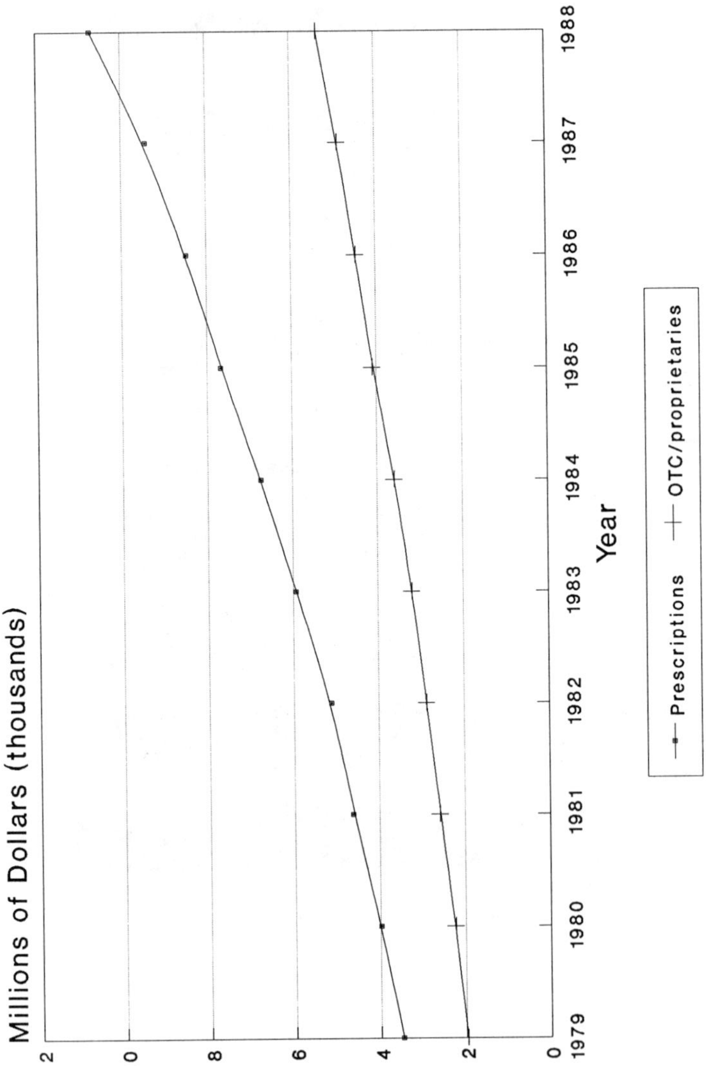

Source: Drug Store News 1989 survey of drug chains.

Drug Store Pharmaceutical Purchases: Total Rx vs. Total OTC

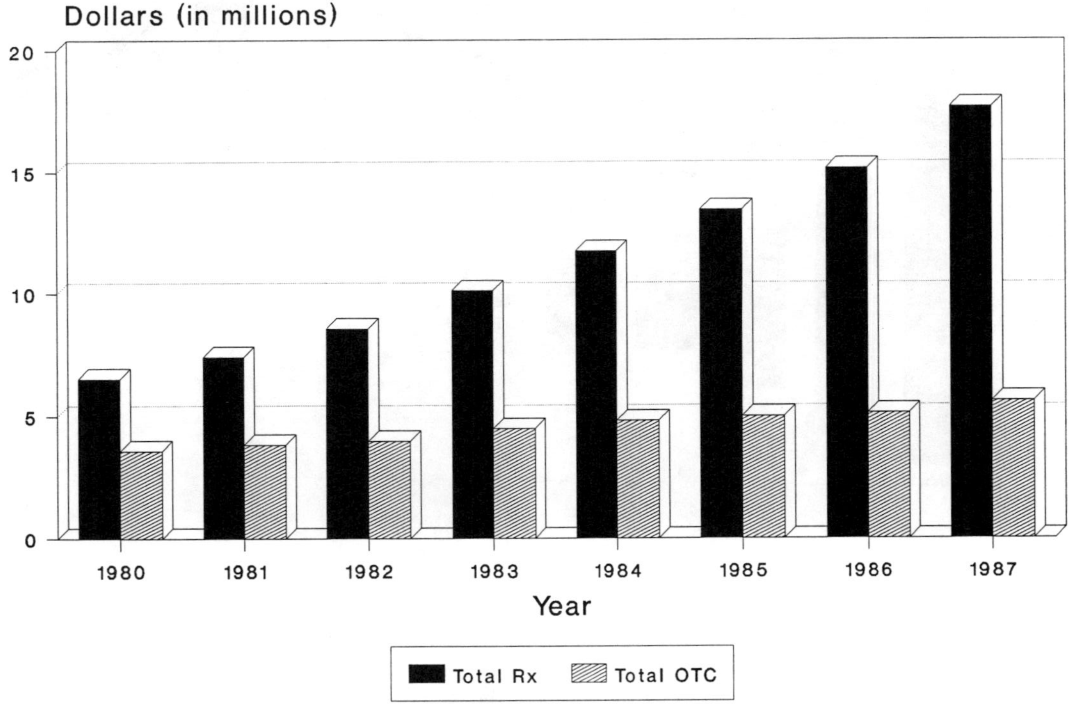

Source: Year In Review, 1987
IMS America, LTD., 1988.

Sales Growth in Independent Community Pharmacies: 1970-1988

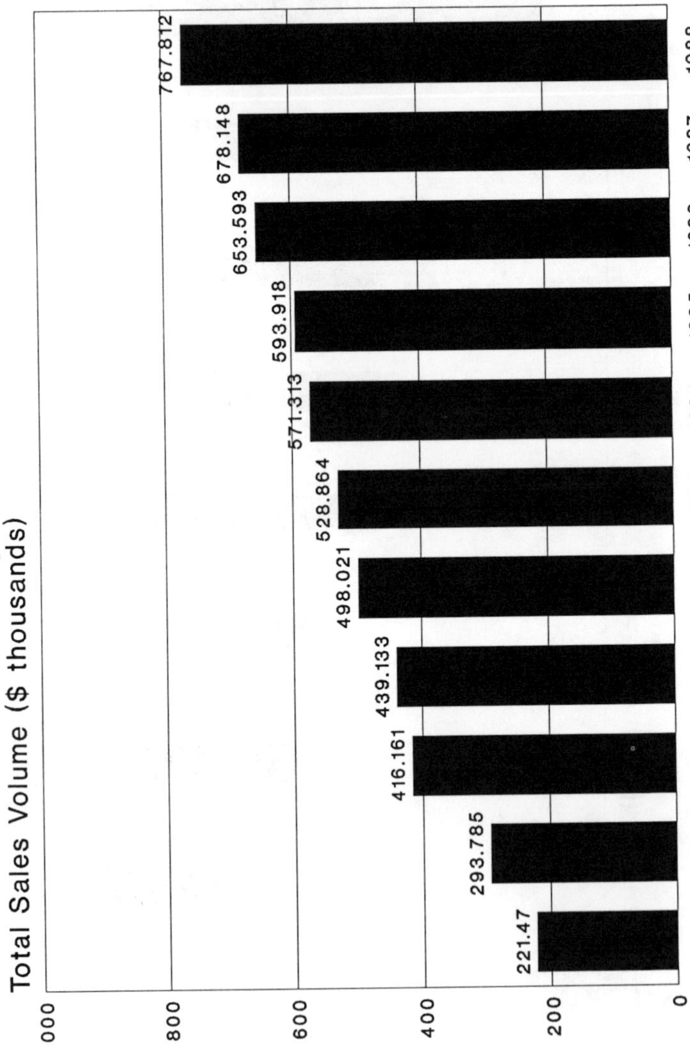

Source: Lilly Digest, 1989

Retail Pharmacies' Shrinking Share of the Nation's Prescription Sales
1985 and 1988

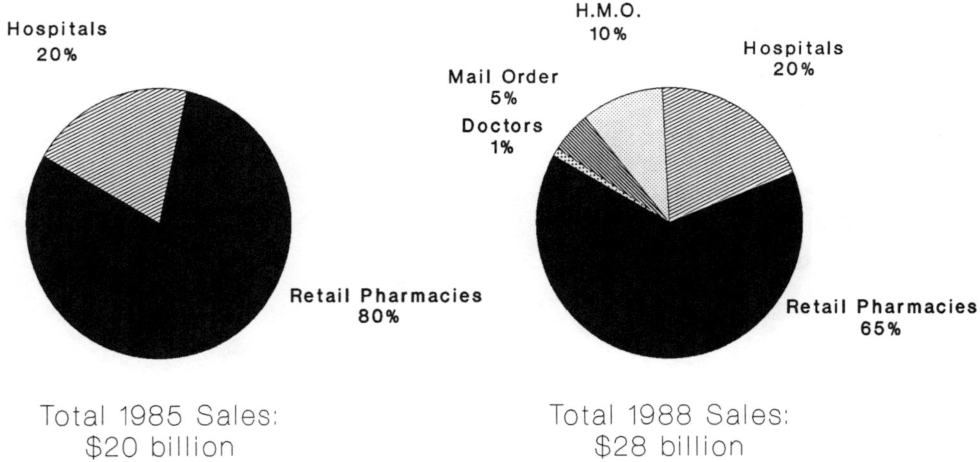

Source: Arthur D. Little, Inc.

Prescription Sales Dollar Distribution (Average Retail Rx Price = $15.37)

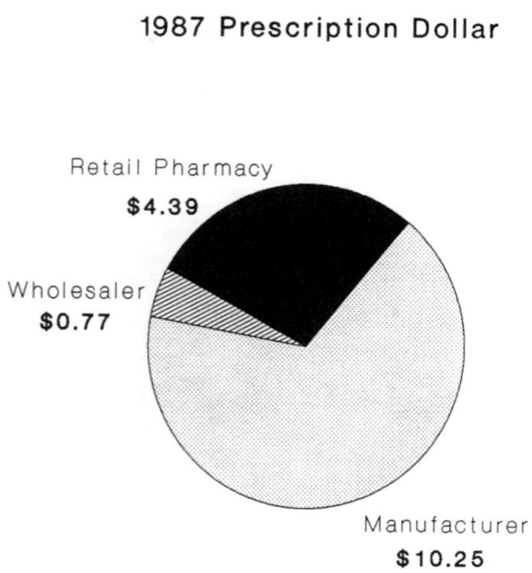

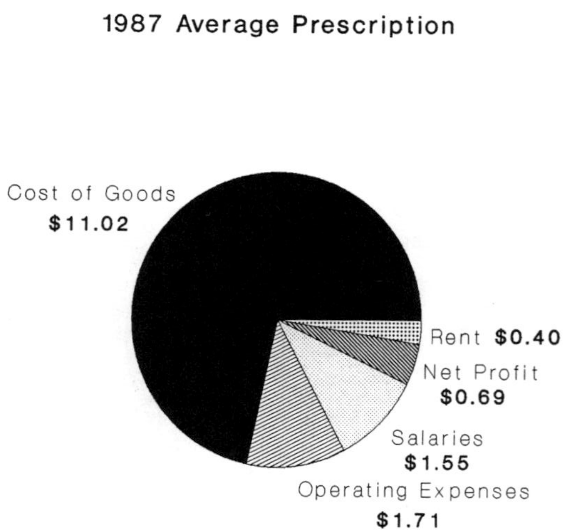

Average Prescription Price from The Lilly Digest: 1988 (Indianapolis: Eli Lilly and Company, 1988), p.3.

Pharmaceutical Purchases: Drug Stores vs. Hospitals

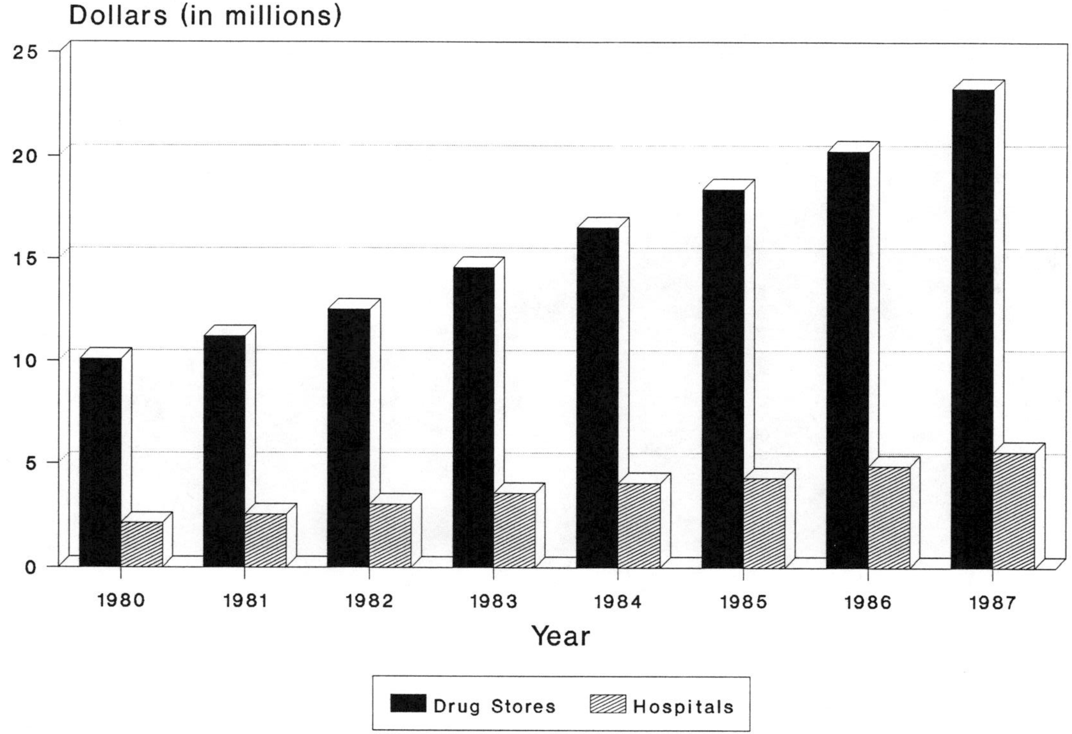

Source: Year In Review, 1987

Chapter 7

HOSPITALS AND LONG TERM CARE

Includes trends in utilization, services, and ownership

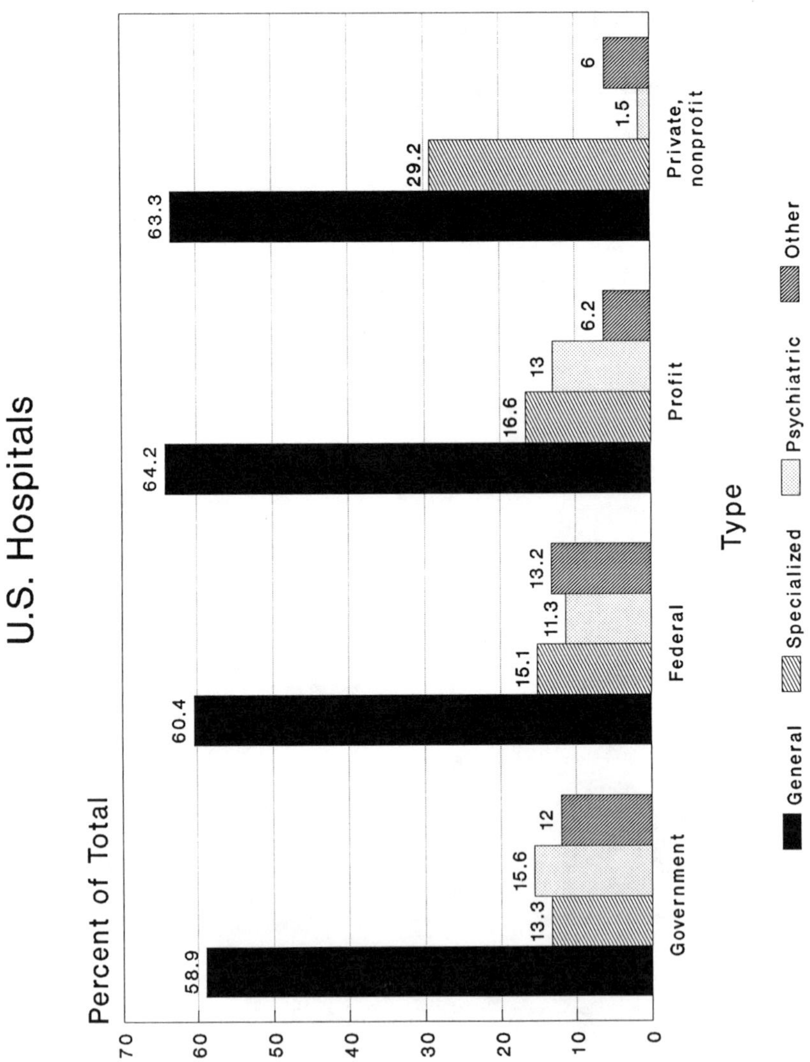

Source: 1989 Lilly Hospital Pharmacy Survey.

Allocation of Beds According to Hospital size: 1987

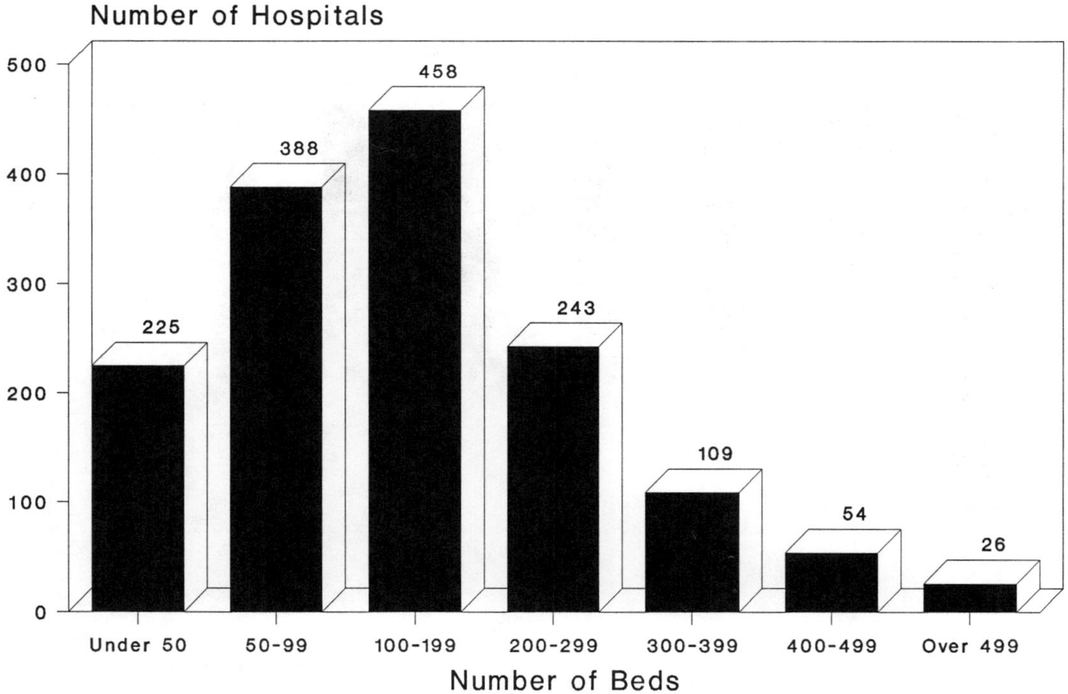

Source: Lilly Hospital Pharmacy Survey, 1988

Total Expenditures of Community Hospitals by Bed-Size

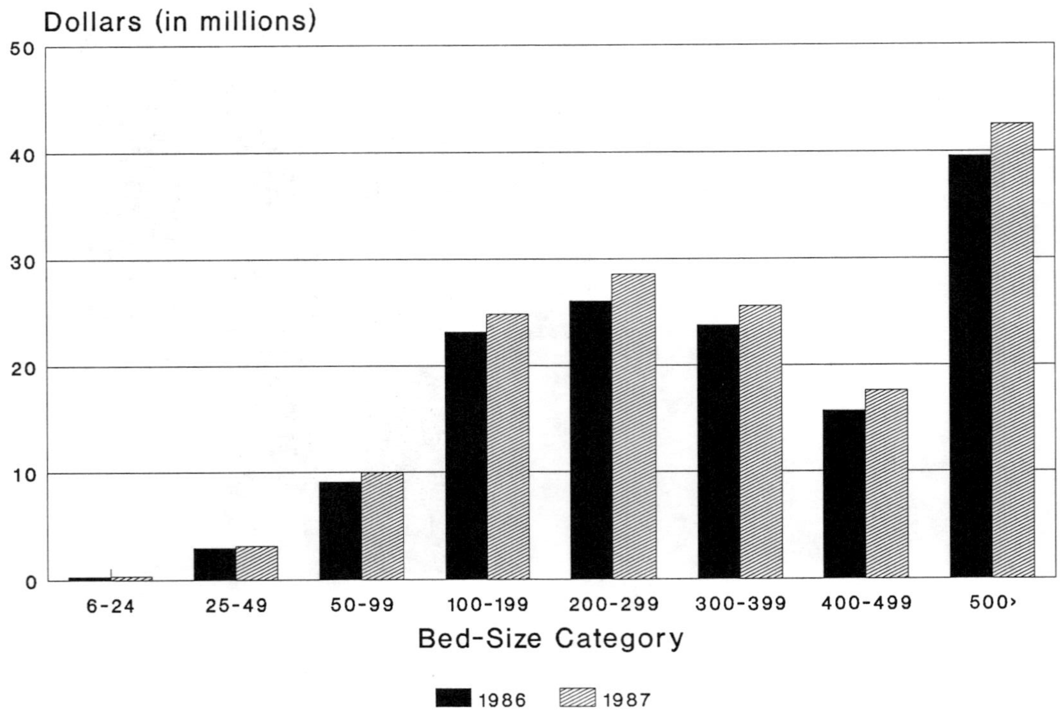

Source: Hospital Statistics, 1988

Trends Among Noncommunity Hospitals

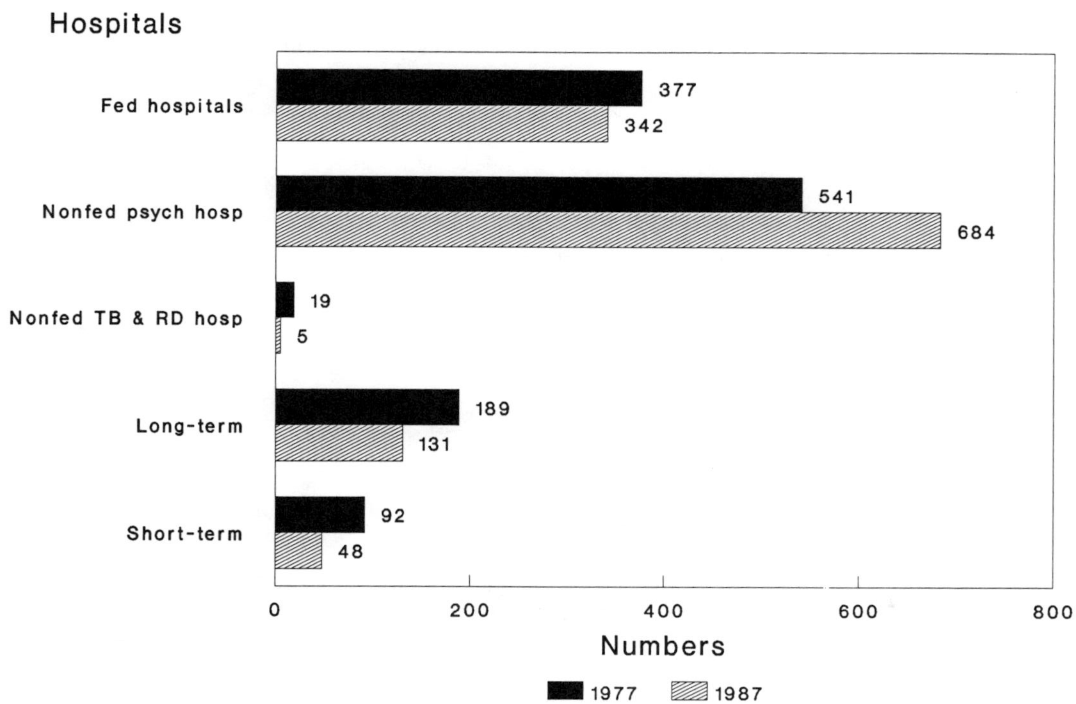

Source: Hospital Statistics 1988.

Hospital Staffing by Type of Hospital

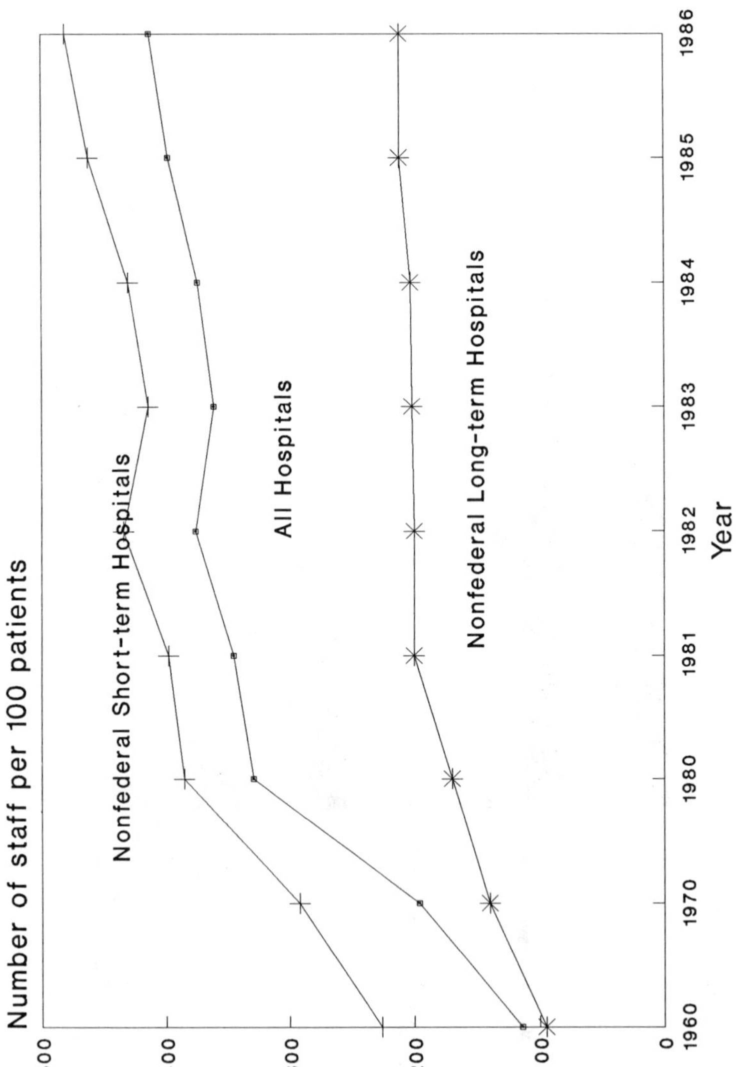

Source: American Hospital Association, Chicago, IL Hospital Statistics, 1986.

Percent of Beds Occupied in Average Private Nonprofit Hospitals

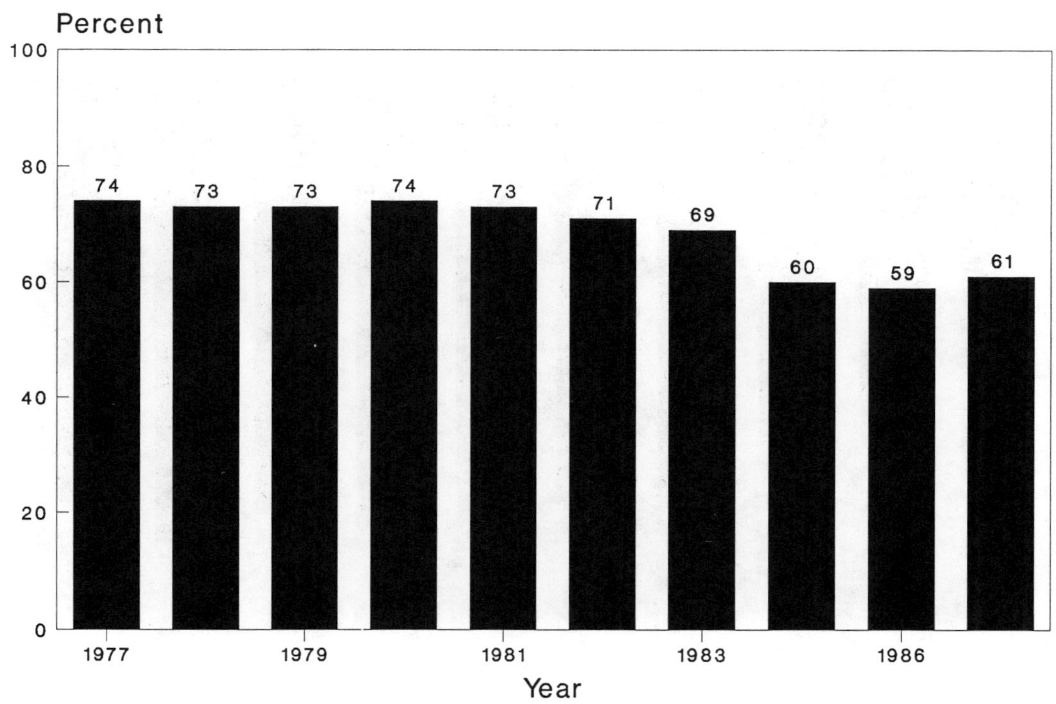

Source: 1988 Lilly Hospital Pharmacy Survey

Length of Stay for Private Nonprofit Hospitals

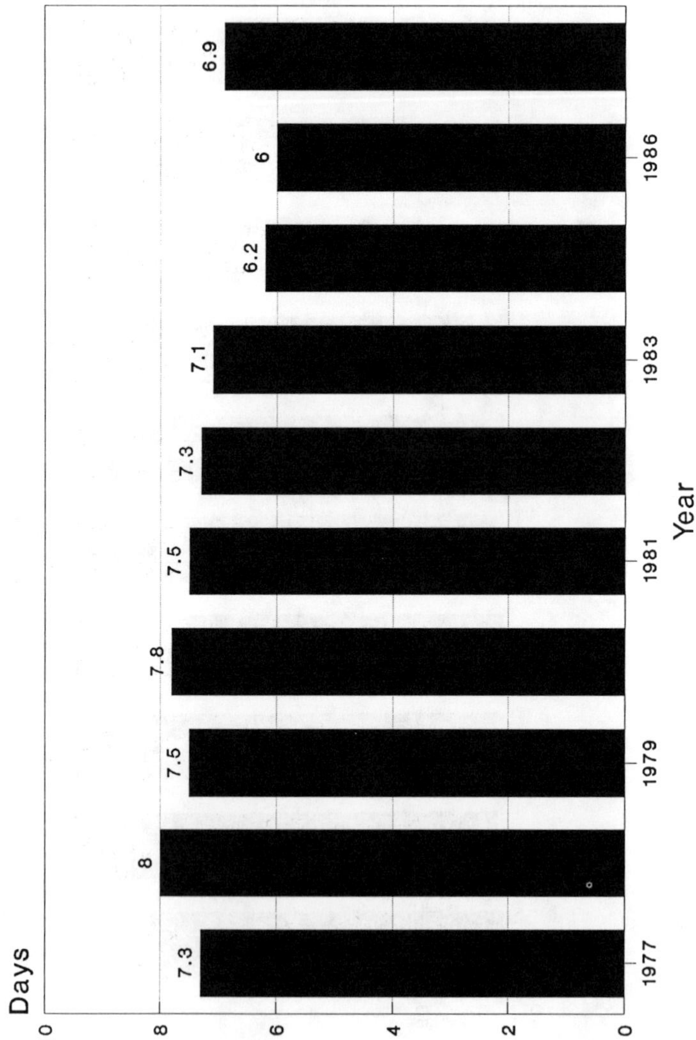

Source: 1988 Lilly Hospital Pharmacy Survey

Average Hospital Discharges per Week and Length of Stay of Discharged Patients (in days) for All Physicians

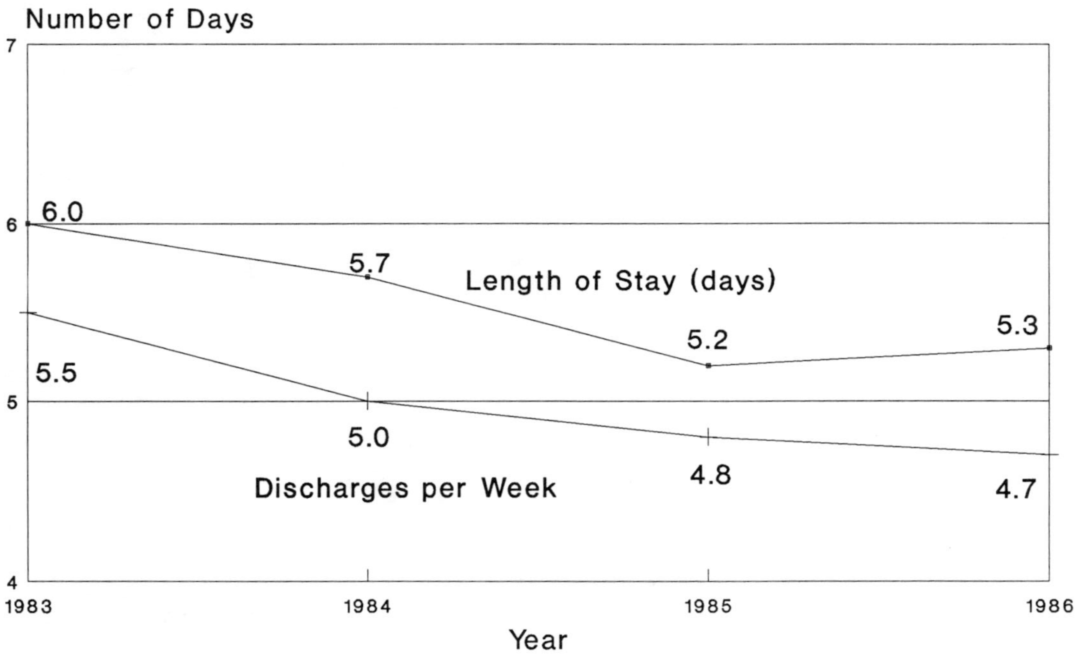

Source: AMA Socioeconomic Monitoring System 1983-1986.

Hospital Operating Statistics: Average Bed Capacity: 1987

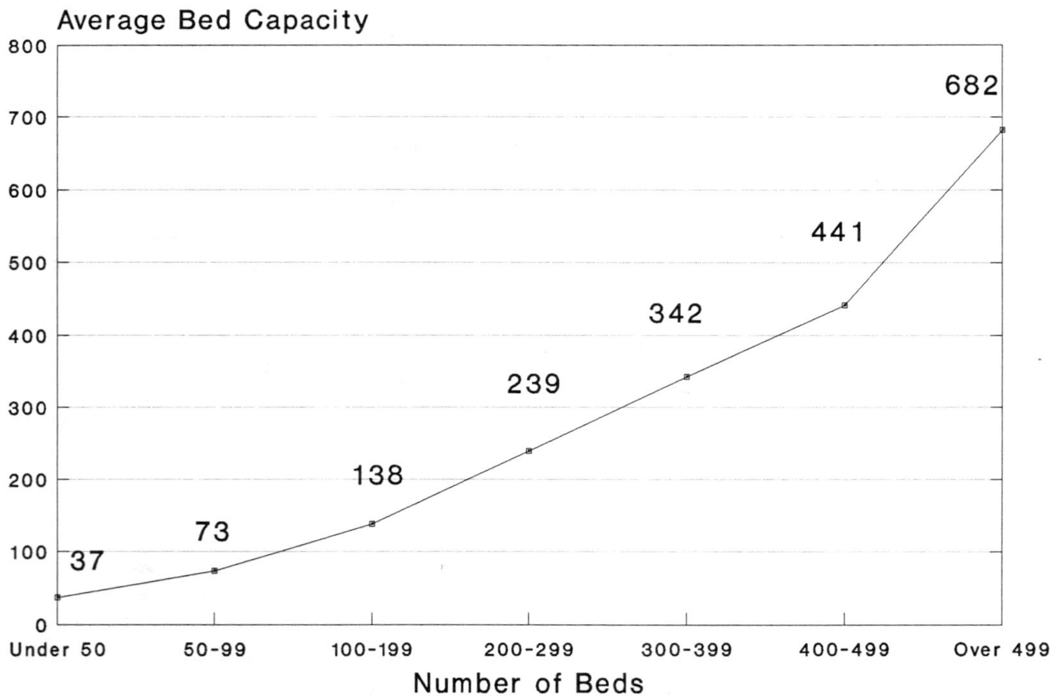

Source: 1988 Lilly Hospital Pharmacy Survey

Average Hospital Prescription Cost 1988

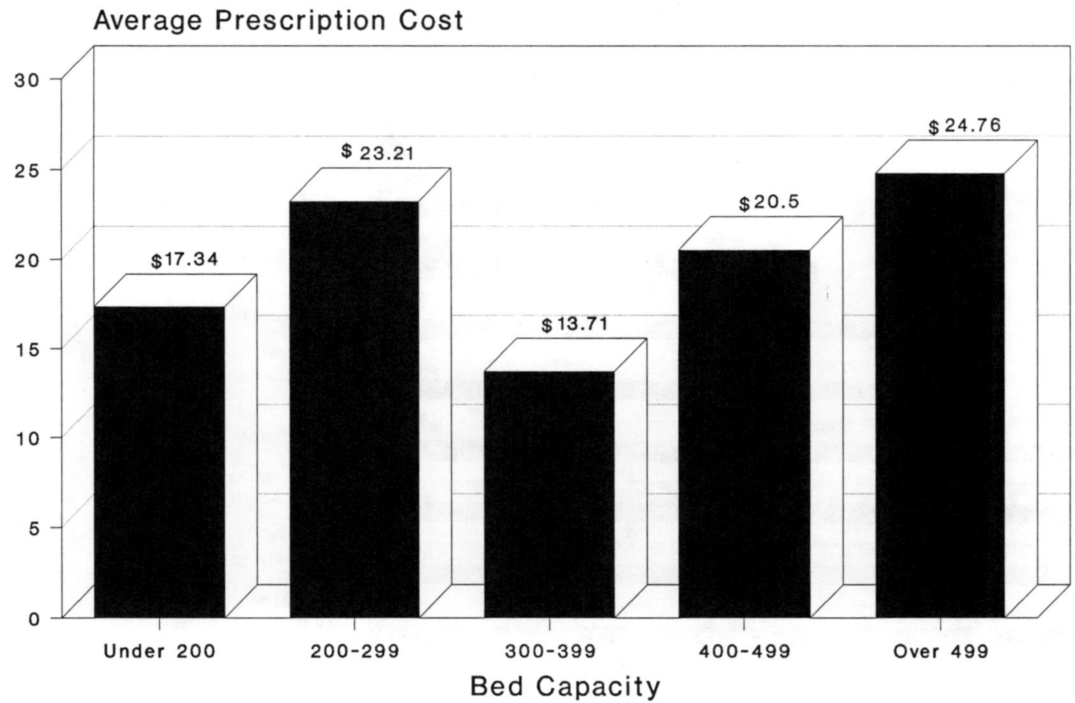

Source: 1989 Lilly Hospital Pharmacy Survey.

Pharmacy Services Offered in Hospitals

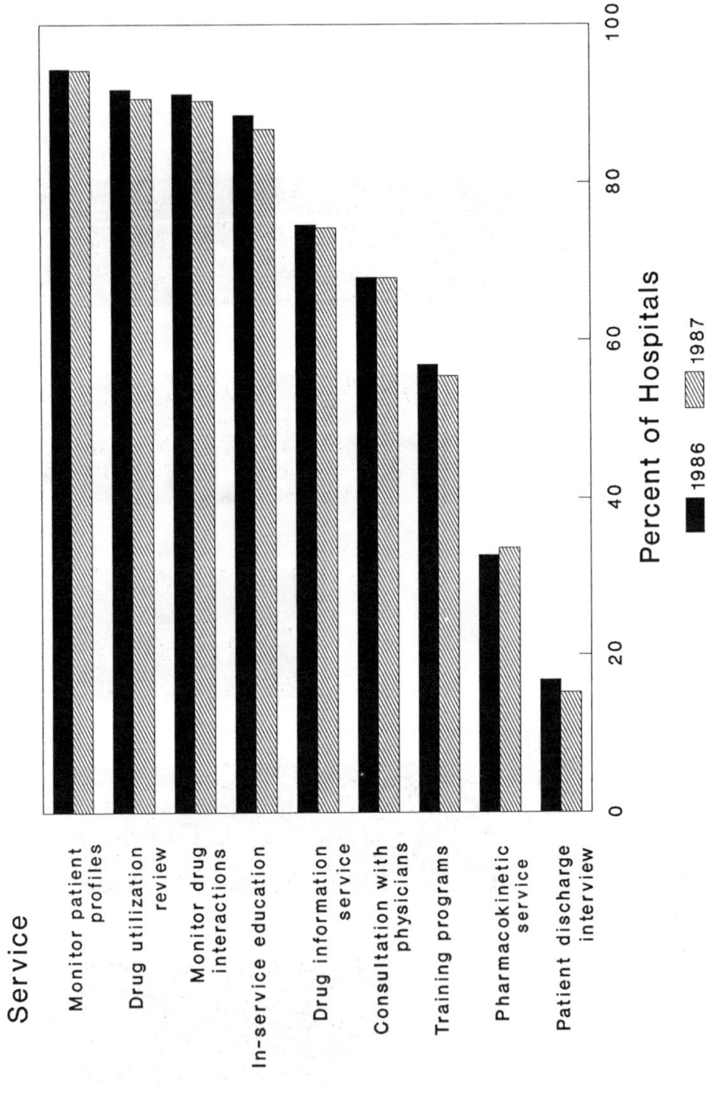

Source: 1988 Lilly Hospital Pharmacy Survey

Average Hospital Pharmacy Admissions

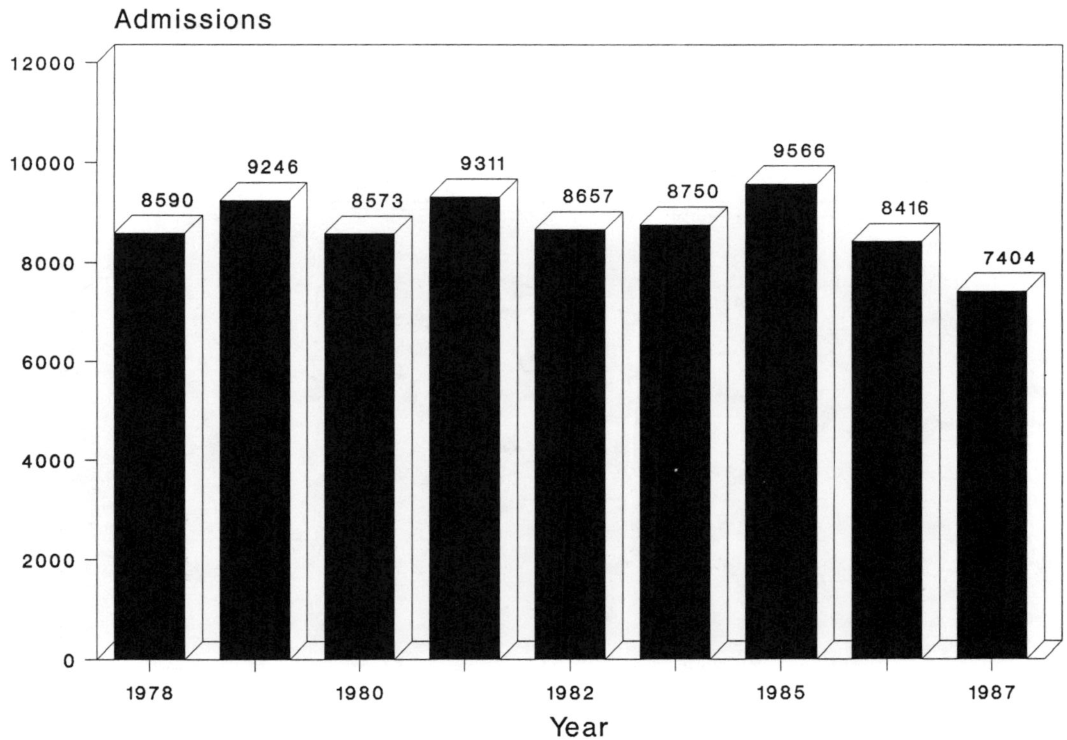

Source: 1988 Lilly Hospital Pharmacy Survey

Hospital Pharmacy Inventory and Purchases by Bed Capacity: 1988

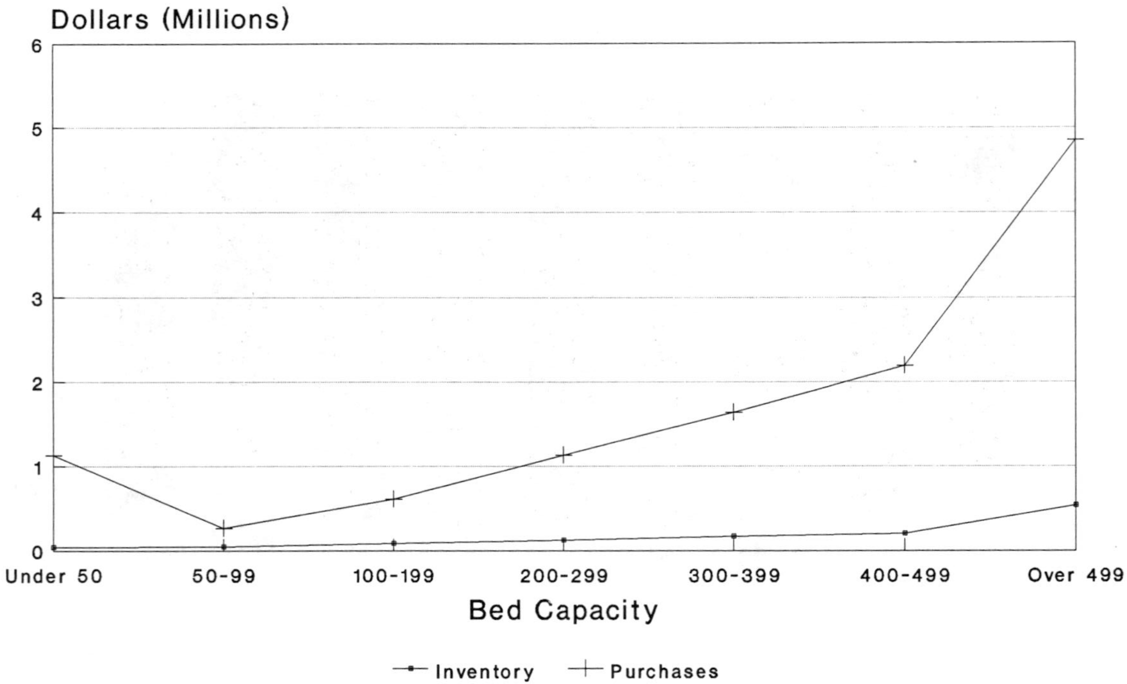

Source: 1989 Lilly Hospital Pharmacy Survey.

Average Hospital Pharmacy: Inventory and Purchases 1978-1987

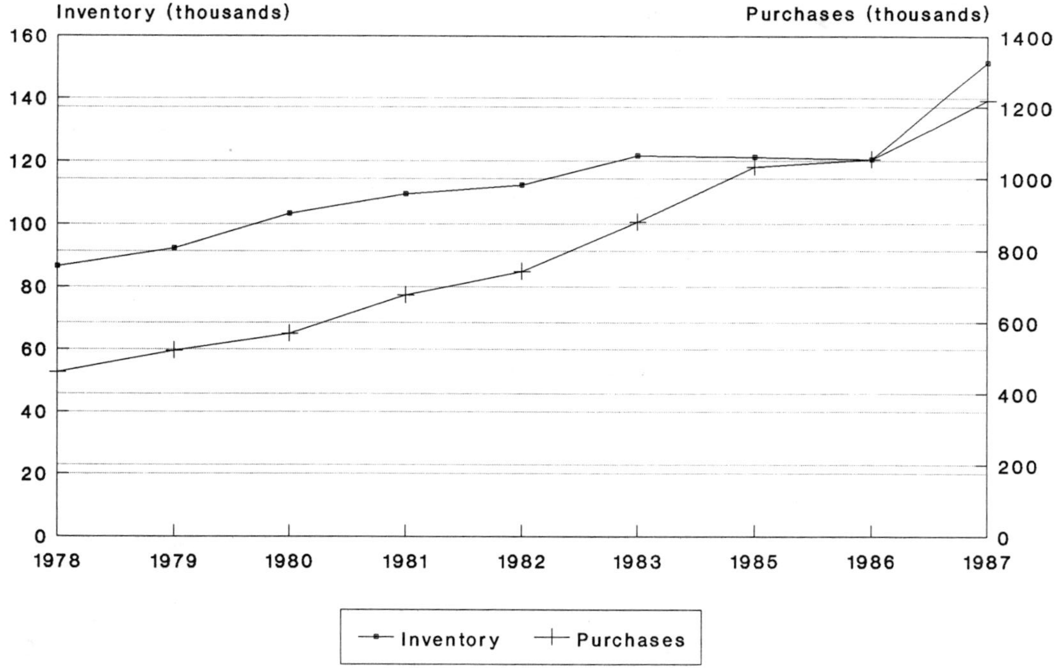

Source: I988 Lilly Hospital Pharmacy Survey

Hospital Pharmacy: Nonparenteral and Parenteral Orders/Week: 1987

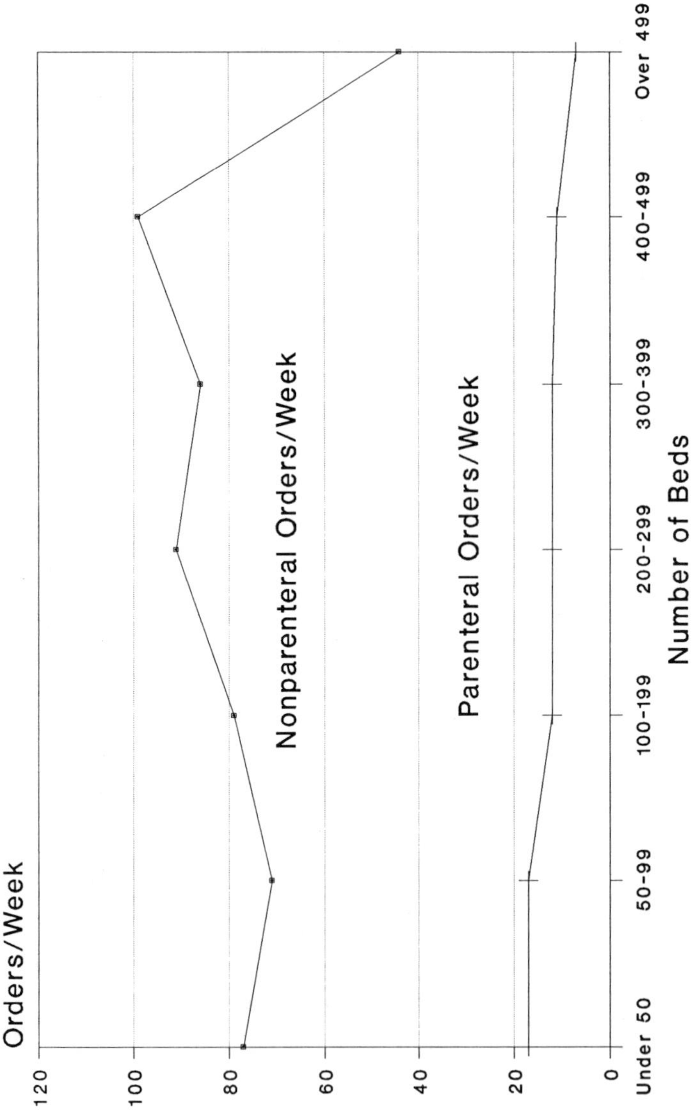

Source: 1988 Lilly Hospital Pharmacy Survey

Chemical Entities Most Frequently Dispensed in Hospitals, Patients Ages 65 Years and Older: 1987.
(Estimated U.S. Hospitalizations)

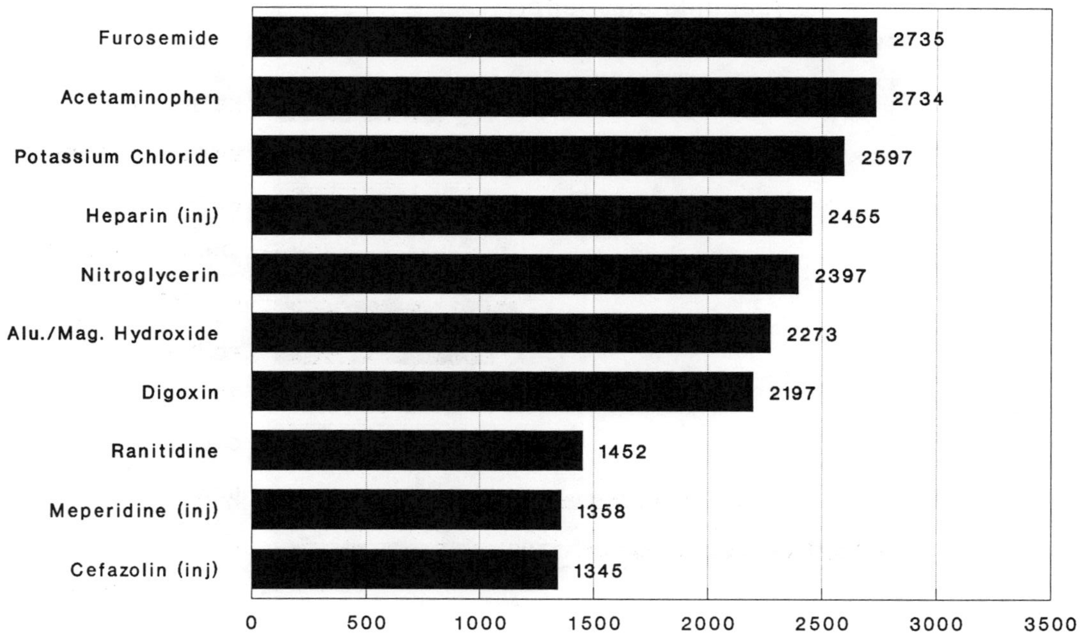

Source: IHS Hospital Pharmacy Data Base
International Health Services, LTD

Ethical Pharmaceutical Sales: Leading Companies for Hospitals

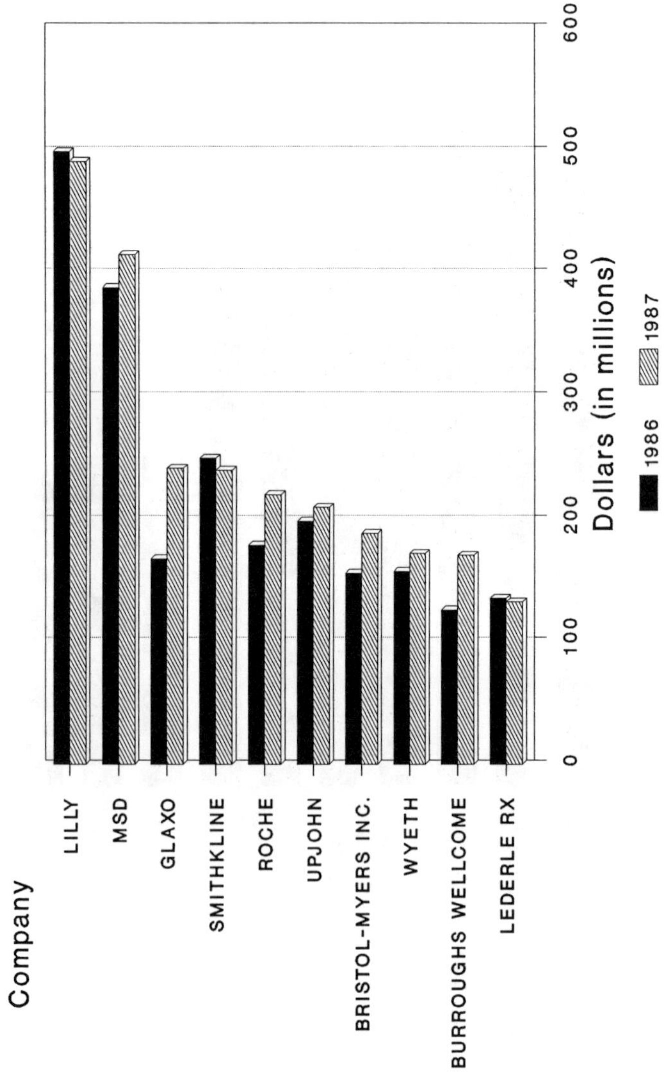

Source: Year in Review, 1987: IMS America, Ltd., 1988.

Trends in Hospital Surgery

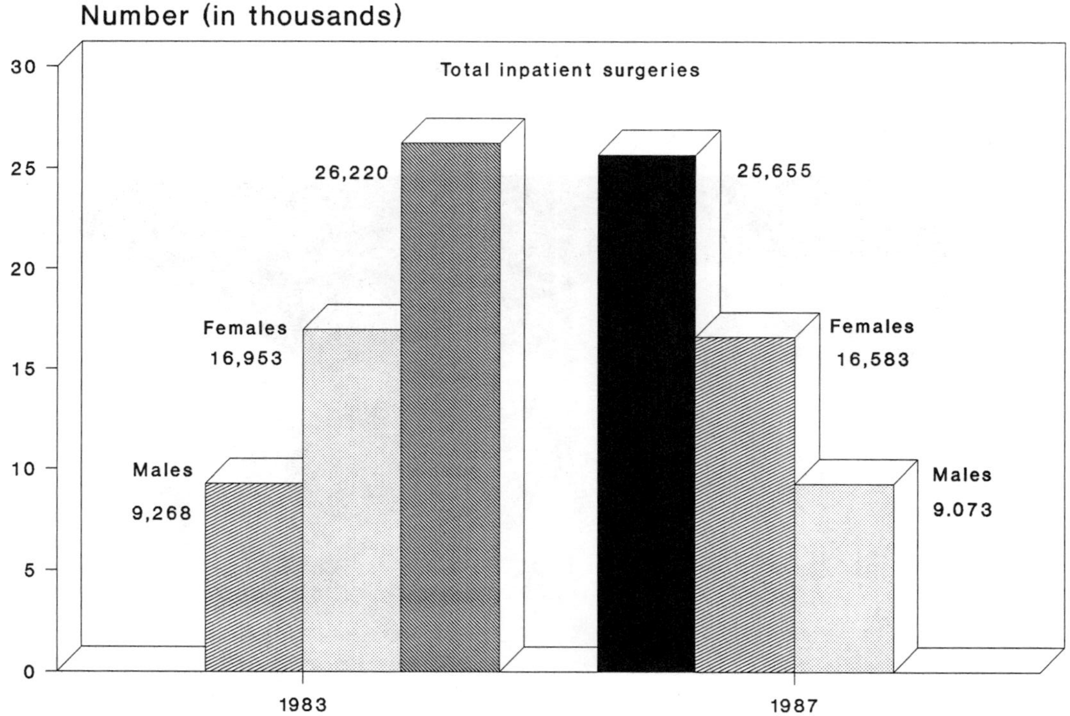

Data from National Hospital Discharge Survey. Published in "Hospital Inpatient Surgery: United States, 1983-1987", National Center for Health Statistics.

Trends in Hospital Surgery by Age Group

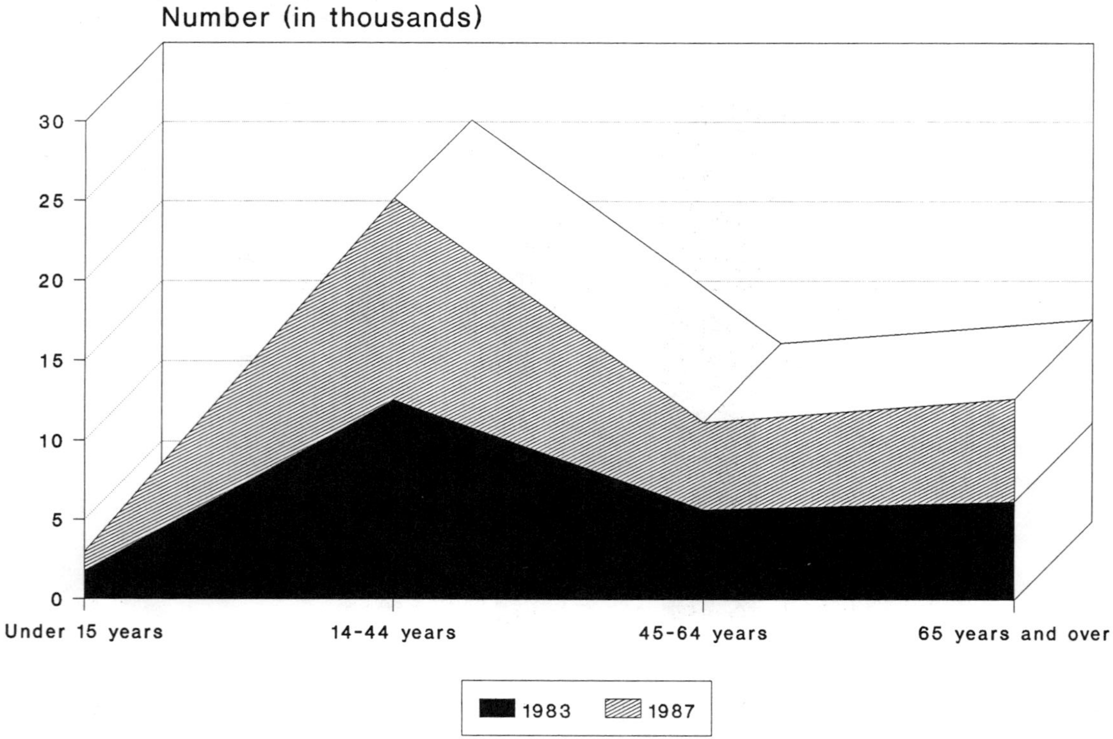

Data from National Hospital Discharge Survey. Published in "Hospital Inpatient Surgery: United States, 1983-1987", National Center for Hospital Statistics.

Source of Payment for Hospital Surgery

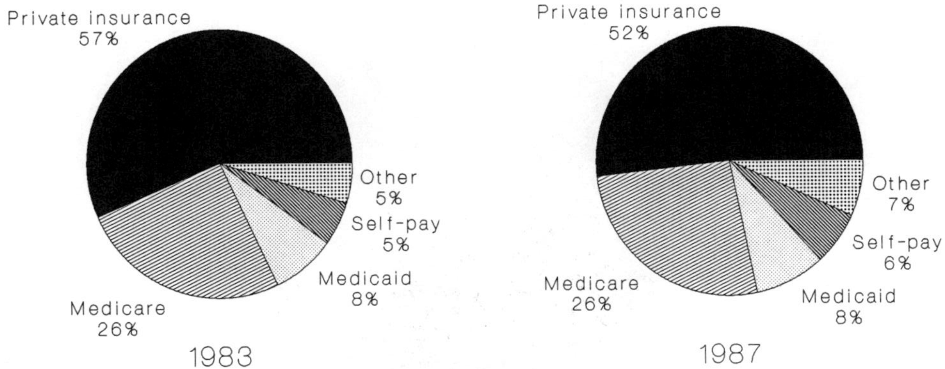

Data from National Hospital Discharge Survey. Published in "Hospital Inpatient Surgery: United States, 1983-1987", National Center for Health Statistics.

Planned Involvement of Hospitals in Retirement Communities

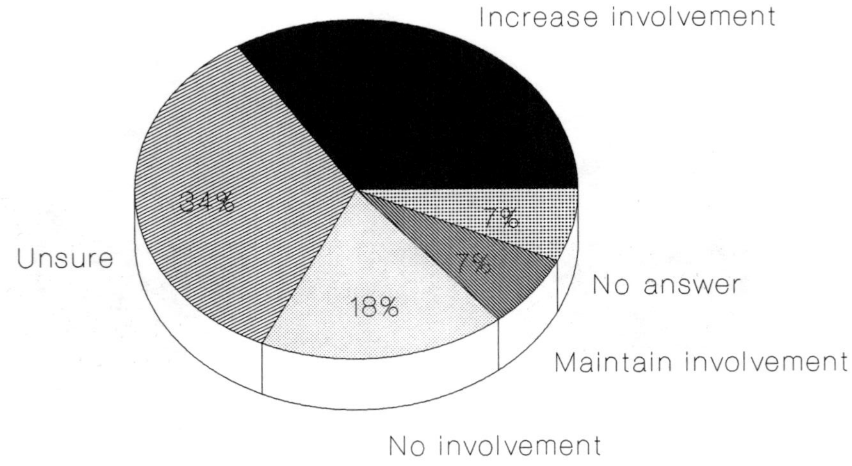

Source: Witt Associates, 1988

Hospitals and Nursing Homes

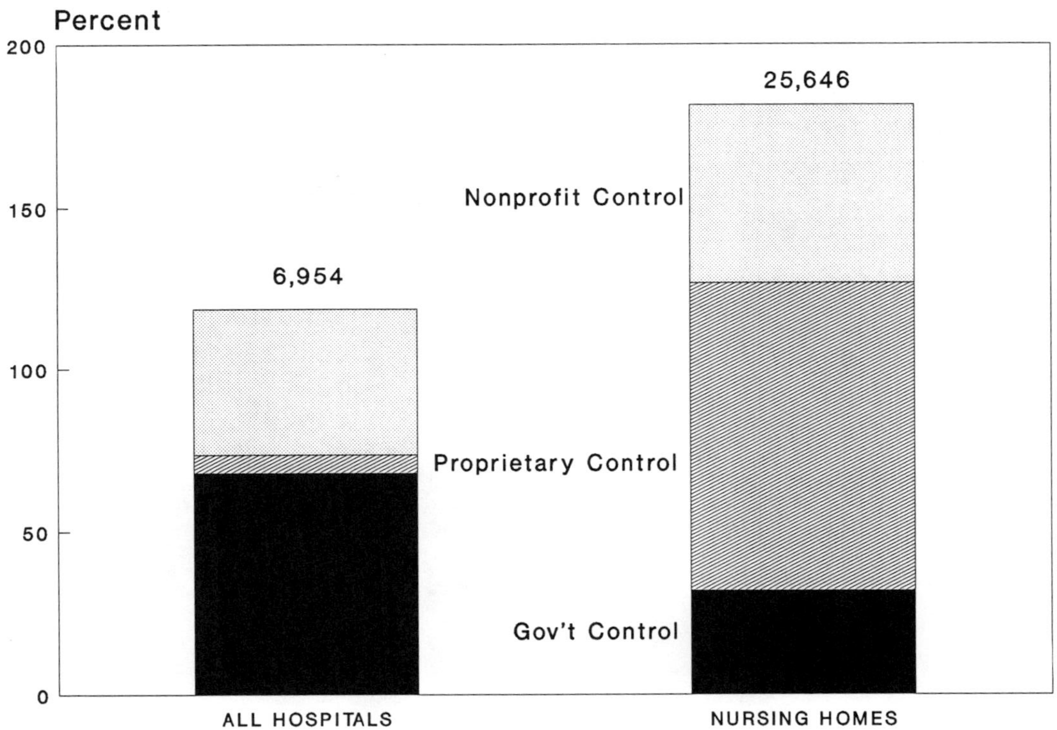

Source: U.S. National Center for Health Statistics, 1986.

Nursing Homes by Type of Ownership

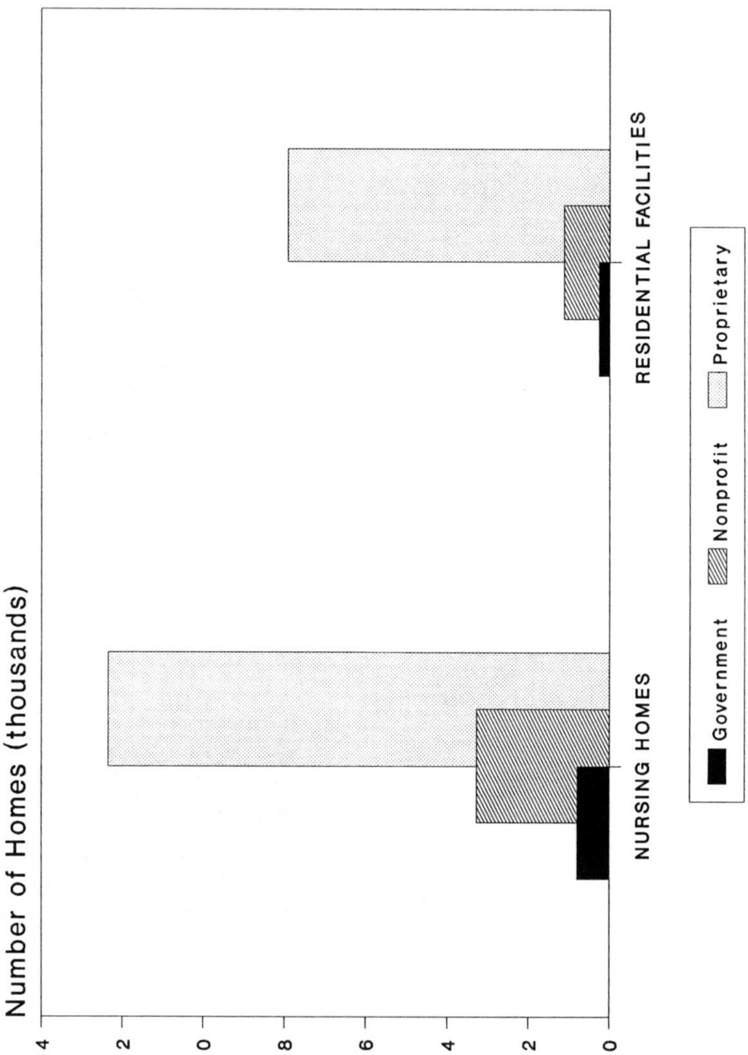

Source: U.S. National Center for Health Statistics

Chapter 8

PHARMACEUTICAL HUMAN RESOURCES

Includes trends in retail manpower, hospital manpower, degree rise, influx, dropout, and productivity

U.S. Health Industry Personnel

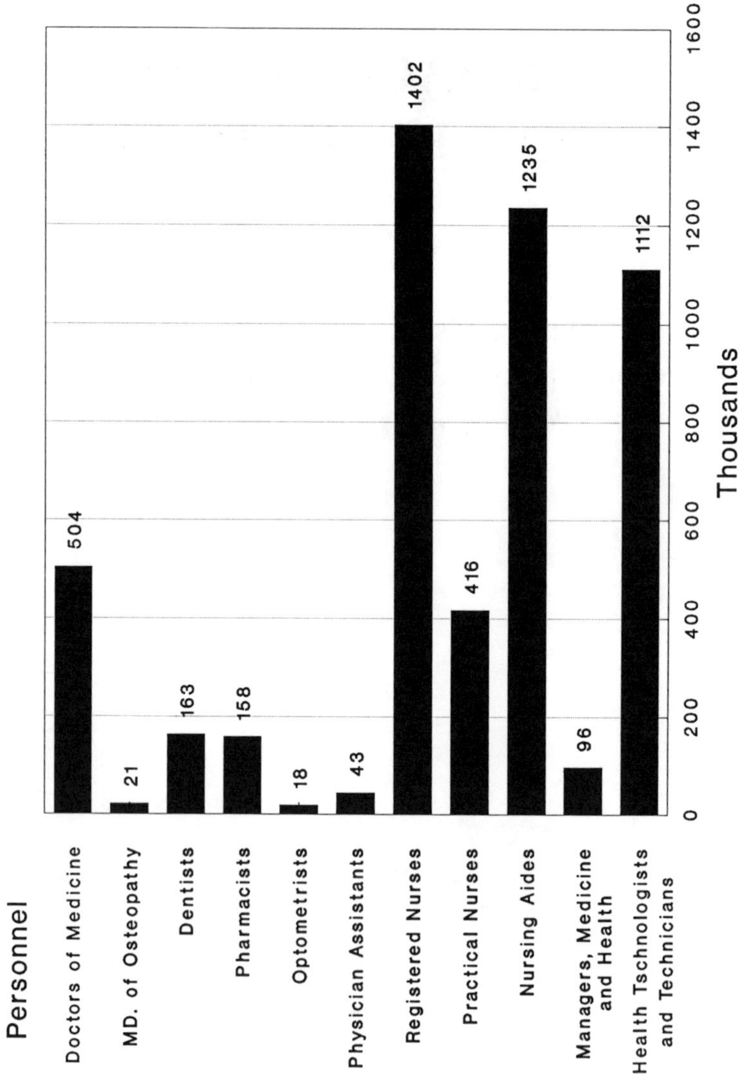

Source: Business Mailers, 1986
1986 Statistical Abstract of U.S.

Total Health Care Employment: No Direct Patient Care

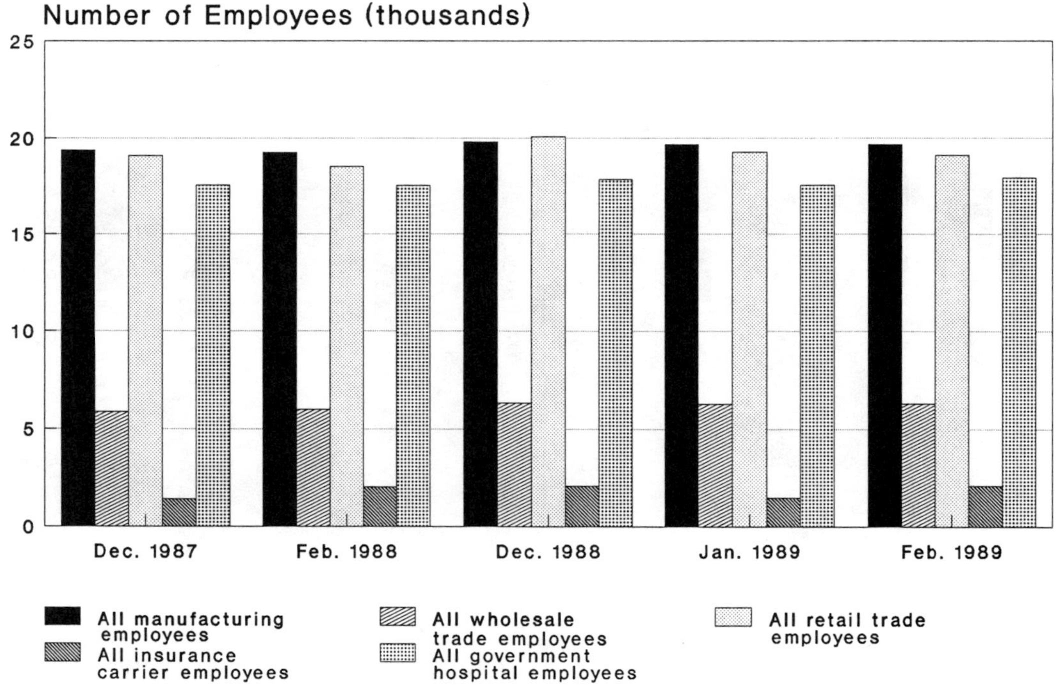

Sources: U.S. Department of Labor, Bureau of Labor Statistics, "Employment and Earnings", Table C-2, April 1989 and earlier issues.

Health Care Employment: Direct Patient Care

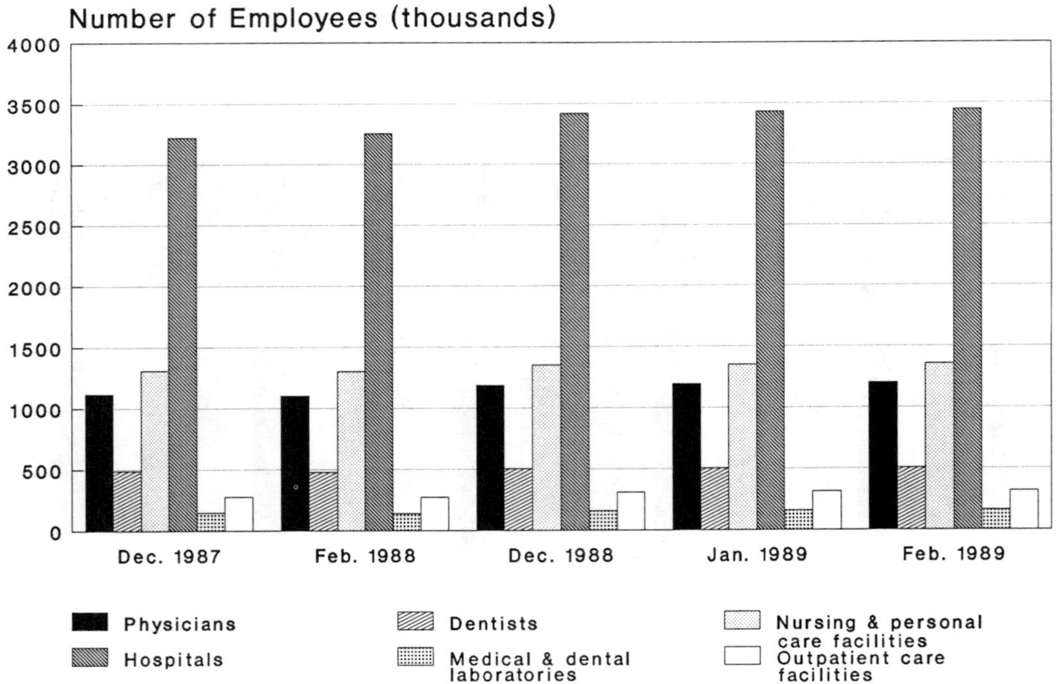

U.S. Department of Labor, Bureau of Labor Statistics, " Employment and Earning", Table C-2, April 1989 and earlier issues.

Food and Drug Administration Staffing Levels

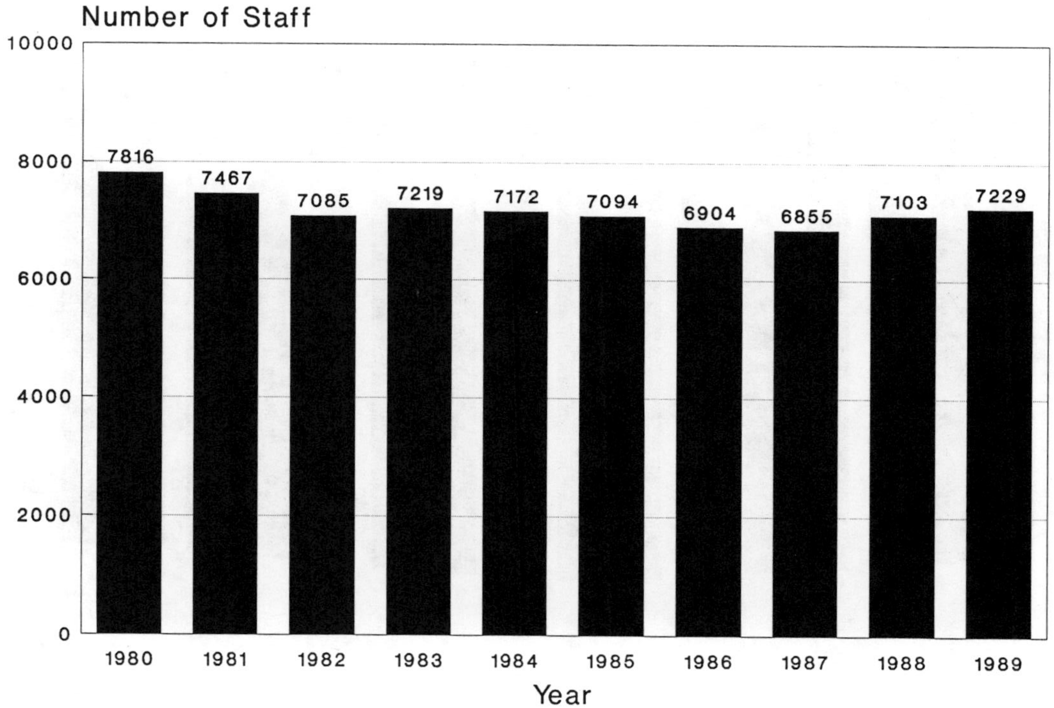

Source: GAO/HRD-89-142 FDA Resources, September 1989.

Pharmacy Manpower
1975-1990

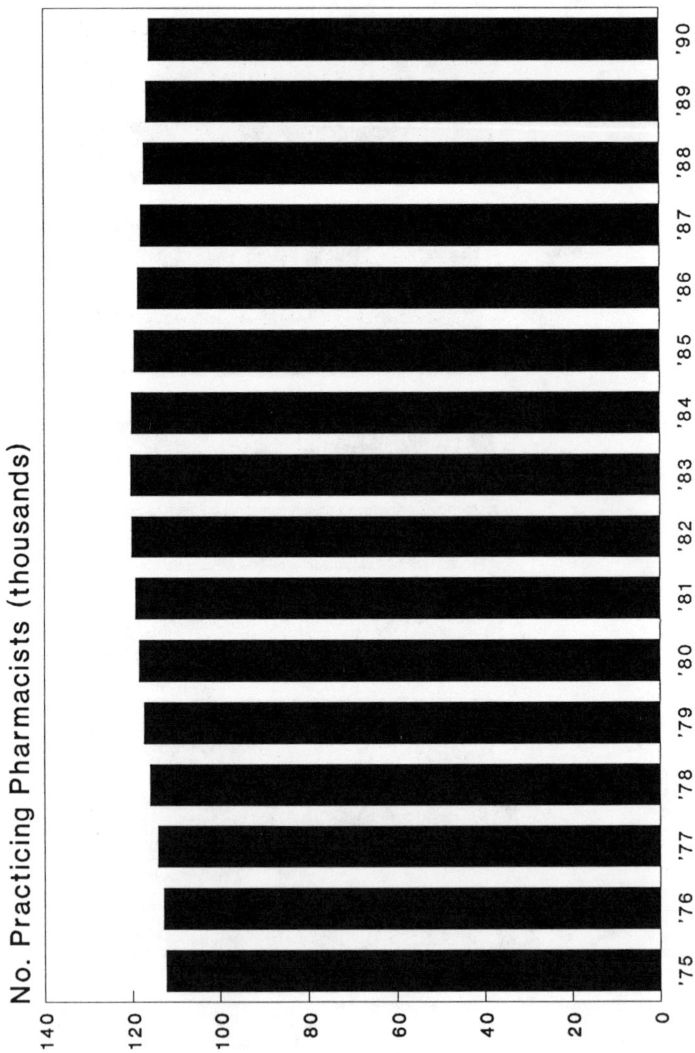

Source: American Journal of Hospital Pharmacy, Vol.45, Oct. 1988.

Pharmacist Employment (1st Qtr. 1989)

Total No. 62,194

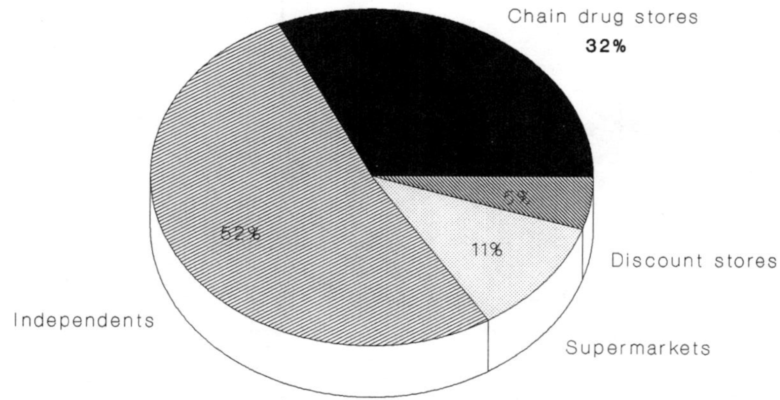

Source: Chain Drug Review July 3, 1989.

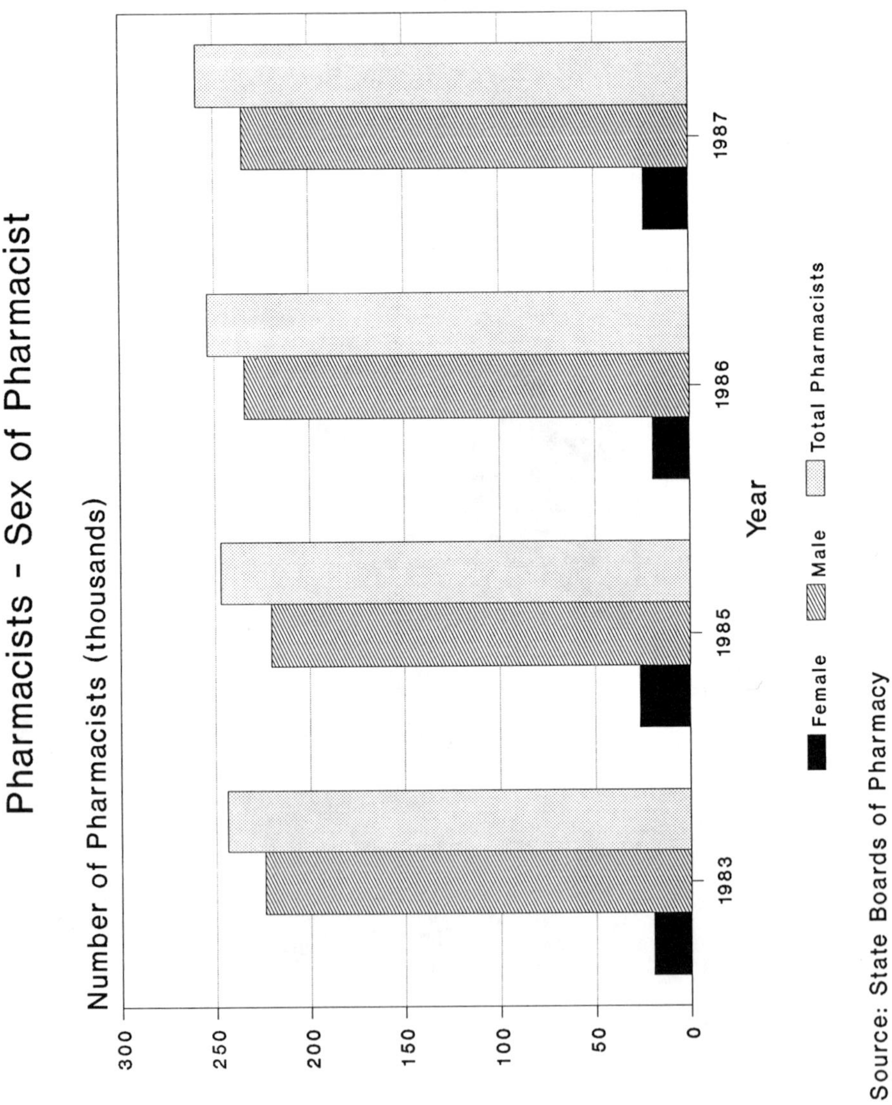
Pharmacists - Sex of Pharmacist
Number of Pharmacists (thousands)
300
250
200
150
100
50
0
1983
1985
1986
1987
Year
Female
Male
Total Pharmacists
Source: State Boards of Pharmacy

Chain Drug Store Personnel: 1987

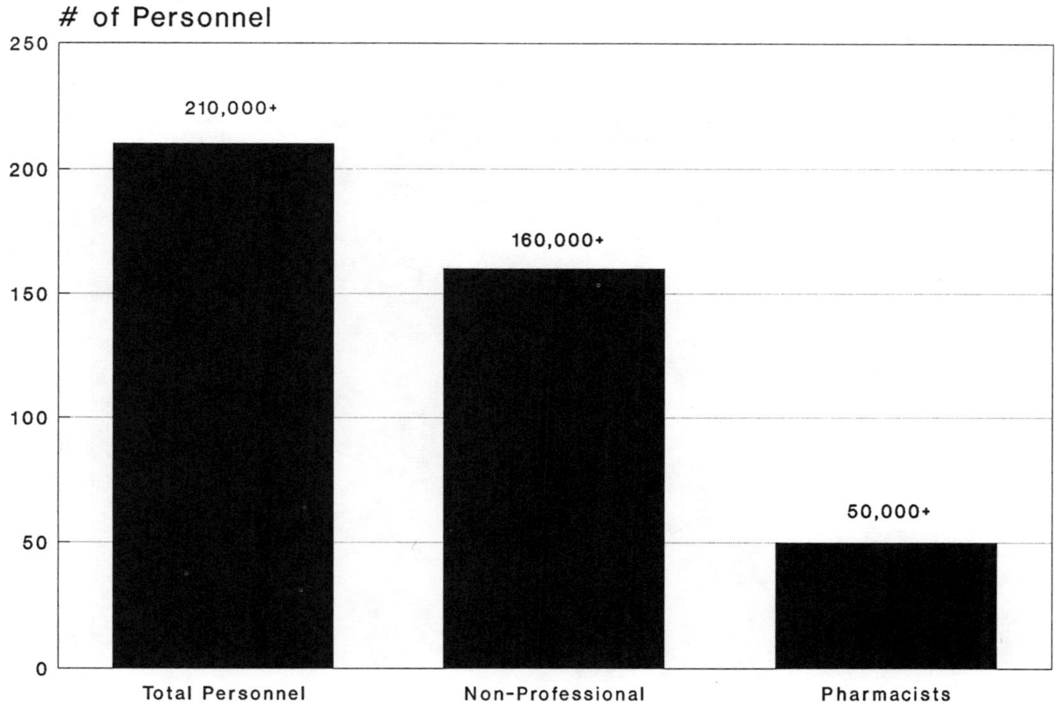

NACDS Resource Guide, The Chain Drug Store Industry and the Retail Prescription Market.

Pharmacists - Licensing Status Trends

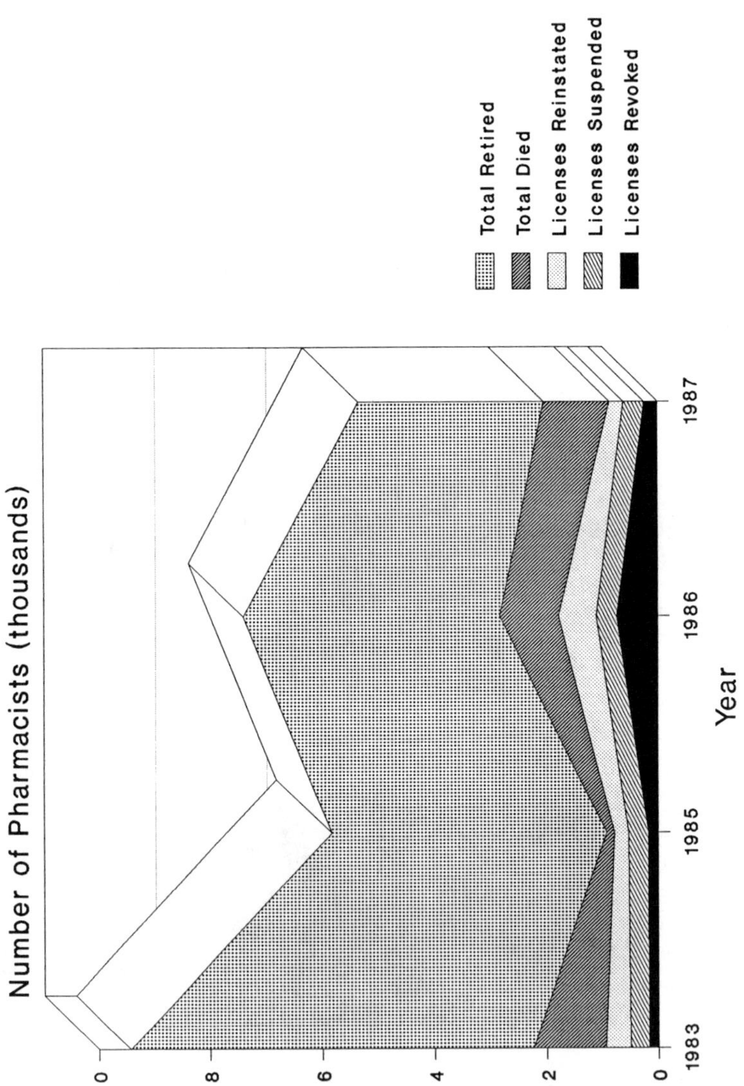

Source: State Boards of Pharmacy, 1983-1987.

Pharmacists - Total Number Licensed

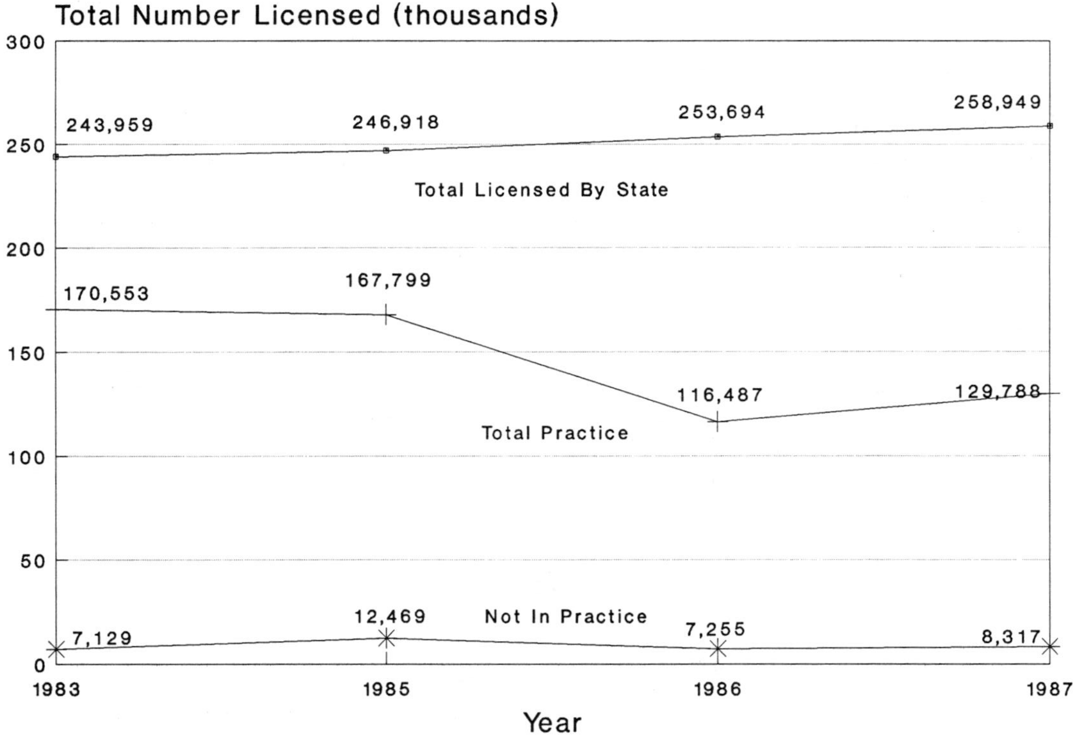

Source: State Boards of Pharmacy, 1983, 1985-1987.

Licensed Pharmacies (1983-1987)

Number as of Decembers 31 each year

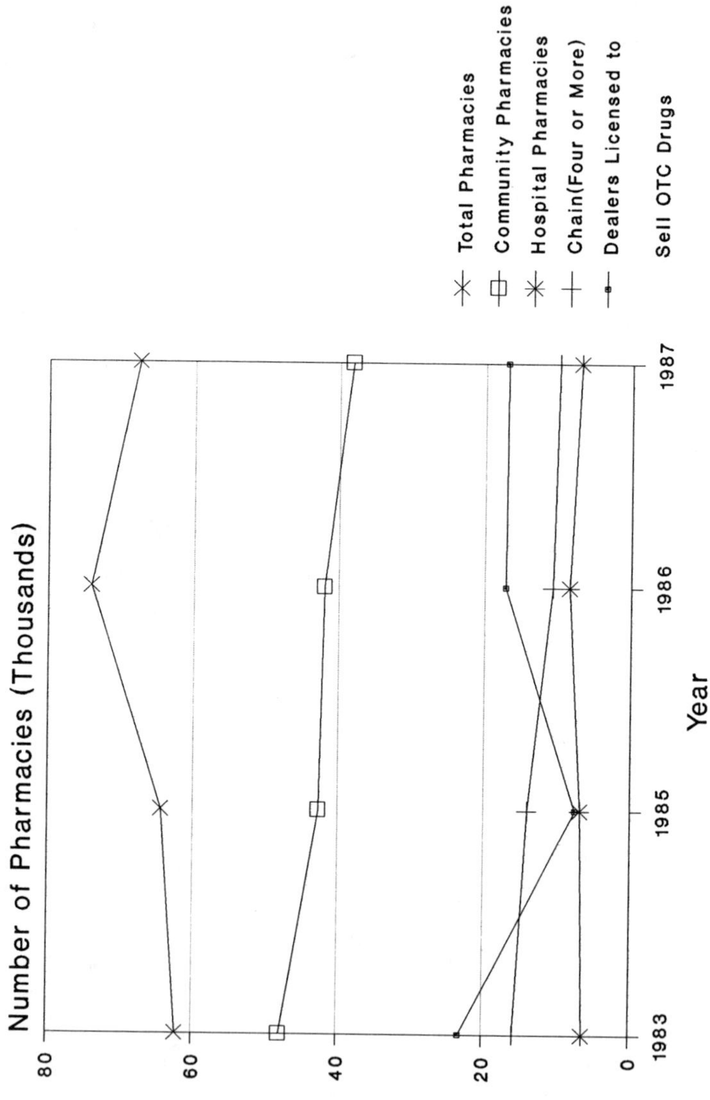

Source: State Boards of Pharmacy, 1983-1987.

Pharmacists - Total Number by Practice
(1987)

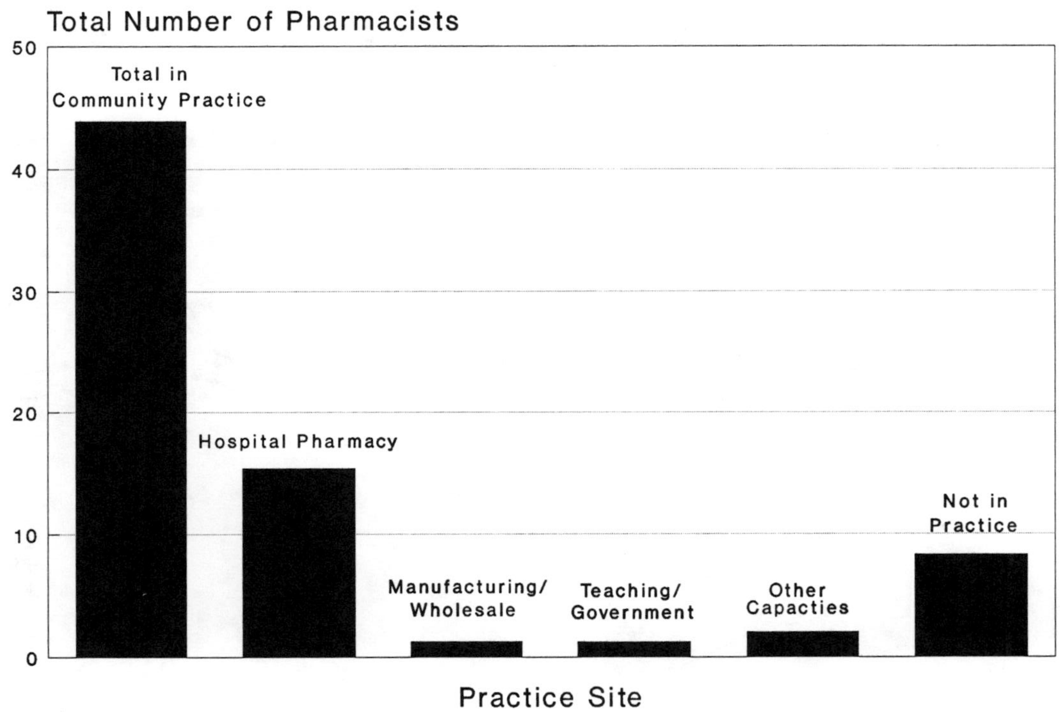

Source: State Boards of Pharmacy, 1983-1987.

Bachelor of Science Degrees Conferred

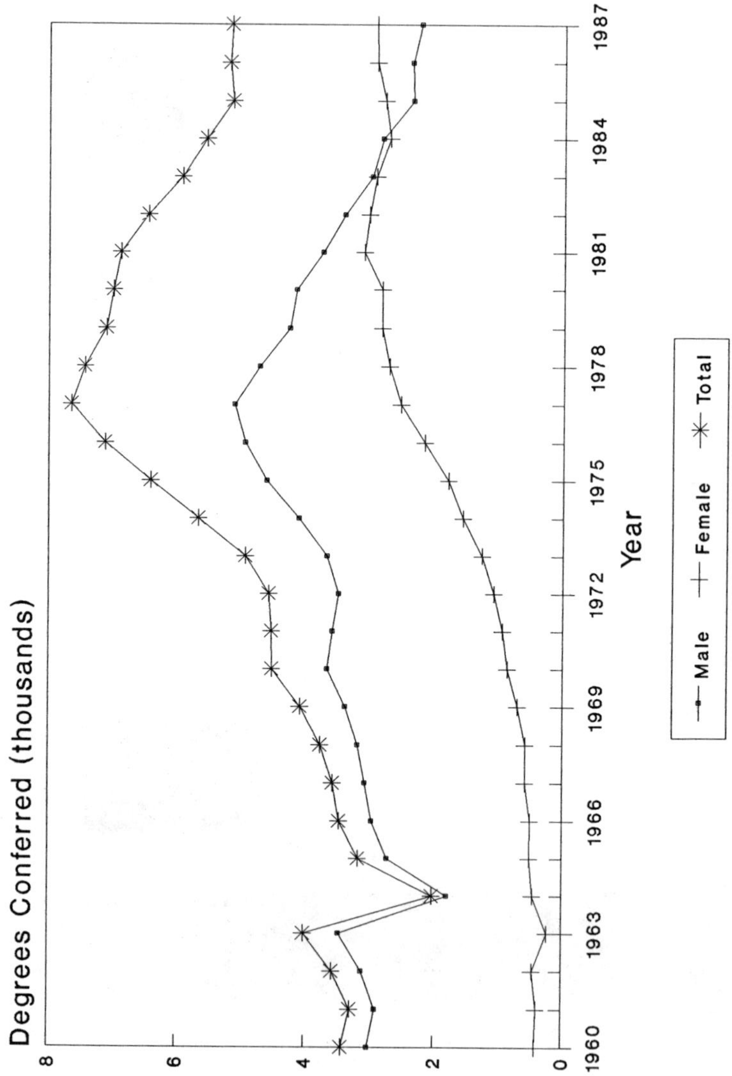

Source: American Journal of Pharmaceutical Education, Vol. 52, Fall 1988

Doctor of Pharmacy as the First Professional Degree Conferred, 1960-1987

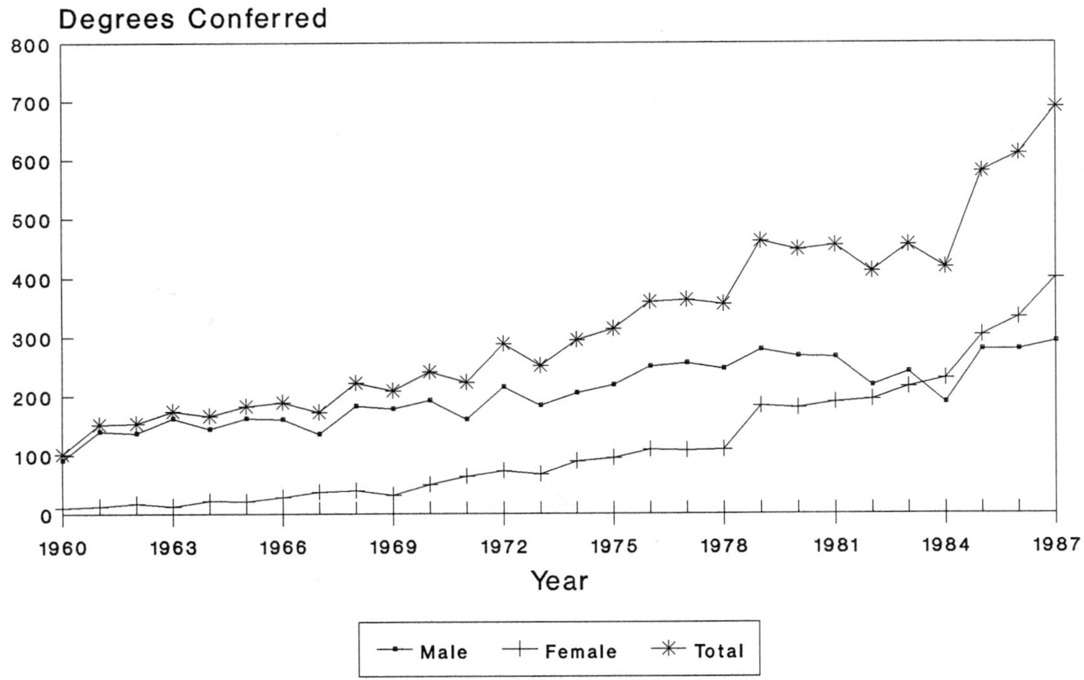

Source:American Journal of
Pharmaceutical Education, Vol.52
Fall 1988

Master of Science Degrees Conferred

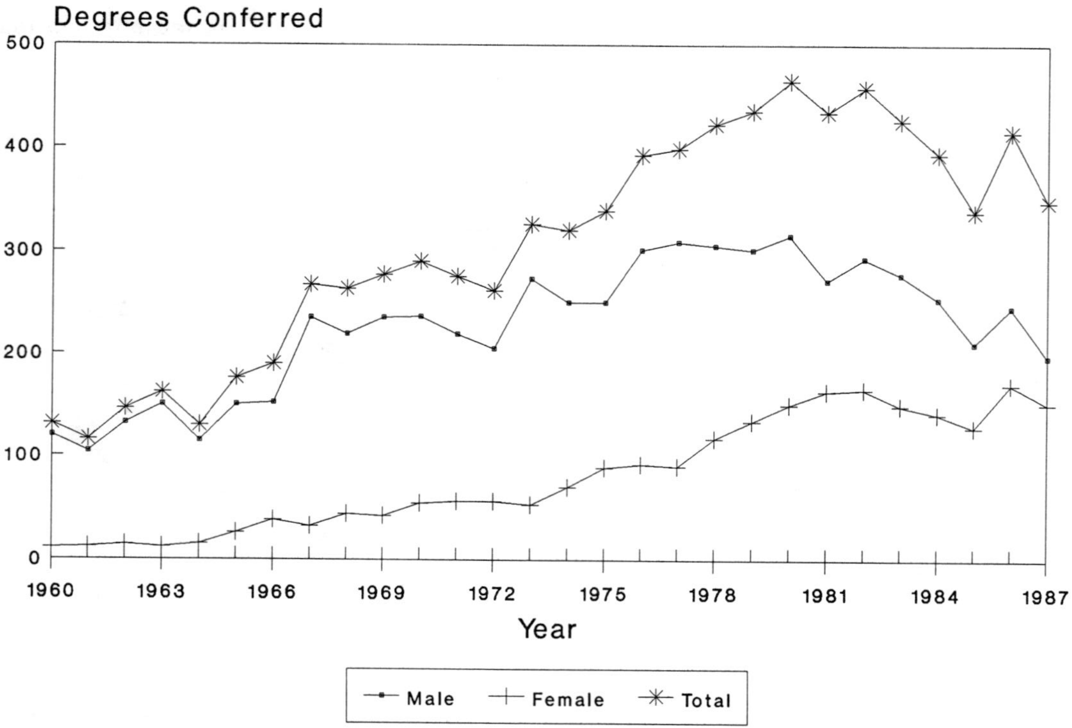

Source: American Journal of Pharmaceutical Education, Vol.52, Fall 1988

Doctor of Philisophy Degrees Conferred

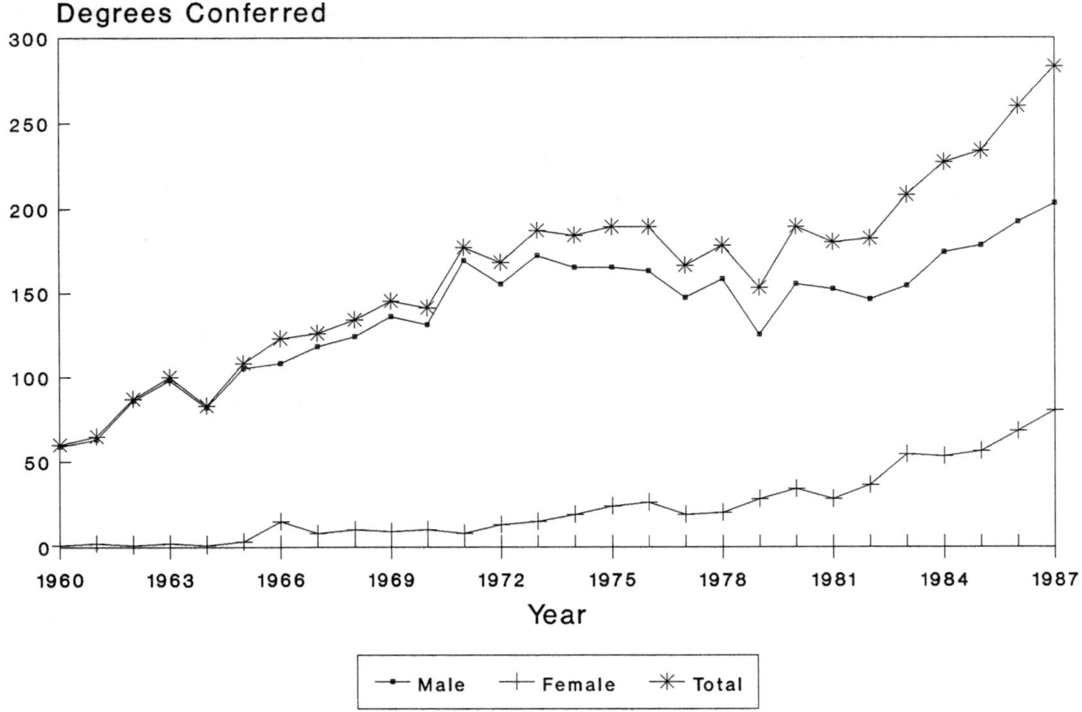

Source: American Journal of
Pharmaceutical Education, Vol.52
Fall 1988

Total Pharmacy Degrees Conferred

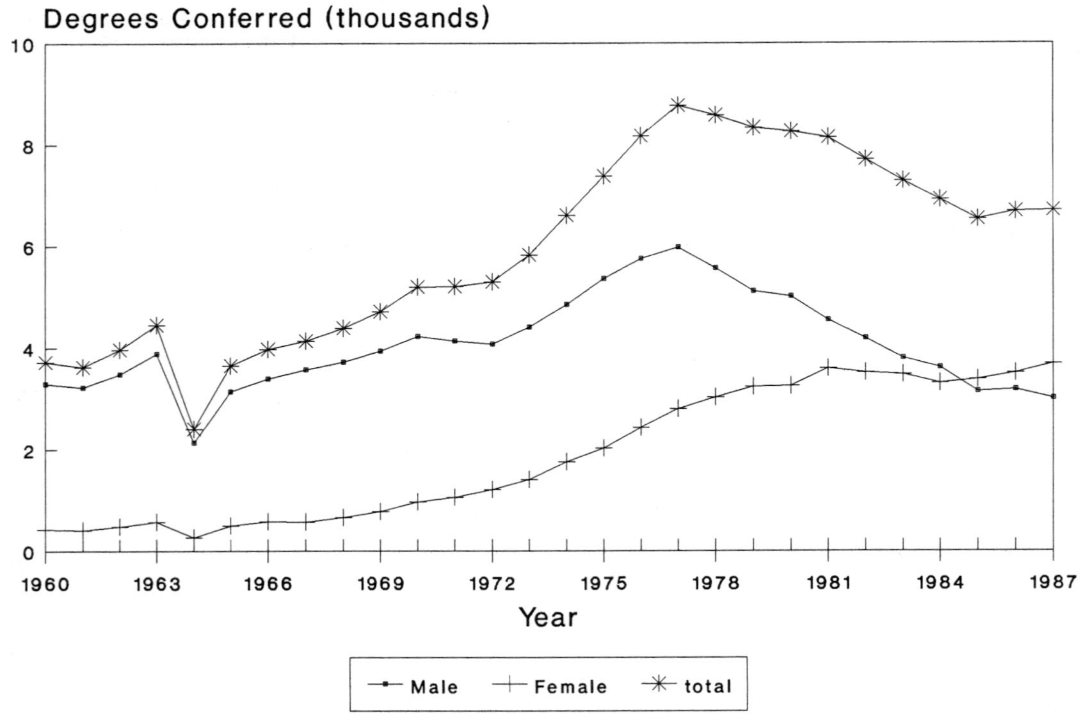

Source: American Journal of
Pharmaceutical Education, Vol.52
Fall 1988

Pharmacy Degrees Conferred by Ethnic Group, 1976-1987

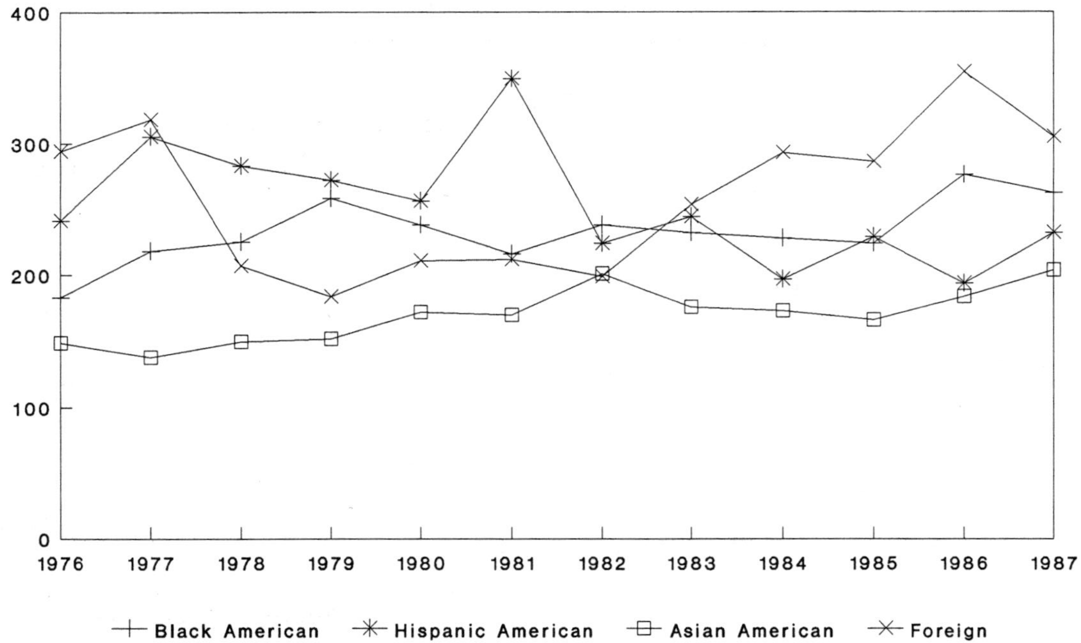

Source: American Journal of Pharmaceutical Education, Vol.52 Fall 1988

Entry Level Degrees Conferred in the Northeast, South, Midwest and West Regions, 1976-1987

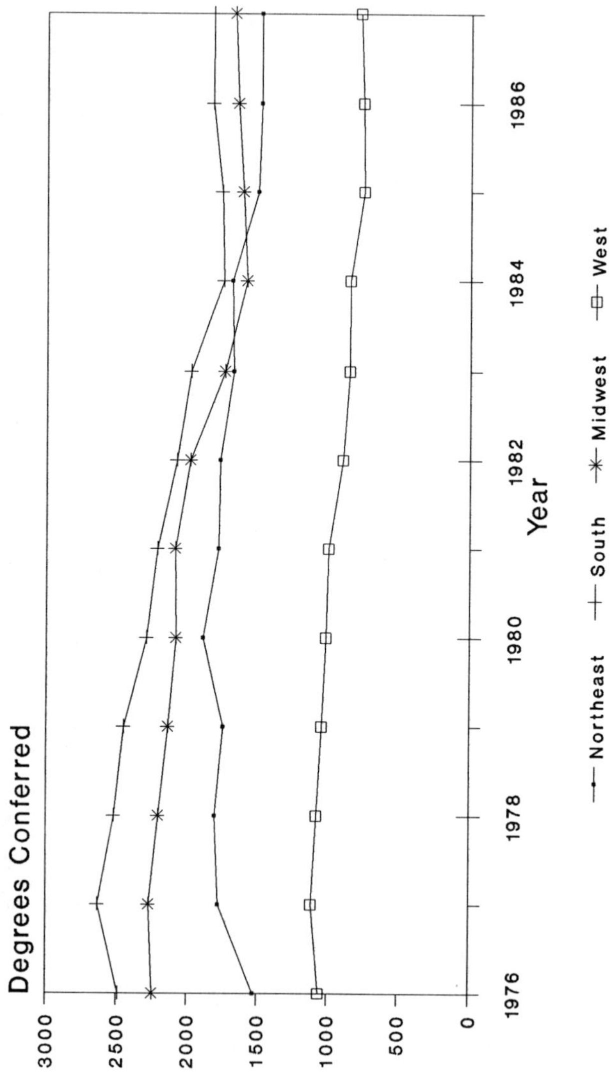

Source: American Journal of Pharmaceutical Education, Vol.52, Fall 1988

Pharmaceutical Science Graduate Studies: Enrollment of Pharmacists

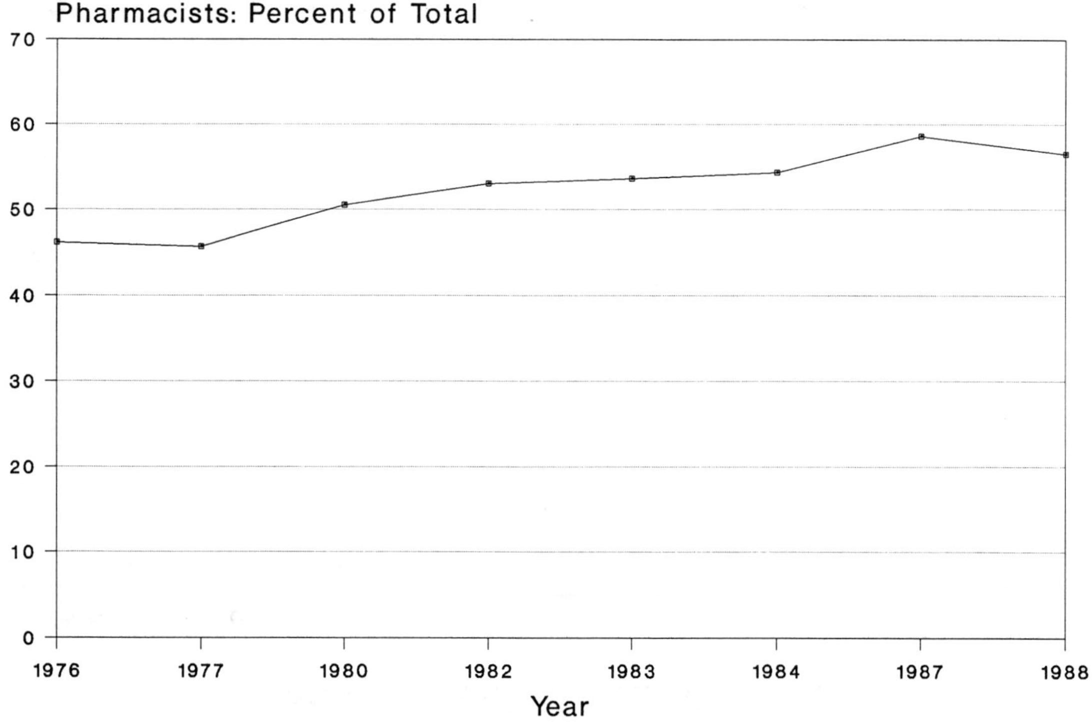

Source: AJPE (Fall, 1988) and AACP 1989.

Pharmaceutical Science
Ph.D. Degrees Granted to Non-Americans as a Percent of Total Degrees

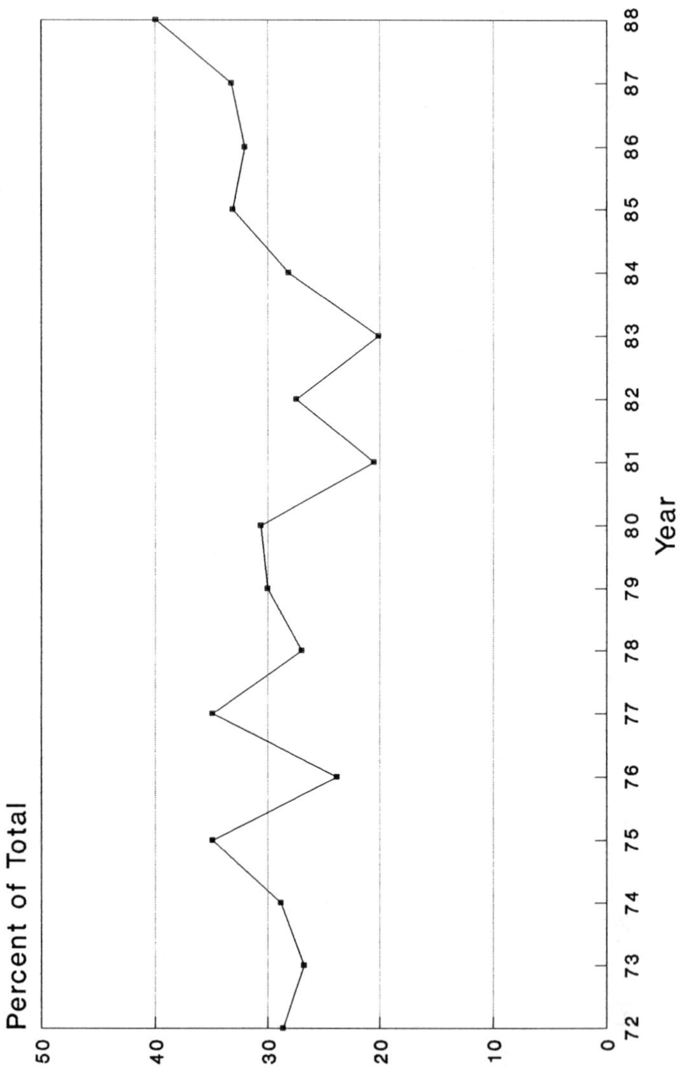

Source: AJPE (Fall, 1988) and AACP 1989.

Total Pharmaceutical Science Ph.D. Degrees Granted

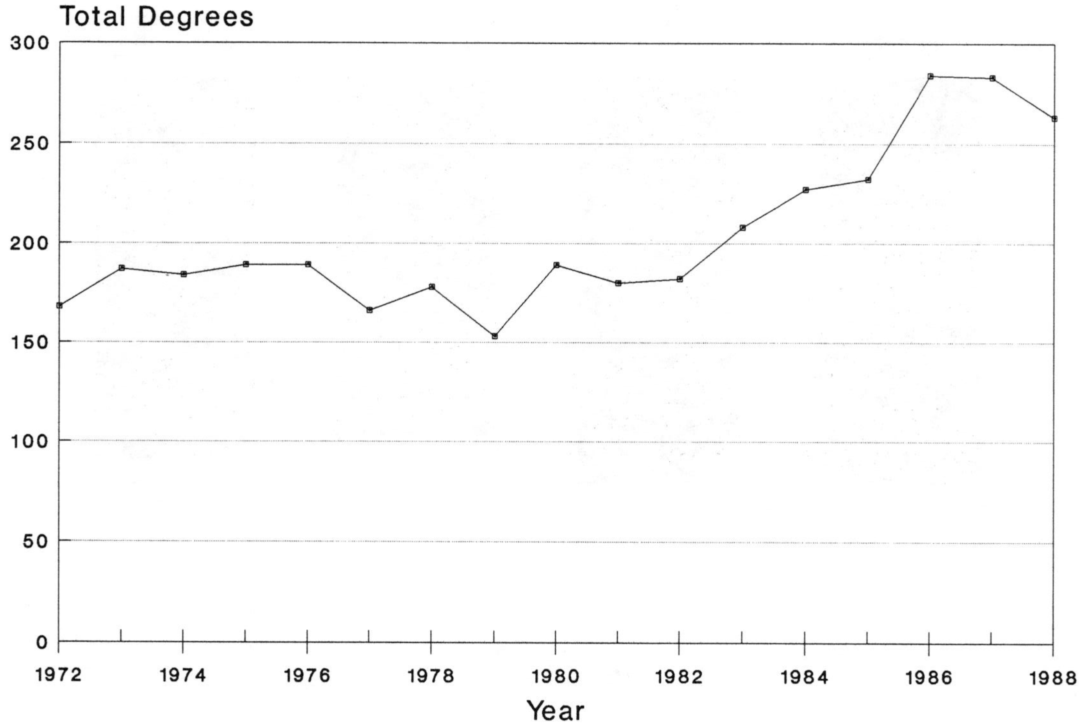

Source: AJPE (Fall, 1988) and AACP 1989.

Average Base Salaries for Pharmacists-How the Practice Settings Stack Up.

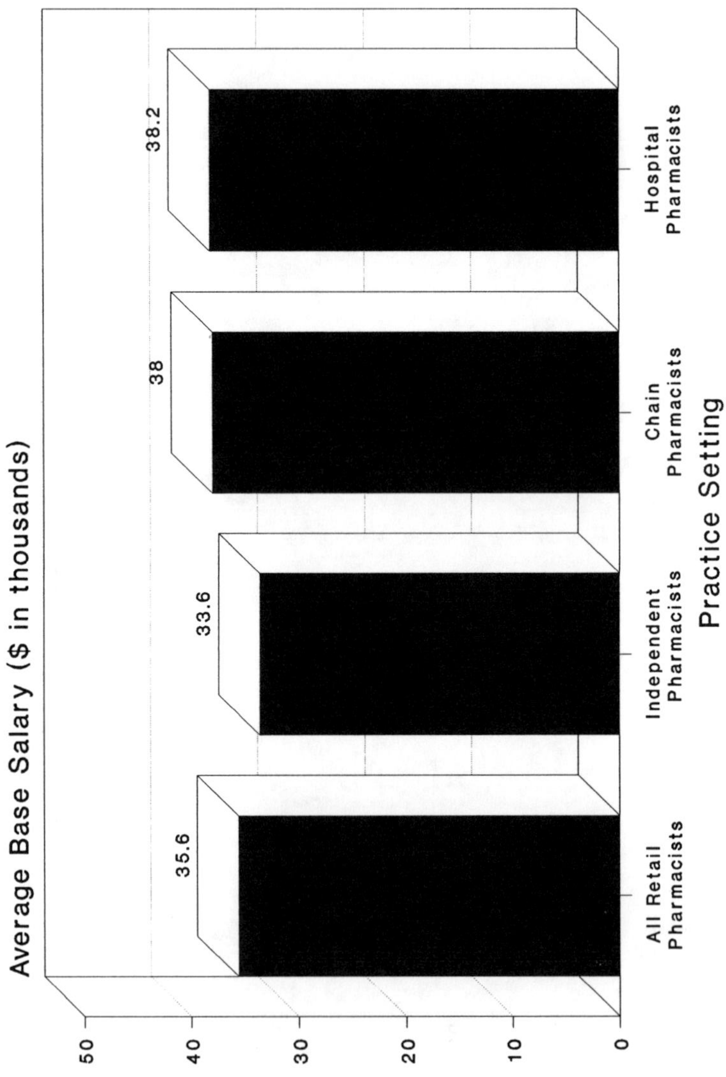

Source: Drug Topics, October 5, 1987

Average Total Compensation

By practice setting	Independents	Chains	Hospitals
	$41,546	$46,276	$43,894
By sex			
	$42,450	$47,105	$44,724
	37,266	43,313	41,293
By job title			
Store manager	$42,822	$48,017	
Chief/ supervising R.Ph.	43,764	46,807	
Staff	37,477	43,990	$40,427
Director			$45,486
By age			
Under 36	$40,932	$45,217	$42,129
36-45	43,005	48,088	45,338
46-plus	40,798	45,798	44,385
By store volume*			
Low	$38,964	$43,088	
Medium	40,255	45,653	
High	44,132	48,810	

*In the case of independents, low volume is under $500,000 per year; medium is $500,000-$749,000; and high is $750,000-plus. Among chains, low is under $750,000; medium is $740,000-$1,249,999; high is $1,250,000-plus.

Source: Drug Topics June 5, 1989

Average Overtime Earnings of Employee Pharmacists

By practice setting	Independents	Chains	Hospitals
	$6.614	$5,694	$4.061
By sex			
	$7,322	$5,652	$3,437
	3,021	5,216	6,838
By job title			
Store manager	$6,708	$6,328	
Chief/ supervising R.Ph.	7,264	5,496	
Staff	5,429	5,502	$2,683
Director			6,510

Source: Drug Topics June 5, 1989

Total Average Compensation by Region
1989

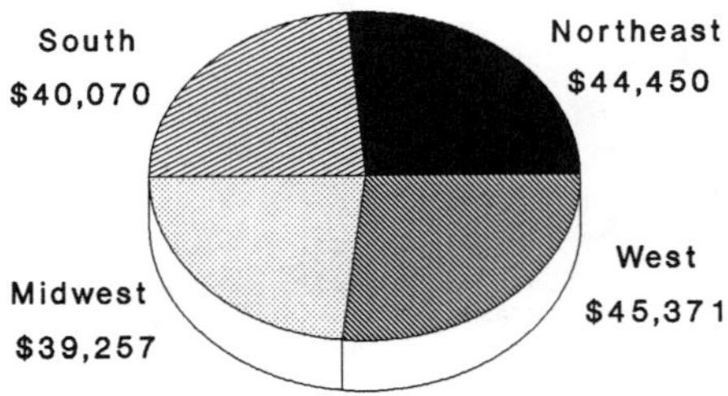

Independents

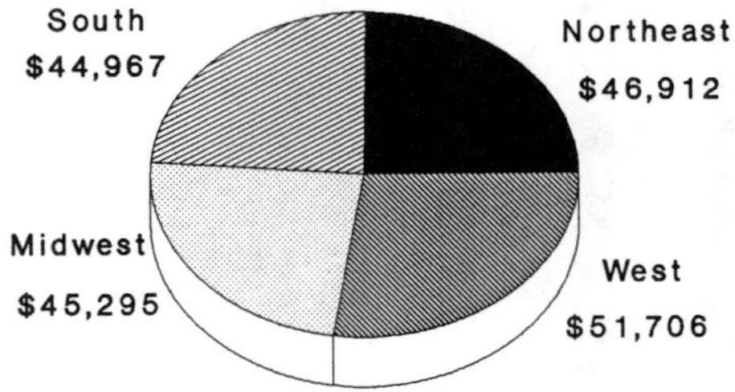

Chains

Source: Drug Topics June 5, 1989

HOURS WORKED BY EMPLOYED PHARMACISTS: 1986 AND 1987

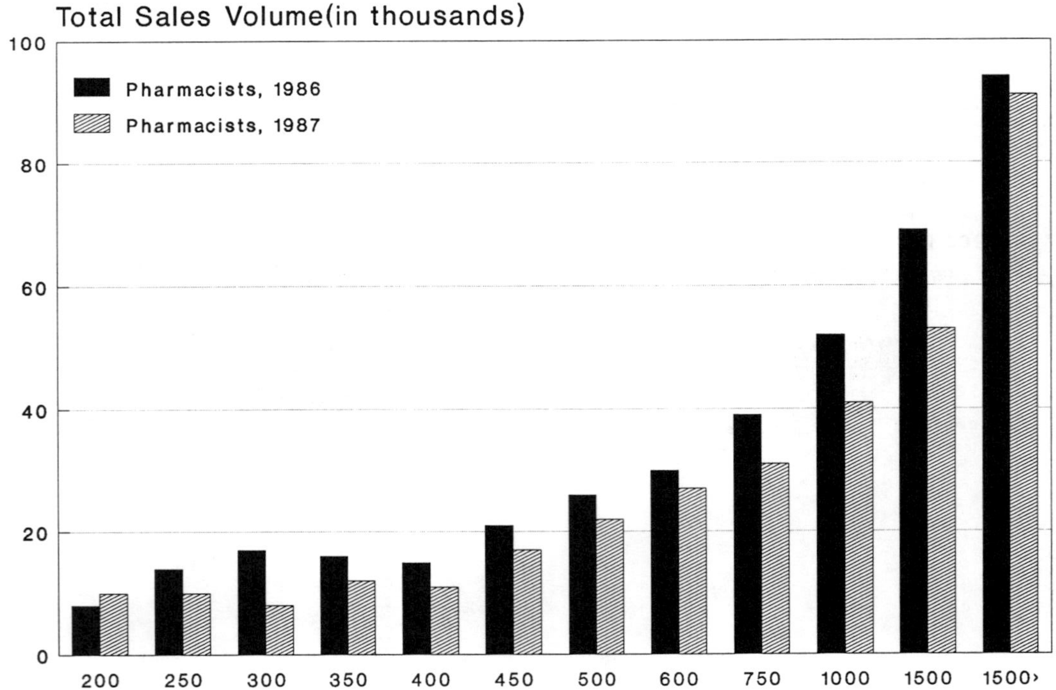

Source: Lilly Digest, 1987 & 1988

Fringe Benefits-
How Widespread Are They ?

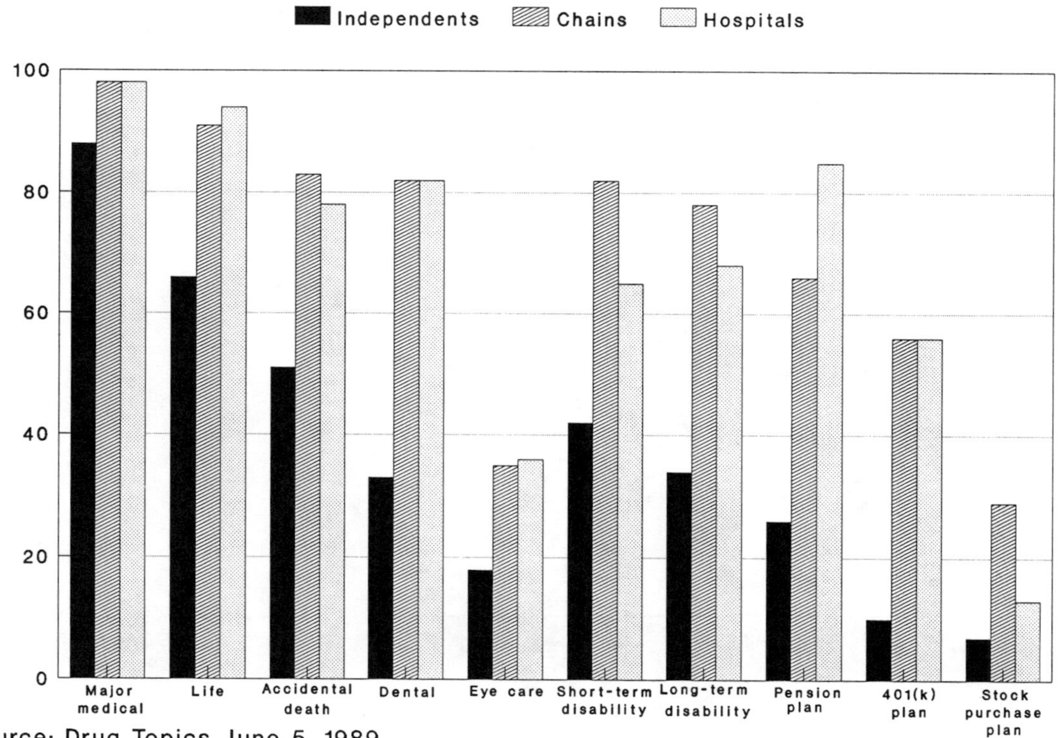

Source: Drug Topics June 5, 1989

Hospital Pharmacy: Pharmacist, Technician, and Support Personnel Hours/Week, 1987

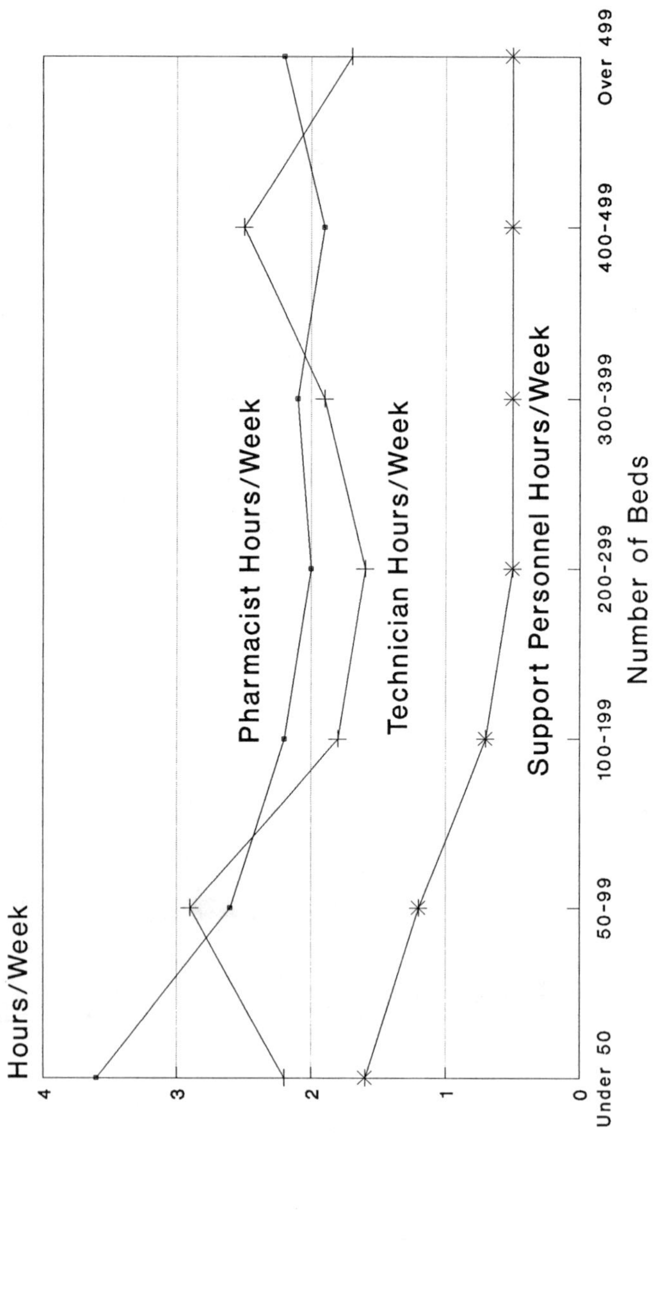

Source: 1988 Lilly Hospital Pharmacy Survey

Pharmacy Personnel Hours in Average Private Nonprofit Hospital

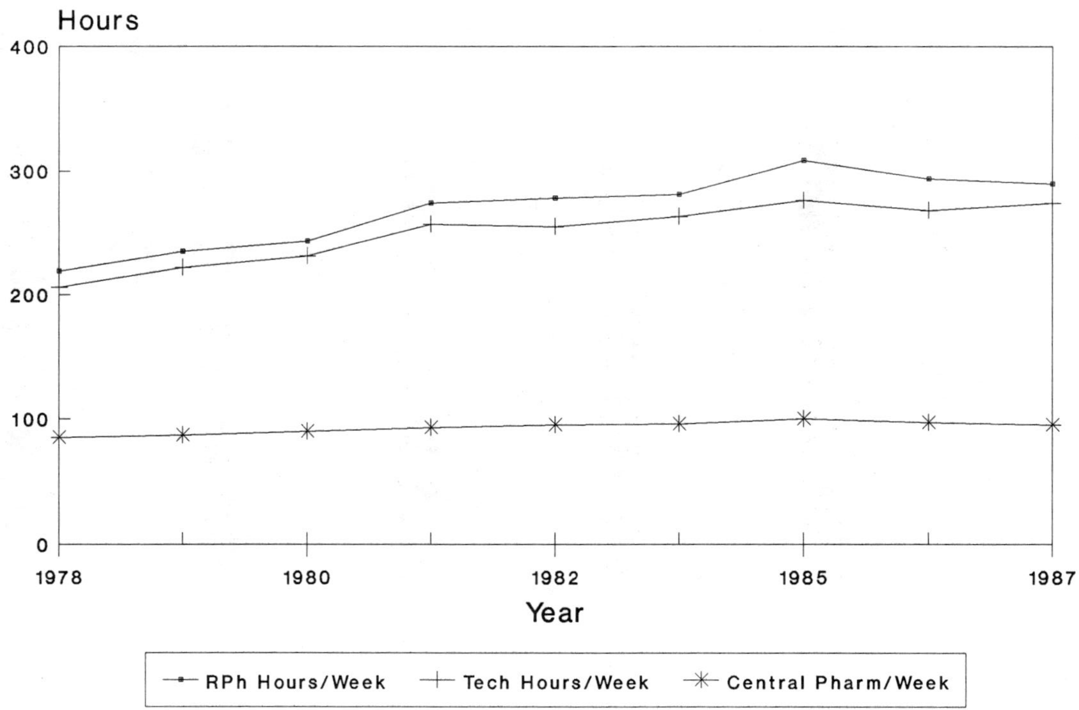

Source: Lilly Hospital Pharmacy Survey, 1988

Average Hourly Earnings of Health Care Production and Nonsupervisory Workers

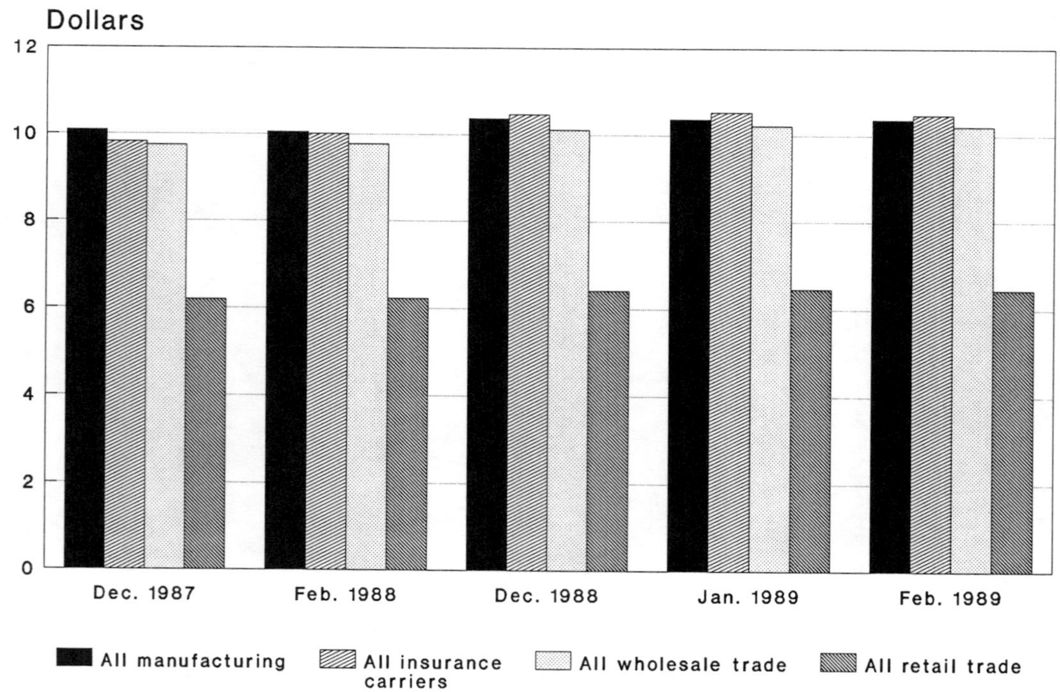

Sources: U.S. Department of Labor, Bureau of Labor Statistics, "Employment and Earnings", Table C-2, April 1989 and earlier issues.

Average Hourly Earnings of Health Care Production and Nonsupervisory Workers: Health Services

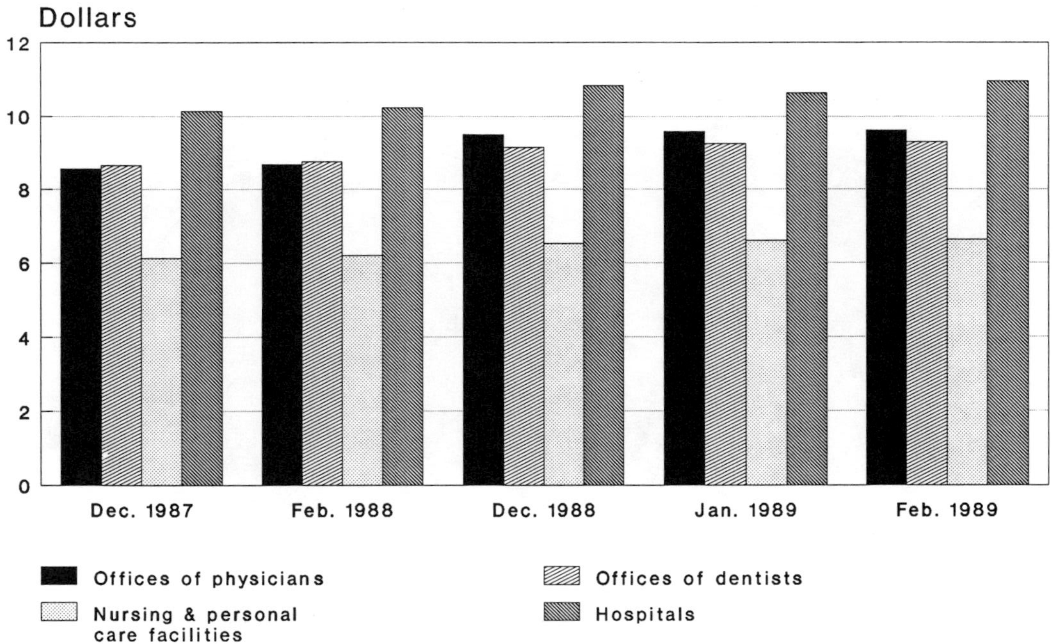

Sources: U.S. Department of Labor, Bureau of Labor Statistics, "Employment and Earnings", Table C-2, April 1989 and earlier issues.

Indexes of Productivity U.S. Pharmaceutical Industry and U.S. Private Non-Farm Business

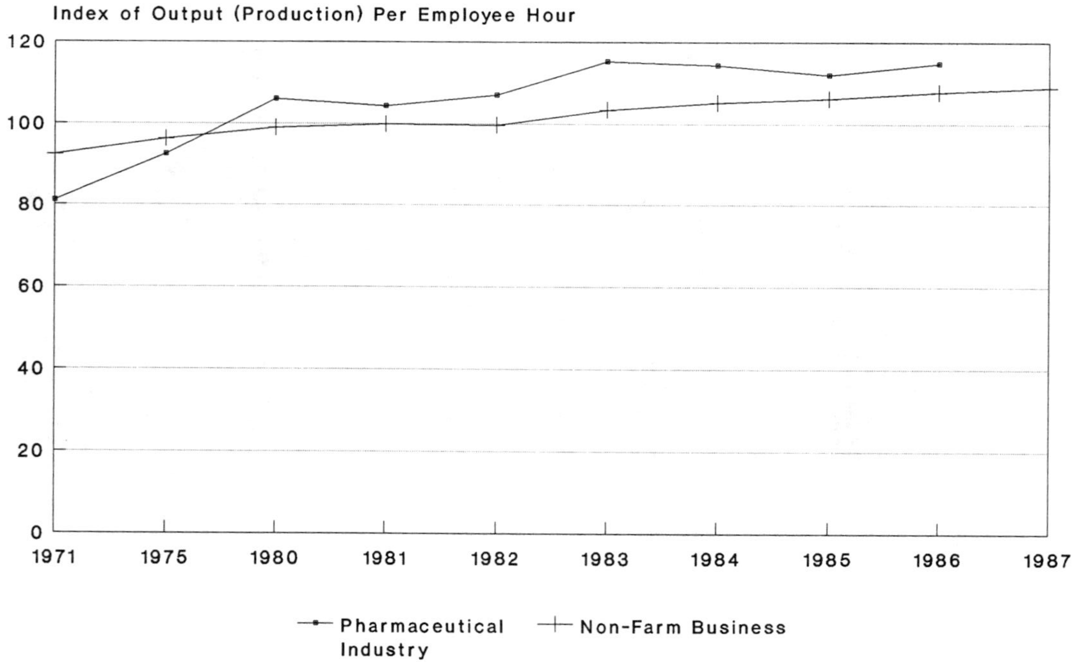

Source: Office of Publications, U.S. Bureau of Labor Statistics, U.S. Department of Labor, (various series).

1987 Pharmaceutical Industry data not available

Annual Percent Change in Employment

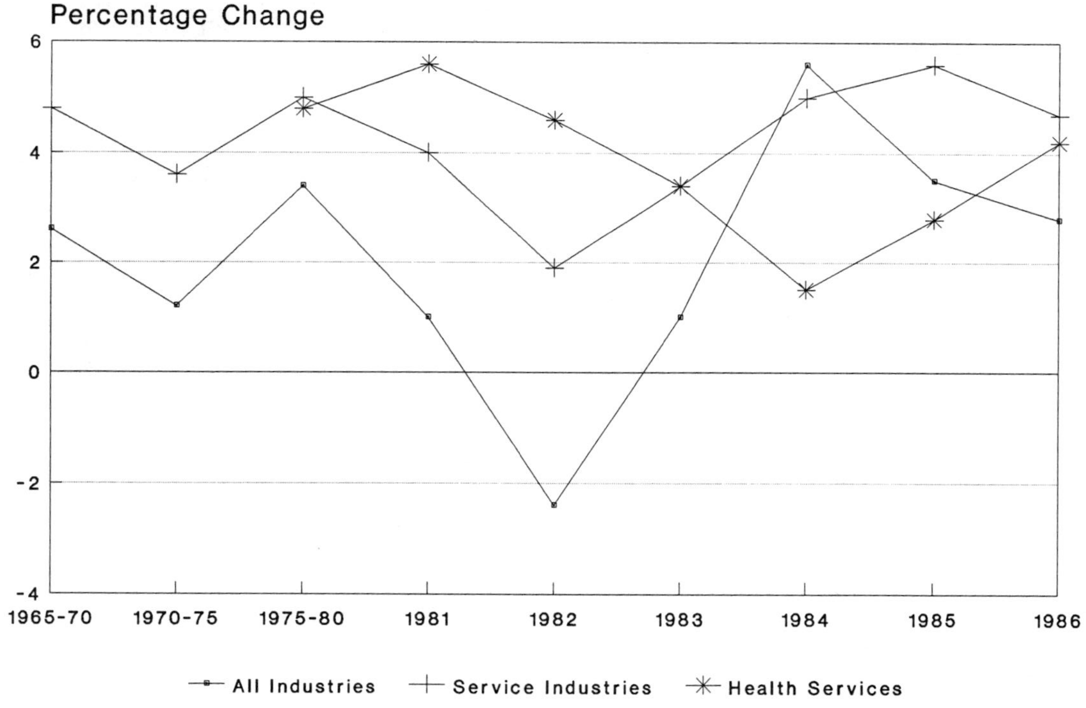

Source: Bureau of Labor Statistics:
Employment and Earnings. Washington.U.S.
Government Printing Office, 1986 & 1987.

Annual Percent Change in Workhours

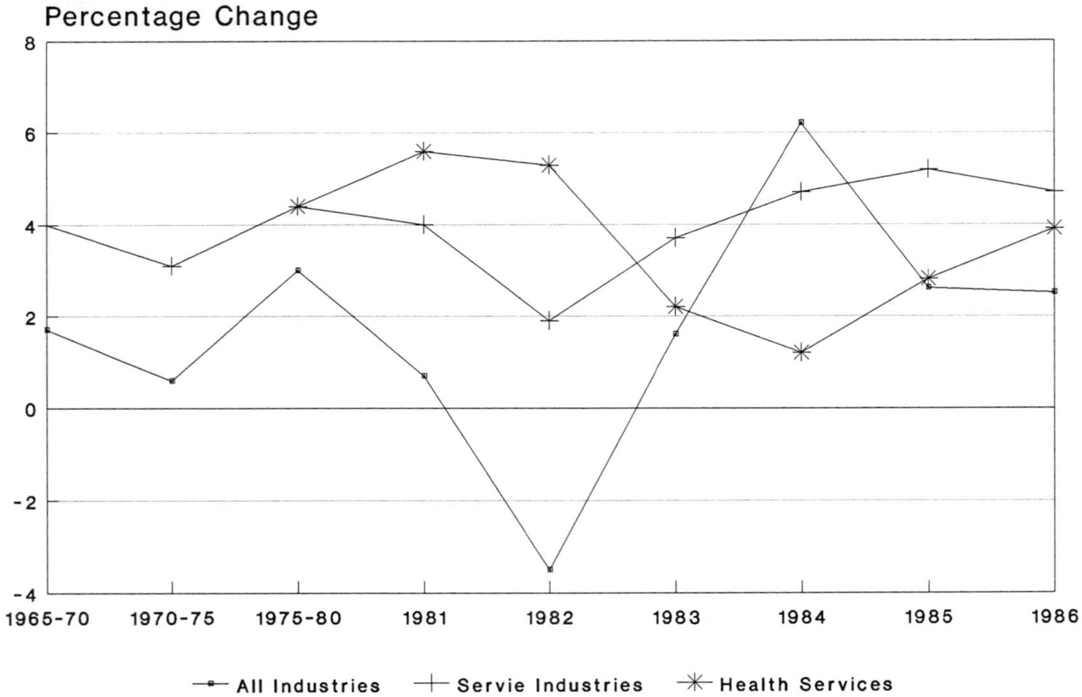

Source: Bureau of Labor Statistics:
Employment and Earnings. Washington.U.S.
Government Printing Office, 1986 & 1987.

Annual Percent Change in Earnings

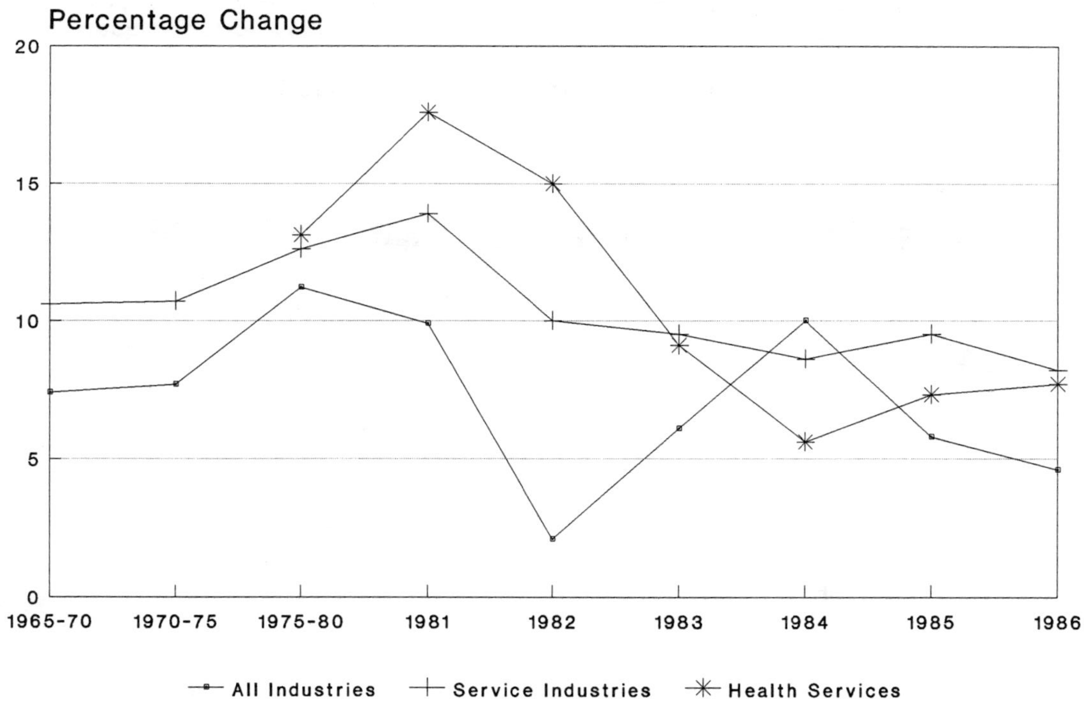

Source: Bureau of Labor Statistics:
Employment and Earnings. Washington.U.S.
Government Printing Office, 1986 & 1987.

Physicians, Dentists and Nurses: 1960 to 1986

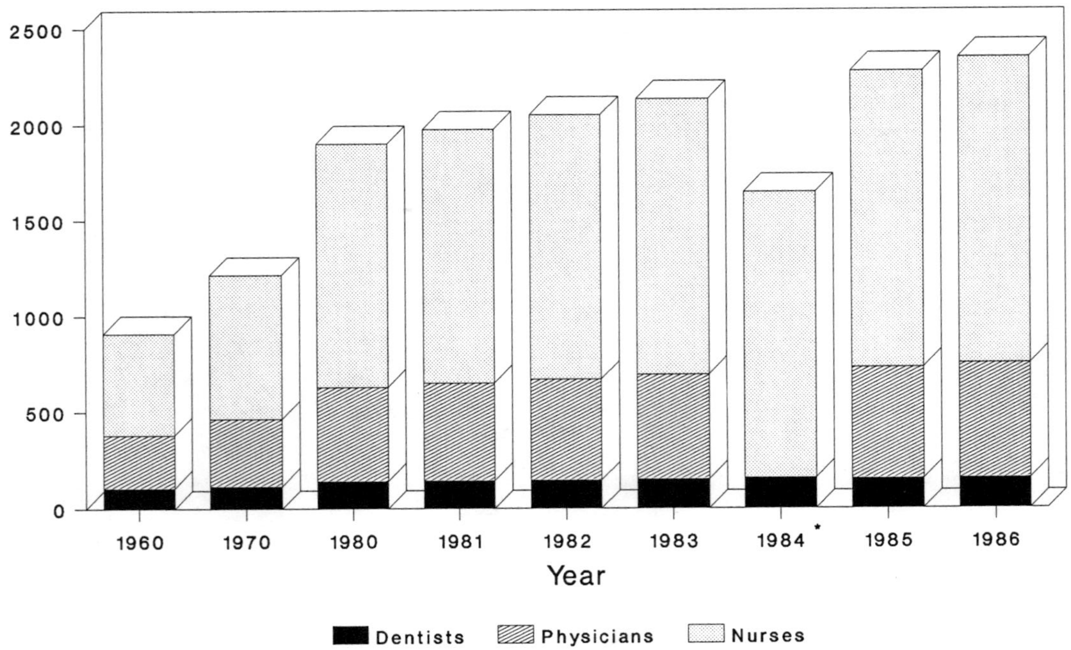

Source: U.S. Department of Health and Human Services, 1989 Statistical Abstract.

* 1984 physician data unavailable

Active U.S. Physician Population

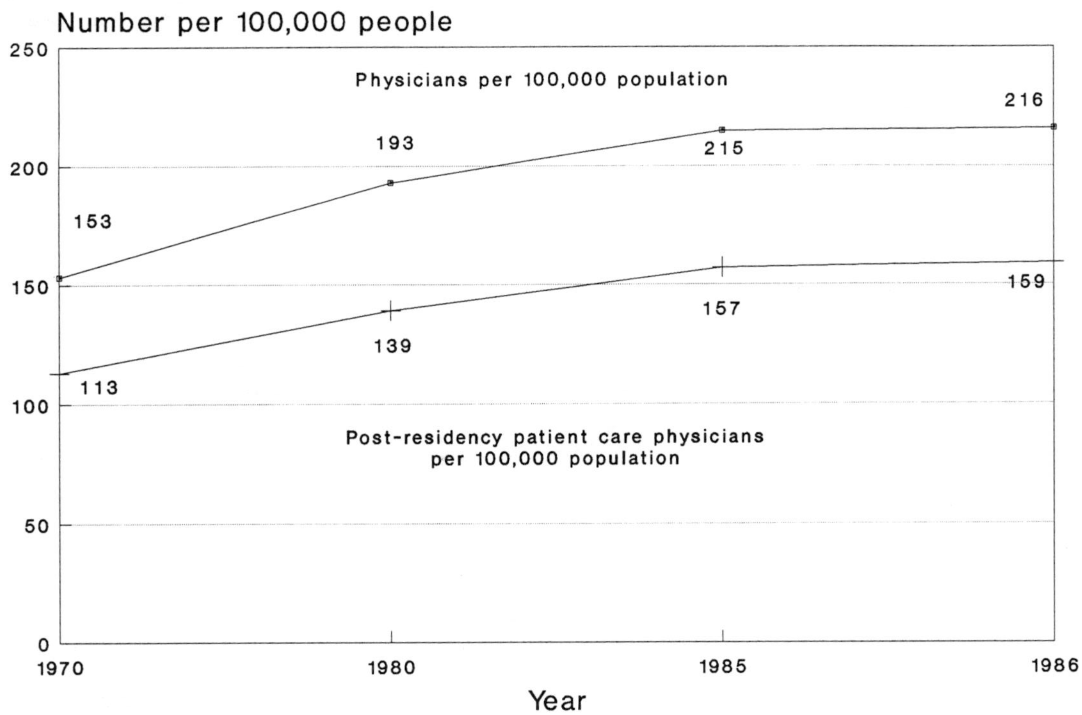

Source: AMA Physician Masterfile 1970-86, Department of Data Release Services

Active U.S. Physician Population for Selected Years: 1970-1986

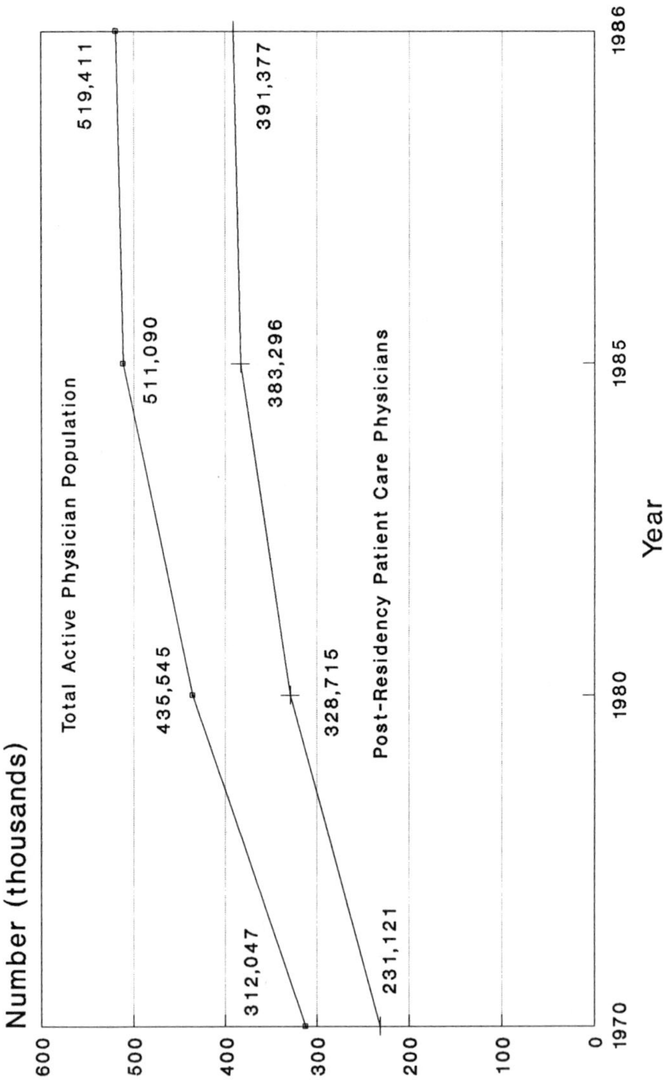

Source: AMA Physician Masterfile, 1970-1986, Department of Data Release Services

Projected Percent Distribution of U.S. Active Physician Population 1986-2010

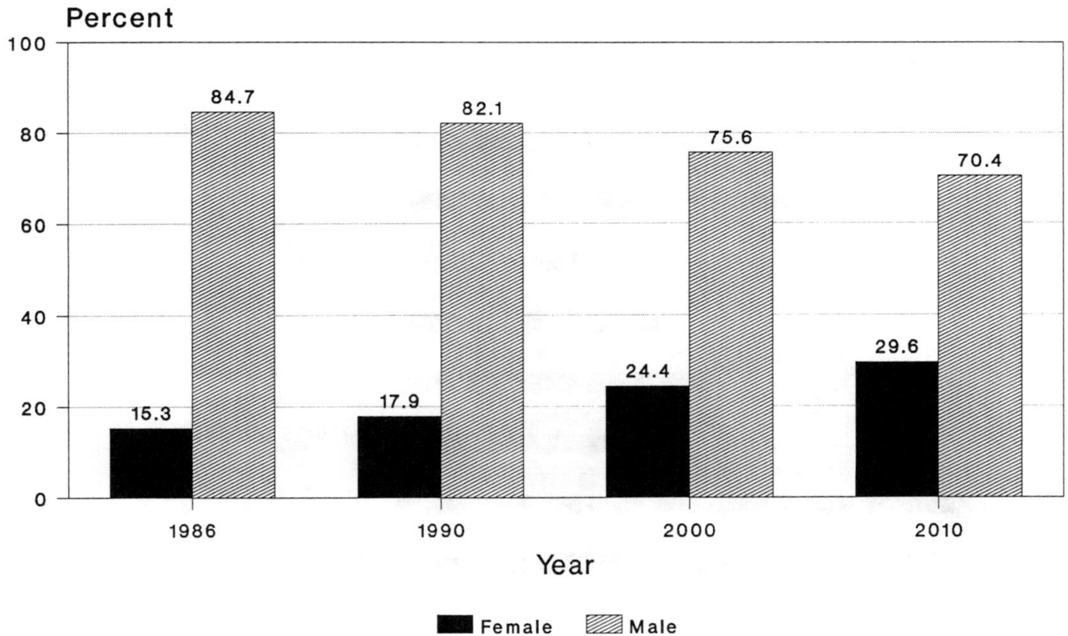

Source: AMA Demographic Model of the Physician Population

Projected Percent Distribution of Active Physician Population by Specialty

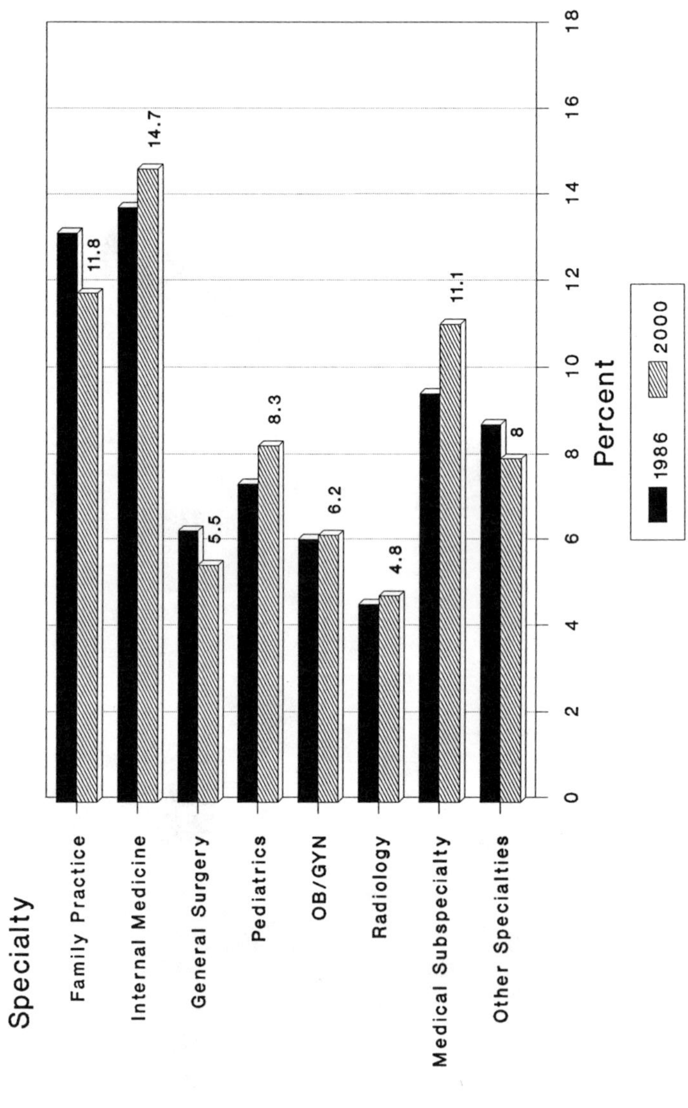

Source: AMA Demographic Model of the PPhysician Population, 1988

Post-Resident U.S. Physician Population in Direct Patient Care by Specialty

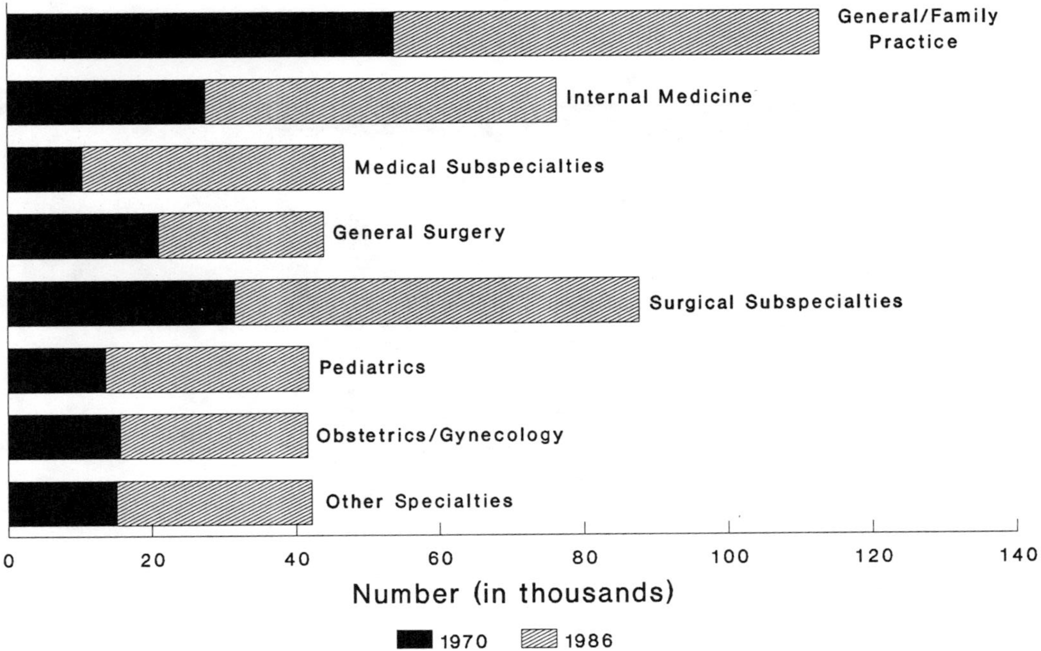

Source: AMA Center for Health Policy Research, 1988

Post-Resident U.S. Physician Population in Direct Patient Care

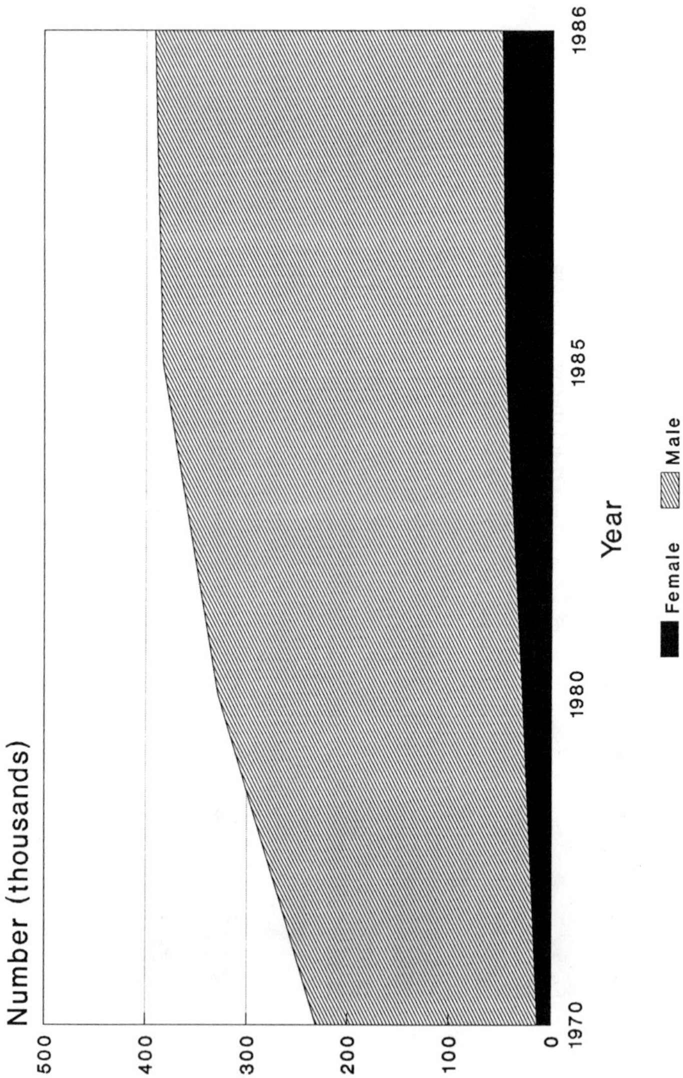

Source: AMA Center for Health Policy Research, 1988

Physician and Dental Visits Per Person by Sex: 1970-1986

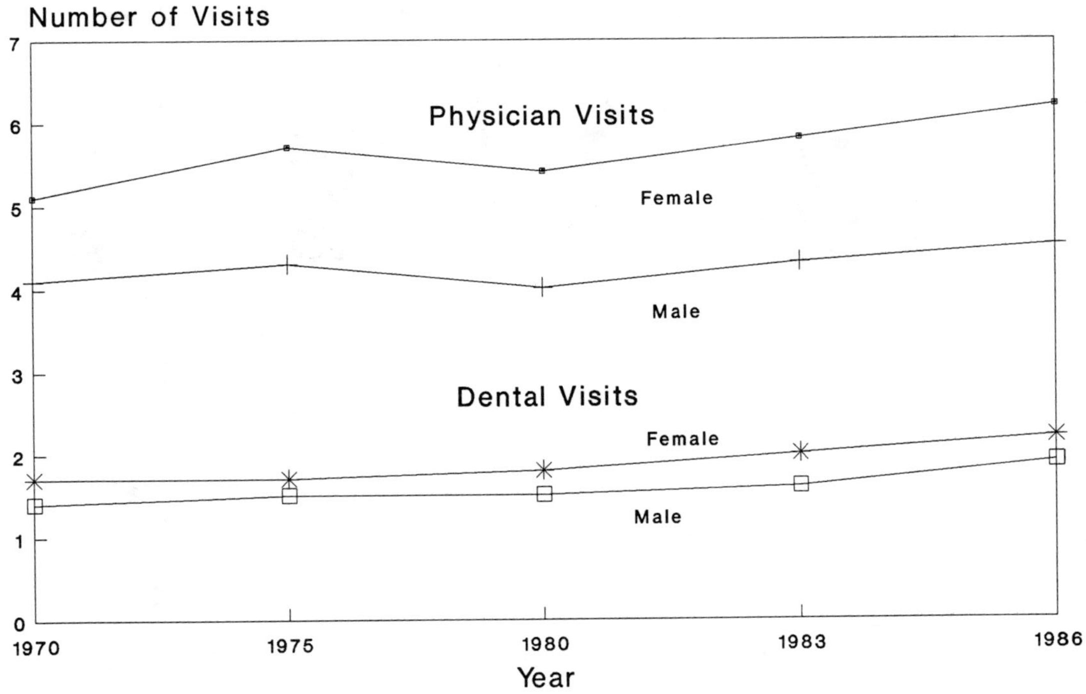

Source: U.S. National Center for Health Statistics, 1989 Statistical Abstracts.

Percent Change in Average Fees for Physician Visits: 1982-1986

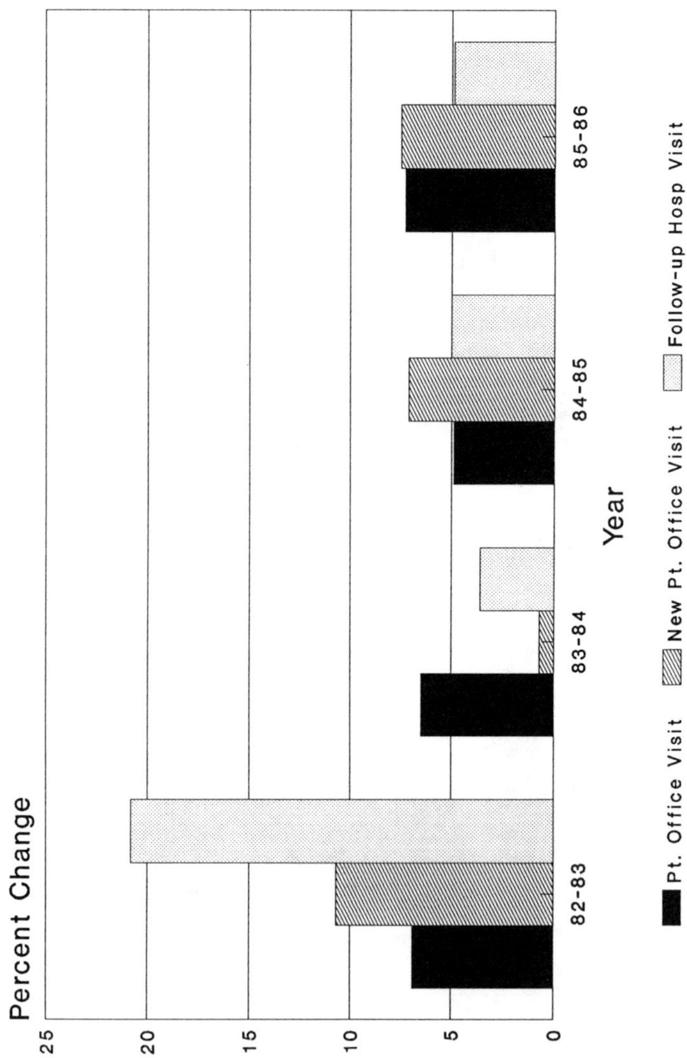

Source: AMA Socioeconomic Monitoring System 1982-1986

Mean Expenditure on Medical Supplies per Self-Employed Physician: 1986

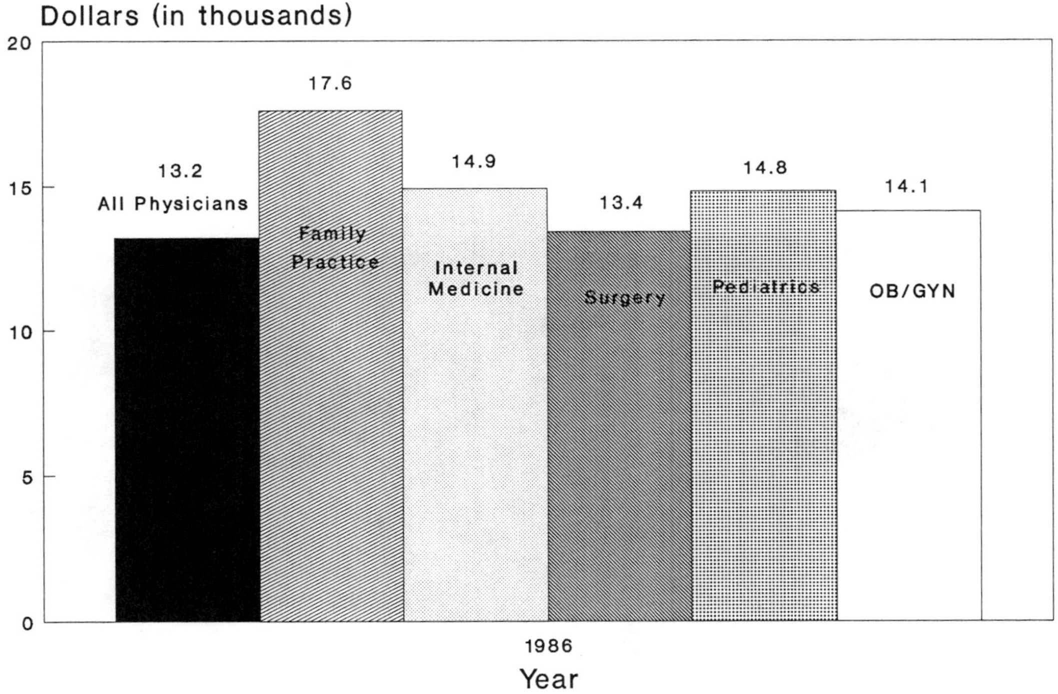

Source: AMA Socioeconomic Monitoring System 1983-1987 core surveys

Distribution of Average Professional Expenses of Self-Employed Physicians 1982 and 1986

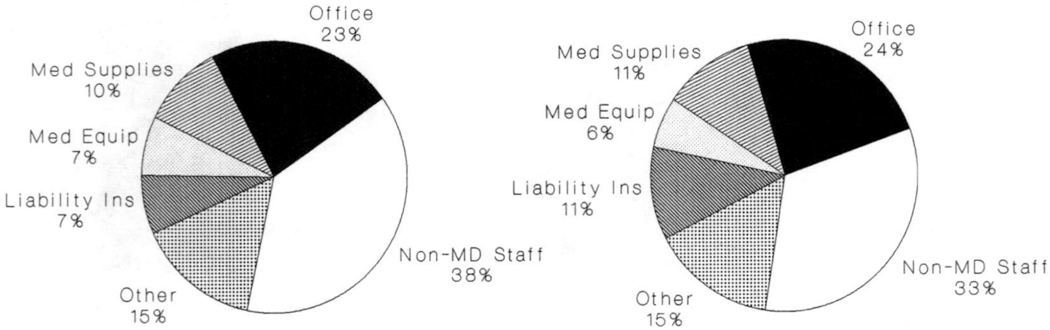

Source: AMA Socioeconomic Monitoring System 1983 and 1987 core surveys

Office-Based Physicians' Net Earnings from Practice, by Specialty: 1986

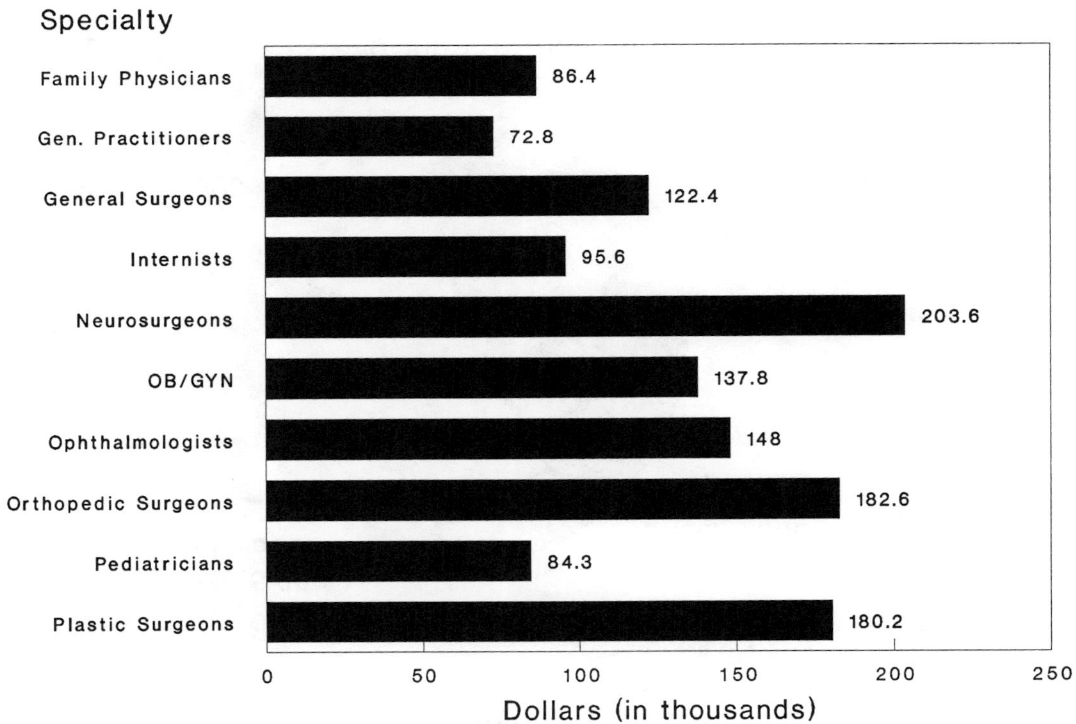

Source: Medical Economics

Companies with Flexible Benefit Plans, by Size

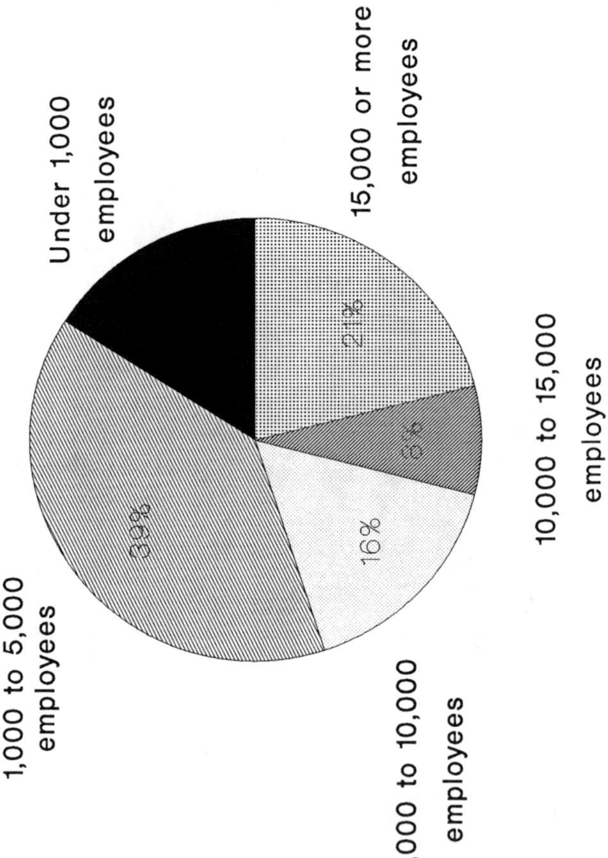

Source: Hewitt Associates;
Managed HealthCare, October 10, 1989.

Flexible Benefit Plan Coverage
(257 Companies Surveyed)

Health Benefits:	
Fee-for-service medical care	97%
HMO medical care	85%
Dental care	88%
Vision care	19%
Disability benefits:	
Short term	21%
Long term	54%

Hewitt Associates; Managed HealthCare, 1989.

Percent of Employers Providing Retiree Health Coverage
(by employer size)

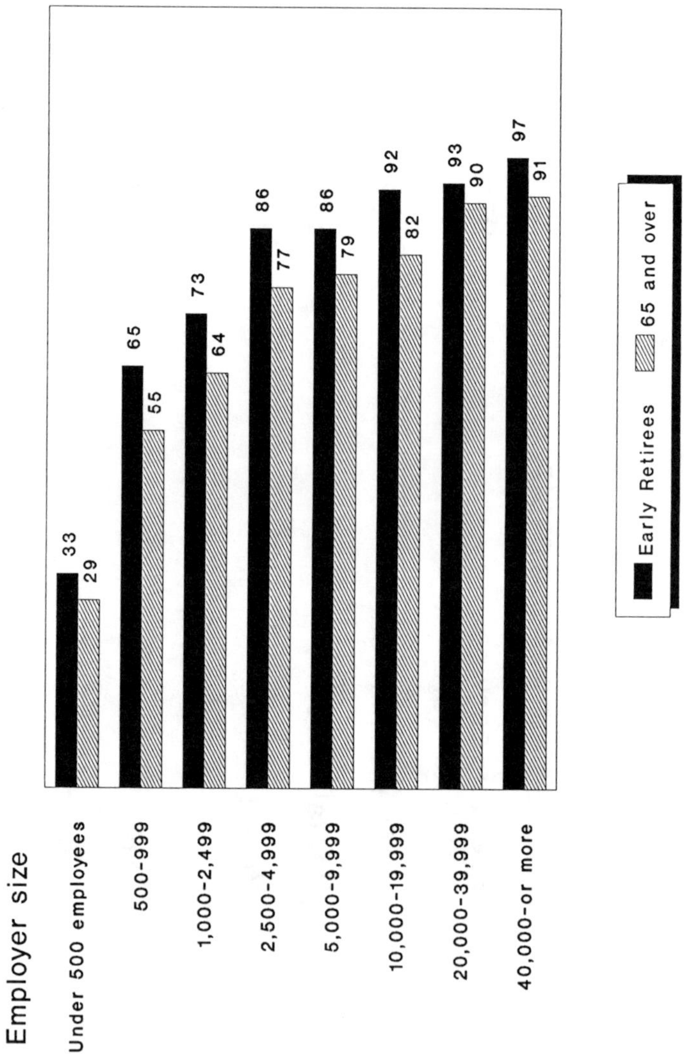

Source: Foster Higgins, 1988

Percent of Employers Providing Retiree Health Coverage
(by region)

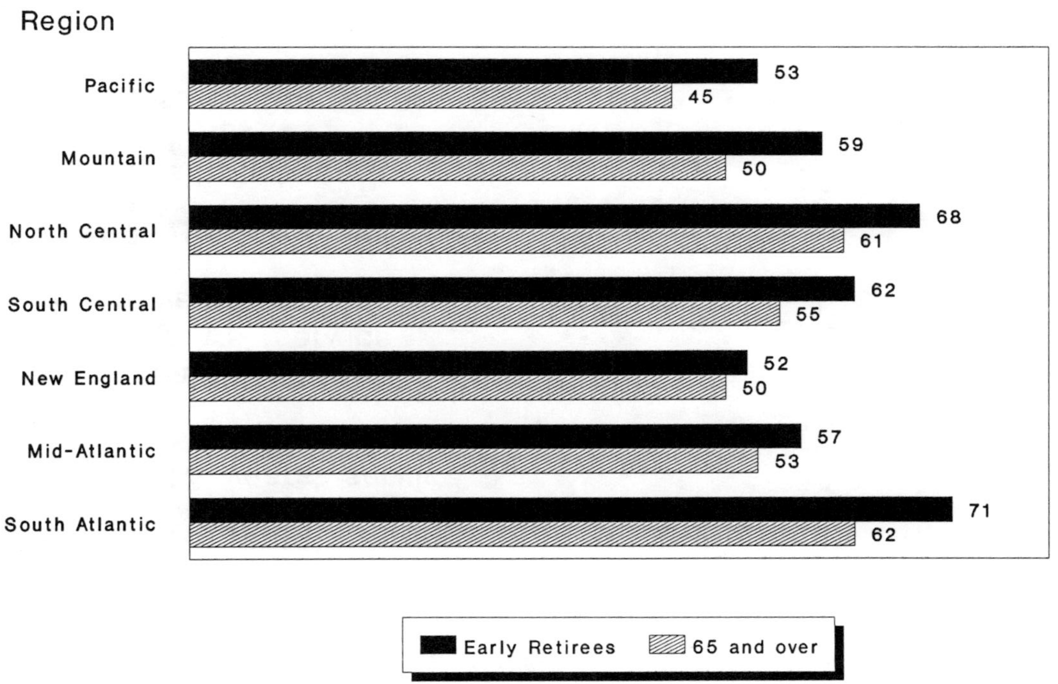

Source: Foster Higgins, 1988.

Percentage of Defined-Benefit Plans Under Which Employees Can Retire Early with Full Benefit

	1988
Age 50 with 10 years' service	2%
Age 50 with 15 years' service	1
Age 55	12
with 5 years' service	9
with 10 years' service	37
with 15 years' service	6
Age 60 with 10 years' service	1
Two or more alternatives (e.g., earlier of age 55 and 10 years, or 30 years)	23
Other	9

Source: Hewitt Associates, 1988

Flexible Benefit Plans Among Major Employers
(500+ employees)

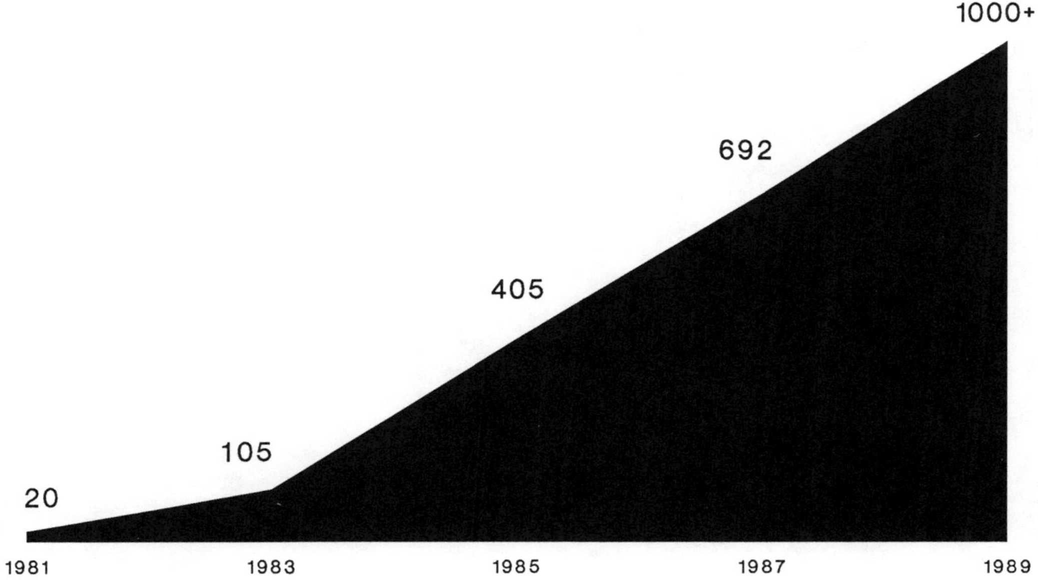

Source: Hewitt Associates; Managed Health Care, October 1989.

INDEX

A

ACE inhibitors, 79, 80, 82, see also specific types
Acquired immunodeficiency syndrome (AIDS), 14—16
Acute conditons, 13, see also specific types
Adverse drug reactions, 46
Age
  acute conditions by, 13
  AIDS cases by, 15, 16
  hospital days of care by, 15
  hospital discharges by, 16
  life expectancy by, 7
  Medicare enrollees by, 106
  prescription drug use by, 45
  psychotropic drug use by, 39—42
  surgery trends by, 258
  of U.S. population, 3, 4
Aged, see Elderly
AIDS, see Acquired immunodeficiency syndrome
Ambulatory care, 157, 158
Amoxil, 35
Analgesics, 37, 72, see also specific types
Anaprox, 34
Ancef, 36
Annuities, 99
Antiarrhythmics, 82, see also specific types
Antiarthritics, 38, 78, see also specific types
Antibiotics, 38, see also specific types
Antidepressants, 38, 73, see also specific types
Antihistamines, 73, see also specific types
Antihypertensives, 38, 74, 82, see also specific types
Anti-infectives, 74, 164, 191, 192, see also specific types
Antilipemics, 83, 84, see also specific types
Anti-metabolics, 37
Anti-neoplastic agents, 164, 191, 192, see also specific types
Anti-peptic ulcerants, 37
Antirheumatic non-steroids, 37
Anti-ulcer agents, 38, 76, 77, see also specific types
Asthma, 11
Atherosclerosis, 11
Axid, 38

B

Bachelor of science degrees in pharmacy, 276
Benefit packages, 146—148
  for elderly, 22
  for health care workers, 312, 313, 317
  for pharmacists, 291
Beta-blockers, 37, 82, see also specific types
Biological products, 66, 164, 182—186, 188
Biotech firms, 195
Births, 5
Blood products, 37
Blood spectrum penicillins, 37
Botanicals, 182—187, 188
Brand name prescriptions, 26, 30, 155
Broad spectrum penicillins, 37

C

Calan, 81
Calcium antagonists, 37, see also specific types
Calcium channel blockers, 81, 82, see also specific types
Capoten, 33, 79, 80, 180, 219
Capozide, 79, 80
Carafate, 76, 77
Cardiovascular agents, 82, 164, 191, 192, see also specific types
Cardizem, 33, 34, 81, 180, 219
Catastrophic drug insurance program, 125
Ceclor, 33, 180
Cefobid, 36
Ceftin, 38
Central nervous system agents, 164, 191, 192, see also specific types
Cephalosporins, 37
Cerebral vasotherapy, 37
Cerebrovascular disease, 11
Chain drug stores, 28, 31, 89, 90
  discount, 214
  expense ratio for, 230
  growth of, 215
  licensed, 274
  net-to-sales ratio for, 229
  number of, 274
  pharmacist fringe benefits in, 291
  pharmacist salaries in, 286, 288, 289
  pharmacists employed by, 269
  prescriptions sold by, 222, 227, 228
  retail sales figures for, 210
  sales gains for, 216
  sales mix for, 221
  sales per average store for, 213
  sales volume for, 210, 212, 214, 220, 221, 223, 225, 226
  staffing of, 271
  top ten, 211, 212

total number of, 224
wholesaler sales to, 207
Charities, 58
Chemical entities, 167, 255, see also specific types
Claforan, 36
Cleocin, 36
Clinoril, 78
Codeine, 35
Cold medicines, 72
Colestid, 83, 84
Collection period, 206
Community hospitals, 242
Consumer Price Index
annual change in, 75
for over-the-counter drugs, 65, 67
for prescriptions, 67, 85
Copayments, 147
Corporate-owned HMOs, 141, 142
Costs
chain drug store, 230
community hospital, 242
distribution of in hospitals, 122
distribution of in retail drug industry, 122
health care, see Health care costs
hospital prescription, 247
labor, 122
medical care, see Health care costs
medical supply, 309
non-labor, 122
operating, 198, 203
pharmaceutical, 71
prescription, 60, 61, 68—70, 120, 124, 236, 247
professional, 310
psychotropic drug, 42
wholesaler, 197, 198
Cough medicines, 72
Cytostatic immunodilators, 37

D

Death, see Mortality
Dental care benefits, 313
Dentists, 264
Consumer Price Index for fees of, 65
health care costs paid to, 61
hourly earnings of workers in offices of, 295
number of, 266, 300
visits to by sex, 307
Dermatologicals, 164, 191, 192
Diabeta, 34
Diabetes therapy, 73
Diagnostic related groups (DRGs), 43
Digestive system disorders, 13
Diphtheria, 12
Disability benefits, 313
Discount stores, 214
pharmacists employed by, 269
prescriptions sold by, 227, 228
Diseases, see also specific types
deaths from, 11
infectious, 12
Diuretics, 37, see also specific types
Doctor of pharmacy degrees, 277
Doctor of philosophy degrees in pharmacy, 279, 284, 285
Doctors, see Physicians
DRG, see Diagnostic related groups
Drug Policy Census Surveys, 132, 134
Drugs, see also specific drugs, types
approval process for, 160, 173, 177, 178
"A"-rated, 169
clinical trials for, 160
exports of, 181, 183, 185, 190, 193
imports of, 181, 182
new, 169—174, 179
over-the-counter, see Over-the-counter drugs
patents for, 165, 166, 188
prescription, see Prescriptions
sales volume by product class, 191, 192
top manufacturers of, 170, 171
Drug stores, 31, see also Pharmacies
chain, see Chain drug stores
daily prescriptions sold by, 231
health care costs paid to, 60
hospitals vs. in sales, 237
hourly earnings for workers at, 294
independent, see Independent drug stores
international sales of, 37
leading products sold to, 219
number of, 274
OTC sales of, 233
pharmaceutical sales to, 92, 217, 218
prescription sales vs. OTC sales of, 233
sales trends for, 232
wholesaler sales to, 207
Dyazide, 35, 219

E

Elderly
annual health care costs for, 113
chemical entities dispensed in hospitals to, 255
HMO premium increases and, 151
income distribution for, 19
income sources for, 20
living arrangements of, 21
medical benefits of, 22

Medicare enrollment by, 104, 106
as percent of population, 9
prescription use by, 45, 115—119
prescription costs for, 114
retirement benefits for, 314, 315
surgery for, 258
Employer dollar outlay for insurance, 95
Employment, see Staffing
Endocrine agents, 164, 191, 192, see also specific types
Expenditures, see Costs
Exports of drugs, 181, 183, 185, 190, 193

F

FDA, see Food and Drug Administration
Fee-for-service, 126, 127, 313
Feldene, 70, 78, 180
Females
dental visits by, 307
life expectancy of, 8
mortality rates for, 10
as pharmacists, 270, 280, 288
as physicians, 303, 306
physician visits by, 307
psychotropic drug use by, 39—42
surgery for, 257
Flexeril, 34
Food and Drug Administration (FDA)
approval process of, 160, 175, 177, 178
staffing of, 267
therapeutic classifications of, 170
Food stores, 207, 227, 228, 269
Forane, 36
Free-choice health plans, 126
Freestanding ambulatory centers, 157

G

Gamma globulin, 37
Gastrointestinal agents, 164, 191, 192, see also specific types
GDP, see Gross Domestic Product
Generic prescriptions, 26, 30, 155
Genitourinary agents, 164, 191, 192, see also specific types
Glucotrol, 34
Government health insurance, 93, 94, see also specific types
Grocery stores, 207, 227, 228, 269
Gross Domestic Product, 57
Gross National Product, 52, 56
Group life insurance, 95
Growth of U.S. population, 2

H

Health and beauty aids, 208
Health-care aids, 61
Health care costs, 50—54, 56
per capital, 68
changes in, 55
Consumer Price Index for, 65
containment measures for, 64
distribution of, 59—61
household income and, 62
international, 63, 68
for Medicare beneficiaries, 113
as percent of GDP, 57
sources for payment of, 58, 59, 88
Health insurance
claims payments for, 98
coverage rates for, 94
coverage status of, 93
employer dollar outlay for, 95
free-choice health plans and, 126
government, 93, 94, see also specific types
premium increase causes in, 103
private, see Private health insurance
Health maintenance organizations (HMOs), 91, 98, 127
agreements among, 144
benefit plans and, 313
characteristics of, 145
copayments and, 147
corporate-owned, 141, 142
distribution of membership in, 139
diversification of activities of, 144
enrollment in, 128, 135—138, 148
Medicare, 143
number of, 129, 130, 132
ownership of, 141
premium increases at, 151—154
prescriptions sold by, 155, 235
preventive services and, 146
provider counts for, 133
rating method of enrollees in, 140
by region, 131
total membership in, 128
total number of, 130, 132
transplants and, 150
Heart disease, 11
HMOs, see Health maintenance organizations
Home health care, 111, 112, 156, 208
Hospital pharmacies
admissions to, 251
inventory of, 252, 253
licensed, 274
nonparenteral orders of, 254
number of pharmacists in, 275

parenteral orders of, 254
pharmacist fringe benefits in, 291
pharmacist salaries in, 286, 288
purchases of, 252, 253
staffing of, 292
Hospitals, 96
AIDS patient days of care in, 15
AIDS patient discharges from, 16
bed allocation in, 241, 245
bed capacity of, 248, 252
chemical entities dispensed in, 255
community, 242
Consumer Price Index for costs paid to, 65
Consumer Price Index for services of, 75
control of, 261
discharges from, 16, 43, 247
vs. drug stores in sales, 237
expenditures for, 242
health care costs paid to, 60, 61
HMOs owned by, 141
hourly earnings of workers in, 295
inpatient, 111, 112
labor costs in, 122
leading drugs in, 36
length of stay for, 246, 247
long-term, 243, 244
Medicare and, 111, 112
non-labor costs in, 122
occupancy rates for, 241, 245
outpatient, 111, 112
percent of health care costs paid to, 59
pharmaceutical sales to, 92, 256
pharmacies in, see Hospital pharmacies
pharmacy services in, 250, see also Hospital pharmacies
prescription costs in, 247
prescriptions dispensed by, 235, see also Hospital pharmacies
in retirement communities, 260
short-term, 243, 244
staffing of, 244, 266, 293
therapeutic classes of prescription drugs in, 37
types of, 240, 243
wholesaler sales to, 207
Hypertension, 11

I

Immunodilators, 37, see also specific types
Imports of drugs, 181, 182, 184
Income
distribution of, 18, 19
health care costs and, 62
of health care workers, 299
insurance premiums costs ratio to, 99
life insurance policy value and, 100
of pharmacists, 286—289
of physicians, 311
sources of, 20
IND, 160
Independent drug stores, 89, 90
number of, 274
pharmacist fringe benefits in, 291
pharmacist salaries in, 286, 288, 289
pharmacists employed by, 269
prescriptions sold by, 227, 228
sales volume for, 223, 225, 226, 234
total number of, 224
wholesaler sales to, 207
Inderal LA, 35
Individual practice associations (IPAs), 91, 138
Indocin, 78
Infant mortality, 5, 6
Infectious diseases, 12; see also specific types
Influenza, 11
Injuries, 13
Inpatient hospital care, 112
Insurance, see also specific types
catastrophic drug, 125
health, see Health insurance
liability, 102
life, see Life insurance
premium cost ratio to personal income, 99
unemployment, 95
worker's compensation, 95
Inventory trends, 206
IPAs, see Individual practice associations
Isoptin, 81
IV solutions, 37

K

Kidney infections, 11

L

Labor costs, 122
Labor-intensive industries, 122
Lanoxin, 35
Length of stay for hospitals, 246, 247
Liability insurance for physicians, 102
Licensing
of pharmacies, 274
of pharmacists, 272, 273
Life expectancy, 7, 8
Life insurance, 95
average size of policies of, 101
policy value for, 100
premiums for, 99
Life insurance companies, 97
Live births, 5
Living arrangements for elderly, 21

Long-term hospitals, 243, 244
Lopid, 83, 84
Lorelco, 83, 84

M

Mail order prescriptions, 235
Males
  dental visits by, 307
  life expectancy of, 8
  mortality rates for, 10
  as pharmacists, 270, 280, 288
  as physicians, 303, 306
  physician visits by, 307
  psychotropic drug use by, 39—42
  surgery for, 257
Managed care, 91, 126, 129, 130, see also Health maintenance organizations (HMOs); Preferred provider organizations (PPOs); specific types
  copayments and, 147
  expected growth of, 127
  prescription utilization in, 155
  by region, 131
  transplants and, 150
Marital status, 17
Mass merchandisers, 207
Master of science degrees in pharmacy, 278
Measles, 12
Medicaid, 58, 59, 88, 89, 93, 99
  HMOs and, 139, 145
  prescriptions and, 120, 121
  surgery paid for by, 259
Medical benefits for elderly, 22
Medical care costs, see Health care costs
Medicare, 58, 59, 88
  allowed charge per user of, 110
  annual health costs for beneficiaries of, 113
  catastrophic drug insurance effects of, 125
  enrollment in, 104—106
  growth of, 107
  HMOs and, 139, 143, 145
  physician services per user of, 108
  physician visits per week and, 109
  prescriptions and, 113—119
  reimbursement for services under, 112
  surgery paid for by, 259
  utilization of, 111
Medications, see Prescriptions
Medicinals, 182—185, 187, 188
Mefoxin, 36
Meningitis, 11
Mevacor, 83, 84
Micronase, 34
Mortality
  disease specific, 11
  infant, 5, 6
  rates of by sex, 10
Motrin, 78

N

Nalfon, 78
Naprosyn, 33, 78, 180, 219
National Institutes of Health (NIH), 161
National Wholesale Druggists' Association, 201, 205, see also Wholesalers
NDA, see New drug applications
Net worth, 194
Neuroleptics, 37
New drug applications (NDA), 160, 175
New molecular entities (NME), 173—177
NIH, see National Institutes of Health
NME, see New molecular entities
Non-labor costs, 122
Non-narcotic analgesics, 37
Nurses, 264, 266, 300
Nursing aides, 264
Nursing homes, 111, 112, 156
  control of, 261, 262
  health care costs paid to, 60, 61
  hourly earnings of workers in, 295
  ownership of, 261, 262
  percent of health care costs paid to, 59
Nutrients, 191, 192

O

Operating expenses, 198, 203
Optometrists, 264
Ortho novums, 219
Orudis, 78
Osteopathy, 264
OTC, see Over-the-counter drugs
Out-of-pocket payment, 58, 59, 88, 139, 259
Outpatient hospitals, 111, 112
Over-the-counter drugs, see also specific types
  Consumer Price Index for, 67, 85
  vs. prescriptions in sales volume, 233
  Producer Price Indexes for, 72
  sales trends for, 232
  sales volume for, 220, 221, 233

P

Parasitic disease, 13
Patents, 165, 166, 180
Penicillins, 37
Pensions, 20, 97
Pepcid, 76, 77
Peripheral vasotherapy, 37

Personnel, see Staffing
Pharmaceutical industry, 169—171
  drug store sales by, 217, 218
  hospital sales of, 256
  hourly earnings for workers at, 294
  international, 174, 181—185, 190, 192, 193
  net worth of, 194
  patent expirations and, 180
  productivity indexes of, 296
  sales volume of, 190, 191
  therapeutic breakthroughs of, 172
Pharmaceutical Manufacturers Association (PMA), 190, 193
Pharmaceuticals, see also Drugs; Over-the-counter drugs; Prescriptions; specific types
  exports of, 183, 185
  imports of, 182, 184
  as percent of wholesaler product mix, 208
  Producer Price Indexes for, 71
  R&D costs for, 163
  sales by class of customer, 92
  shipments of, 66, 188
  trends in, 66
Pharmaceutical wholesalers, see Wholesalers
Pharmacies, see also Drug stores
  contracted, 91
  daily prescriptions sold by, 231
  fees of, 123
  in HMOs, 133
  hospital, see Hospital pharmacies
  in-house, 91
  Medicaid reimbursement to, 121
  number of, 274
  in PPOs, 133
  staffing of, 268
Pharmacists
  education of, see Pharmacy education
  employment of, 269
  fringe benefits of, 291
  hours worked by, 290
  licensing of, 272, 273
  Medicaid and, 121
  number of, 264, 268, 270, 272, 273, 275
  patients' rating of communication of, 47
  practice types of, 275
  salaries of, 286—289
  sex of, 270
Pharmacy education
  bachelor of science degrees, 276
  doctor of pharmacy, 277
  doctor of philosophy degrees, 279, 284, 285
  ethnic groups and, 281
  graduate studies, 283
  master of science degrees, 278
  by region, 282
  total degrees conferred, 280
Pharmacy services in hospitals, 250, see also Hospital pharmacies
Physician assistants, 264
Physicians
  Consumer Price Index for fees of, 65
  Consumer Price Index for services of, 75
  fees of, 65, 308
  health care costs paid to, 60, 61
  in HMOs, 133
  hourly earnings of workers in offices of, 295
  income of, 311
  liability insurance paid by, 102
  medical supply expenditures of, 309
  Medicare and, 108—110, 112
  networks of, 126
  number of, 264, 266, 300—306
  patients' rating of communication of, 47
  patient visits per week to, 109
  percent of health care costs paid to, 59
  in PPOs, 133
  prescriptions dispensed by, 235
  professional expenses of, 310
  by sex, 303, 306
  specialties of, 304, 305, 311
  visits to by sex, 307
Platinol, 36
PMA, see Pharmaceutical Manufacturers Association
Pneumonia, 11
Polio, 12
Population, U.S.
  age of, 3, 4
  change in, 4
  death in, 5
  elderly, 9
  HMO enrollment as percentage of, 137
  income distribution in, 18, 19
  infant mortality in, 5, 6
  life expectancy of, 7, 8
  live births in, 5
  managed care and, 127
  marital status of, 17
  mortality rates in, 10
  projected growth of, 2
  psychotropic drug use in, 39
PPOs, see Preferred provider organizations
Practical nurses, 264
Preferred provider organizations (PPOs), 91, 127, 134
  HMO diversification and, 144
  provider counts for, 133
  by region, 131
  total number of, 130
Premarin, 35
Prescriptions, see also Drugs

for ACE inhibitors, 79
adverse reactions to, 46
by age, 45
for antilipemics, 84
for anti-ulcer agents, 77
brand name, 26, 30, 70, 155
chain drugstore sales of, 28, 31, 32, 222, 227, 228
Consumer Price Index for, 67, 85
costs of, 60, 61, 68—70, 120, 124, 236, 247
daily output of, 227
daily sales of, 231
decline in number of, 27
distribution of, 91
drugstore sales of, 31, 32
elderly use of, 45, 115—119
generic, 26, 30, 155
health care costs paid for, 60, 61
hospital sales of, 36, 247
independent drugstore sales of, 227, 228
international costs of, 68, 69
international sales of, 37
leading products, 33, 35
Medicaid and, 120, 121
Medicare and, 113—119
new, 25—27, 31, 32, 38
number of, 24, 27, 29, 30
OTC sales volume vs., 233
patents for, 165, 166, 180
patients' rating of communication on, 47
per capital expenditure on, 68
Producer Price Indexes for, 73, 74
psychotropic drugs as percent of, 41
refill, 25, 27, 31
retail sales of, 33—35, 209, 235
sales trends for, 232
sales volume for, 89, 90, 220, 221, 233, 236
sources for payment of, 88—90
therapeutic classes of, 37
trends in, 66
wholesale, see Wholesalers

Preventive services, 146
Price Indexes, see Consumer Price Index; Producer Price Indexes
Prinivil, 38
Private health insurance, 58, 59, 88, 93, 94
employer dollar outlay for, 95
surgery paid for by, 259
Procardia, 33, 81, 180, 219
Producer Price Indexes, 71—74
Product-intensive industries, 122
Productivity indexes, 296
Profits, 194, 199—201, 203
Proventill, 34
Prozac, 38
Psychotropic drugs, 39, 40, see also specific types
cost of, 42
as percentage of all prescriptions, 41
sources of payment for, 42
Public assistance, 20, see also specific types
Public health insurance, see Government health insurance

Q

Questran, 83, 84

R

Railroad pensions, 20
R&D, see Research and development
Registered nurses, 264
Research and development, 163, 176
cost of as percentage of sales, 162
cost of by product class, 164
for molecular entities, 173
national support for costs of, 161
top companies in, 168
Residential facilities, 262
Respiratory agents, 164, 191, 192, see also specific types
Respiratory conditions, 13
Retin-A, 34
Retirees, see Elderly
Retirement benefits, 314—316
Retirement communities, 260
Rhematic diseae, 11
Rocephin, 36
Rogaine, 38

S

Seldane, 34
Self-pay, 58, 59, 88, 139, 259
Sera globulin, 37
Sex, see also Females; Males
dental visits by, 307
life expectancy by, 8
mortality rates by, 10
number of pharmacists by, 270, 280, 288
number of physicians by, 303, 306
physician visits by, 307
psychotropic drug use by, 39—42
surgery by, 257
Short-term hospitals, 243, 244
Skilled nursing facilities, 111, 112
Smallpox, 12
Social Security, 20
Staffing, 264, 266

annual percent change in, 297
of chain drug stores, 271
of FDA, 267
of hospital pharmacies, 292
of hospitals, 244, 293
hourly earnings and, 294, 295
number of employees, 265
of pharmacies, 268
workhours, 298
Supermarkets, 207, 227, 228, 269
Surgeons, 112
Surgery
most frequently performed, 44
sources of payment for, 259
trends in, 257, 258
Syphilis, 12
Systemic antihistamines, 73
Systemic anti-infectives, 74

T

Tagamet, 33, 35, 76, 77, 180, 219
Technicians, 264, 292
Tenormin, 33, 35, 219
Therapeutic breakthroughs, 172
Third-party payments, see specific payees
Tolectin, 78
Tranquilizers, 37, see also specific types
Transderm-Nitro, 70
Transplants, 150
Tuberculosis, 11, 12
Tylenol, 35
Typhoid fever, 12

U

Ulcers, 11
Unemployment insurance, 95
Uninsured, 93, 94, 127
Upper respiratory conditions, 13
U.S. population, see Population, U.S.

V

Vancocin, 36
Vaseretic, 79, 80
Vasodilators, 82, see also specific types
Vasotec, 33, 34, 79, 80, 180
Vasotherapy, 37
Verapamil, 81
Vision care benefits, 313
Vitamins, 164, 191, 192
Voltaren, 38

W

Wholesalers
assets to net worth for, 202
asset turnover for, 204
collection period for, 206
expense trends for, 197
financial leverage for, 202
gross margin of, 198
hourly earnings for workers at, 294
inventory trends for, 206
net worth of, 202
operating expenses of, 198, 203
percentage of sales by, 92
product sales mix for, 208
profit margins for, 199—201, 203
return on net worth for, 201
sales growth for, 196
sales mix for, 207
sales volume for, 197, 206
total assets of, 205
Whooping cough, 12
Worker's compensation insurance, 95
Workhours, 298
Workplace clinics, 61

X

Xanax, 33, 35, 180, 219

Z

Zantac, 33—36, 70, 76, 77, 180, 219
Zestril, 38, 130